CONDITIONING
WITH PHYSICAL
DISABILITIES

Kevin F. Lockette, PT, CSCS
Rehabilitation Hospital of the Pacific

Ann M. Keyes, PT, CSCS
Rehabilitation Institute of Chicago

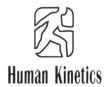

Human Kinetics

Library of Congress Cataloging-in-Publication Data

Lockette, Kevin F., 1966-
    Conditioning with physical disabilities / Kevin F. Lockette, Ann M.
Keyes.
        p.   cm.
    Includes index.
    ISBN 0-87322-614-3
    1. Physical fitness for the physically handicapped.   I. Keyes,
Ann M., 1964-   . II. Title.
    GV482.7.L63   1994
    613.7'087--dc20   93-47606
                                                                                        CIP

ISBN: 0-87322-614-3

Developmental Editor: Mary E. Fowler
Assistant Editors: Anna Curry, Dawn Roselund, Julia Anderson
Copyeditor: Ginger Rodriguez
Proofreader: Chris Little
Indexer: Theresa J. Schaefer
Production Director: Ernie Noa
Typesetter and Layout Artist: Kathy Boudreau-Fuoss
Text Designer: Keith Blomberg
Cover Designer: Jack Davis
Photographer (cover): Oscar Izquierdo
Photographer (interior): Oscar Izquierdo
Illustrators: Gary Bannister (primary), Karen Levy (spot), and David Casement, rehabilitation engineer,
    (technical drawings and equipment designs)
Printer: United Graphics

Human Kinetics books are available at special discounts for bulk purchase. Special editions or book excerpts can also be created to specification. For details, contact the Special Sales Manager at Human Kinetics.

Physical disabilities can vary greatly. Health and fitness are matters that require individual consideration. Readers should consult their physicians regarding their individual needs before engaging in an exercise program. This book is not intended to replace rehabilitation programs through the medical profession. It should be used as a guide to promote and maintain postrehabilitation wellness in conjunction with the medical profession. Any application of the recommendations set forth in the following pages is at the reader's discretion and risk.

Printed in the United States of America   10 9 8 7 6 5 4 3 2

Human Kinetics
Web site: http://www.humankinetics.com/

United States: Human Kinetics, P.O. Box 5076, Champaign, IL 61825-5076
1-800-747-4457

Canada: Human Kinetics, 475 Devonshire Road, Unit 100, Windsor, ON N8Y 2L5
1-800-465-7301 (in Canada only)

Europe: Human Kinetics, P.O. Box IW14, Leeds LS16 6TR, United Kingdom
(44) 1132 781708

Australia: Human Kinetics, 57A Price Avenue, Lower Mitcham, South Australia 5062
(088) 277 1555

New Zealand: Human Kinetics, P.O. Box 105-231, Auckland 1
(09) 523 3462

To the individuals with disabilities we have worked with: Your dedication has proven how exercise can be a way toward a healthier, more active life.

Ann and Kevin

To my family and friends who have supported me throughout this endeavor.

Ann

To my best friend and wife, Ginger, who showed relentless patience and support throughout the entire project, and to my mother and father, who have given me lifelong support.

Kevin

Contents

Preface

This book represents the first practical manual that explains why physical disability need not, and indeed should not, mean physical inactivity. More importantly, it provides conditioning activities and programs specifically designed to help you enjoy and benefit from regular exercise, regardless of your disability.

As a person with a disability, you may be faced with many challenges that reduce your opportunities to participate in and benefit from well-balanced fitness programs and sport-specific training. Your challenges may include your physical impairments, architectural barriers, and limited information on training techniques for people with your disability.

As health care and fitness professionals, we know that a physical disability often limits the capacity for work and may restrict a person from certain activities. However, what we and others have learned is that rarely should a physical disability rule out exercise entirely. To the contrary, most people with disabilities benefit from regular and appropriate physical activity, with results including these:

- Improved stamina and function for activities involved in daily living
- Enhanced self-esteem and confidence through the perception of improved body appearance, control, and function
- Minimized muscle atrophy, joint stiffness, pressure sores, weight gain, and other adverse conditions

- Higher levels of functioning for those with progressive disorders like multiple sclerosis
- Fewer medical complications, including pressure sores and hospitalizations for people who use wheelchairs

Conditioning With Physical Disabilities was written to expand the knowledge base on strength and conditioning for you, coaches, therapeutic recreation specialists, physical educators, and fitness professionals. Medical and health professionals like physical therapists, occupational therapists, and physicians also will find the manual a useful educational tool to initiate postrehabilitation exercise programs. These professionals are often in the best position to initiate an exercise program before someone is discharged from the rehabilitation setting. They can perform initial exercise readiness assessments and identify restrictions, precautions, and appropriate exercise intensity. This care allows people who have physical disabilities to make wise choices about fitness activities and to engage in active, healthy lifestyles.

Several years ago we developed a strength and conditioning program for the physically disabled at the Rehabilitation Institute of Chicago. Most of the information compiled and organized in *Conditioning With Physical Disabilities* was developed from this program. We have learned, from trial and error, what works and what doesn't and how to adapt and apply current exercise concepts to people with disabilities. Hence, this book presents the most current research on exercise for the physically disabled along with practical information on how to begin an exercise program.

In Part I we introduce the elements of a good conditioning program. First, we have shown what steps to take in determining your current fitness status. By the end of chapter 1 you will know your exercise starting point and the areas that need the most attention. Chapters 2 through 4 provide basic information about strength, aerobic, and flexibility training. We explain important training principles and suggest how to design a conditioning program to improve the three components of fitness. In chapter 4 we include a wide selection of stretching exercises.

The sports classifications used by sports organizations for people with disabilities in the United States provides the framework for Part II. This system groups people into classes based on medical and physical characteristics. Within each classification we identify several levels of disability, making the information directly applicable to the exercise readiness status you determined in chapter 1. Each of the four chapters in Part II includes the following:

- Descriptions and charts explaining the class of disability and associated conditions
- Procedures for making a preexercise assessment
- Guidelines for exercise prescription
- Recommended modifications of training programs
- Precautions concerning types of exercise and training programs

- Characteristics of each subclassification in the disability class
- Complete exercise programs for each subclass

These exercise programs specify and illustrate the appropriate choice of exercise, type of equipment, positioning, repetitions, and workout intensity. We also provide convenient training logs for you to copy and use to record your workouts.

In Part III you'll find step-by-step descriptions and illustrations that show precise technique to ensure safe and effective performance for all of the exercises referred to in the exercise programs in Part II. We divided the exercises according to three segments of the body: upper extremities, abdominal and trunk, and lower extremities. We included an exercise finder at the beginning of chapters 9, 10, and 11 to help you quickly locate any exercise. In chapter 12 we suggest how to develop an exercise class that meets your needs.

In the back of the book you'll find two appendixes, one listing accessible exercise equipment and the other listing prominent fitness and sports associations. A glossary of important exercise-related terms and references you can use for further information on a specific topic follow.

Although *Conditioning With Physical Disabilities* is a comprehensive reference, it is also a practical fitness manual. We wrote the book to give you background exercise information and the how-to prescriptions to make sure you do it right. It is both a reference text and an on-site workout companion. Read it at home for background information on exercise and use it at the gym for great results. Most of all, enjoy the challenges and rewards of your efforts.

Acknowledgments

Most of the information in this manual was developed through the Strength and Conditioning Program of the Wirtz Sports Program at the Rehabilitation Institute of Chicago. The photographs throughout depict the athletes of the Wirtz Sports Program. Without the assistance and support from these athletes, sports coordinator Jeff Jones, and the rest of the Wirtz program staff, this project would have been impossible. Pamela J. Redding, MS, also a Wirtz program staff member, deserves recognition for the endless hours she spent at the computer revising our text. Pam helped clarify every page as the manual was written and revised.

The Physical Therapy Department of the Rehabilitation Institute of Chicago showed tremendous support for this project by allowing the use of the physical therapy gymnasium. We would like to extend a special thanks to Karen Ortmann and Bill Keely for approving our flexible schedules. Once again, without the department's support this project would have been impossible.

Additional thanks to the Education and Training Department at the Rehabilitation Institute of Chicago, especially Don Olson, PhD, for coordinating the project until its end stages.

This manual was supported (in part) by a grant from the Paralyzed Veterans of America Spinal Cord Injury Education and Training Foundation.

Reviewers

This manual has been greatly enhanced by the medical contributions and overall content review by Edward R. Laskowski, MD, and Kenneth Richter, DO. Their diverse backgrounds in medicine and sports for the disabled are reflected on every page.

To pull together a manual as comprehensive and in-depth as this, we have required the assistance of many talented people from diverse backgrounds. A special thanks goes to John A. Roberts, PhD, for his work as a reviewer and consultant for the exercise index; and to text reviewers Jim Blas, OTR, MS; David Chen, MD; Kathleen Curtis, PhD, PT; Alan Goldstein; Jeff Jones, MPE; Kristi Kirschner, MD; John Kordich, MEd, CSCS; Norman Lange, BA; Ginger Lockette, PT, CSCS; Ken Lockette, MEd; Claire Orner, PT, ATC; Elliot Roth, MD; Ben Schwartze; James Sliwa, DO; Hillary Vier, BA; Yeongchi Wu, MD; and Gary Yarkony, MD.

Credits

The concentric contraction on page 18 and the isometric contraction on page 19 are from "Flexibility" by K. Rusling. In *Training Guide to Cerebral Palsy Sports* (3rd ed., p. 67) by J.A. Jones (Ed.), 1988, Champaign, IL: Human Kinetics. Copyright 1988 by Jeffery A. Jones. Reprinted by permission.

The figures on page 28 are from "The Use of Strapping to Enhance the Athletic Performance of Wheelchair Competitors in Cerebral Palsy Sports," by R. Burd and K. Grass. In *Training Guide to Cerebral Palsy Sports* (3rd ed., pp. 81-84) by J.A. Jones (Ed.), 1988, Champaign, IL: Human Kinetics. Copyright 1988 by Jeffery A. Jones. Reprinted by permission.

Table 3.5 is from G.V. Borg, "Psychophysical Bases of Perceived Exertion," *Medicine and Science in Sports and Exercise*, **14**, pp. 377-387, © the American College of Sports Medicine, 1982. Reprinted by permission.

The photos on page 53 are from *Facilitated Stretching* (p. 8) by R.E. McAtee, 1993, Champaign, IL: Human Kinetics. Copyright 1993 by Robert E. McAtee. Reprinted by permission.

Table 8.4 on page 145 is adapted from Einarsson (1991); Fillyaw and Ades (1989); Florence and Hagberg (1984); Fowler (1988); Herbison et al. (1973); McCartney et al. (1988); Milner-Brown and Miller (1988); and Vignos and Watkins (1966).

Table 8.5 on page 149 is adapted from Einarsson (1991); Feldman and Soskolne (1987); Grimby and Einarsson (1991); and Halstead and Rossi (1985).

The diagram on page 226 is an original drawing by David Casement, rehabilitation engineer at the Rehabilitation Institute of Chicago. Reprinted by permission.

PART I

Components
of Physical Conditioning

The first part of this manual looks at aspects of a well-rounded fitness program, addressing each component of fitness in a separate chapter.

Chapter 1, "Exercise Readiness Assessment," explains preparations for starting your exercise program, including a medical screening and a general assessment of fitness components.

Chapter 2, "Strength Training," provides the information you need to prescribe a personal exercise program. We also provide practical information, such as how to exercise from your wheelchair and how to choose appropriate exercises.

Chapter 3, "Aerobic Training," provides the information you need to develop your own aerobic exercise program.

Chapter 4, "Flexibility Training," emphasizes the importance of maintaining proper range of motion and provides a full spectrum of flexibility exercises.

Once you have a good handle on these components of fitness, Part II will provide information specific to your disability.

CHAPTER 1

Exercise Readiness Assessment

Congratulations—you have decided to take that first step to living a more active and healthy lifestyle. Despite the many misconceptions regarding the training capabilities and athletic potentials of the physically disabled, researchers have shown that, when administered properly, exercise programs are appropriate and safe for most people with physical disabilities.

This chapter concentrates on how to get started by describing the steps required before you can safely perform regular exercise.

Medical History and Evaluation

A survey of your medical history and a physical examination are the first steps in starting an exercise program. Together they can detect the presence of disease, identify exercise restrictions, and help direct the focus of your exercise program. (A sample athlete medical form appears on pp. 13-14.) Medical approval to participate in exercise programs and sports also helps monitor safety. If you have an unremarkable health history, probably no further examinations or testing will be required before you start your exercise program. But if you have a progressive disorder, such as multiple sclerosis or **muscular dystrophy**, consult with your physician about your special needs. When you survey your health history, ask yourself questions like these:

- Is there any underlying cause of my disability that may restrict my physical activity (cardiovascular disease, diabetes, etc.)?
- Have I sustained any injury, such as a fracture, secondary to my disability that may restrict my physical activity?
- Am I taking any medication that will restrict my ability to perform physical activity or alter my response to exercise?

Check the medical form for other appropriate questions. Some people require further diagnostic and exercise testing before receiving approval for activity. Exercise testing is recommended for people with known cardiovascular, pulmonary, or metabolic diseases, endocrine disorders, renal disease, liver disease, and high coronary risk factors.

Insight Into Your Disability

Once you have received medical clearance and performed your own screening, the next step is identifying any limitations imposed by your disability. Most people with disabilities exercise at community fitness centers or on their own, not under medical supervision, so they must take the responsibility for monitoring their responses to exercise and modify their exercise programs accordingly. You should be aware of your needs and should also have strategies to meet them. For example, if you have multiple sclerosis, you should be careful not to overfatigue or overheat yourself—pace your activities and exercise in a ventilated area, near an open door or window or outdoors.

There is great variation among the limitations imposed by different disabilities. However, whether a disability is static or dynamic and progressive or nonprogressive affects the set-up and performance of your exercise program. (A categorization of several disability groups appears in Table 1.1.)

- With a *static disability*, no physical changes are elicited during physical activity or exercise. For example, someone with an amputation below the knee will not have a change in physical condition no matter what physical activity is undertaken.

- A *dynamic disability* is one that can be influenced or changed during physical activity. For example, fatigue, temperature, and emotional distress can all increase abnormal muscle tone in someone with cerebral palsy. In other words, the physical state, or condition, can change with exercise.

- A *progressive disability* involves a gradual decrease in physical functioning secondary to the disorder (multiple sclerosis, for example). A progressive disorder can be either static or dynamic, especially in the presence of muscle spasticity.

Age-Related Concerns

Adolescents and older adults with disabilities face additional guidelines to consider when setting up exercise programs. Although it is beyond our scope to present specific exercise routines for all ages, we do want you to be aware of some background information and basic exercise parameters if you are an adolescent or are approaching your later years.

Adolescent Training

Research findings increasingly point to a significant role for regular physical activity during growth and maturation. Obesity and other health risk factors can be prevented or delayed if you start a program of regular physical activity during childhood. Many degenerative diseases, especially cardiovascular diseases, have their roots in the formative years. Fundamental motor skills are the foundation of movement, and a variety of sports and activities should be encouraged to develop them during the formative years. Just as cross-training benefits adults, **adolescents** need variety to form a stable fitness base and prevent overuse injuries. Adolescents with disabilities have the same needs and get the same benefits from regular exercise and activity—they need an equal opportunity for physical education.

Table 1.1
Characteristics of Physical Disabilities

Disability	Physical state			
	Static	*Dynamic*	*Progressive*	*Nonprogressive*
Amputation	X			X
Arthrogryposis	X			X
Blindness	X			X
Cerebral palsy		X		X
Dwarfism	X			X
Head injury		X		X
Multiple sclerosis		X	X	
Neuromuscular diseases	X	X	X	
Osteogenesis imperfecta	X			X
Spinal cord injury	X			X
Stroke		X		X

Physical growth and maturation are major factors with children and adolescents. Several changes that take place in adolescent bodies are identical to those resulting from training, so it is not always easy to distinguish them from the effects of training. This is especially true in the case of heart rate (resting and submaximal); as the body matures heart rate decreases, which is the same effect that results from training. In contrast, as the body matures resting and submaximal arterial blood pressure increases, versus regular training, which can produce a lower resting and submaximal arterial blood pressure. **Aerobic** power, muscle strength, and aerobic muscle power are all trainable in the adolescent.

For adolescents, proper use of exercise is the single most important factor in preventing injuries. Adolescents' major problems are inappropriate exercise selection and improper execution of the exercise program. However, when progressive resistive exercise (PRE) is properly selected and performed, there is no question that it is beneficial. PRE has also produced strength gains for adolescents with neuromuscular disorders.

Weight training is a method of physical conditioning using submaximum weights to develop technique, flexibility, and muscle endurance. Proper weight training, along with stretching exercises, uses the full range of motion to ensure range of motion and flexibility are maintained. Experts recommend weight training 2 to 3 days a week for 20 to 30 min. Increase weight in 1- to 3-pound increments when you are able to perform 10 to 15 repetitions in good form. Exercise in sets of 10 to encourage good form and proper breathing technique (breathe deeply and then exhale while lifting). Perform one to three sets of each exercise, depending on the number of exercises.

Prepubescent and adolescent weight training is safe under expert supervision when dynamic concentric contractions are used systematically. Maximum lifts and competition are prohibited until growth is complete, between the ages of 16 and 19, because the growing bone junctions (epiphyseal) are not as strong as the fibrous and ligamentous supports around the joint. If an epiphyseal junction—the weakest link—is injured, bony deformity can result because of subsequent unequal growth. Adolescent bodies are not structurally mature—for instance, the **vertebrae** of the spine are not completely ossified until 25 to 30 years of age. This is significant because the low back region is the

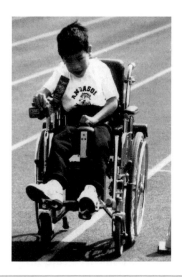

Adolescent training should emphasize a variety of activities and sports.

dominant injury site in powerlifting, and bones that are not completely ossified are at increased risk for injury. No weights greater than 40% of body weight should be used until after 1 year of basic strength development of spinal muscles through a full range of movement. This is to ensure that **trunk** stability is present to prevent low back injuries. Even after growth is complete, a physician or sports medicine specialist should be consulted before beginning weight training.

To avoid injury with exercise, adolescents should follow the same guidelines as adults plus the following:

- They must have the emotional maturity to accept coaching and instruction.
- Weight-training supervision should teach discipline, exercise technique, and safety. Most injuries are the result of immaturity, impaired judgment, or lack of knowledge about training.
- Strength training equipment must accommodate the size and maturity of the body (e.g., adjust the leg machines to height).
- Strength training should only be part of a variety of activities designed to increase coordination and fitness.

Instructor's Note: If you are a coach or instructor, emphasize proper technique and repetitions rather than the amount of weight lifted. During an adolescent growth spurt, it is even more important to decrease the intensity of training and focus on supplementary flexibility **work**.

Exercise Concerns of the Elderly

Odd as it may seem, as you become older than 65, many of the adolescent exercise guidelines apply to you again. Like the adolescent, you also need to focus on exercise technique versus the quantity you lift, stretching exercises through your full range of motion, and aerobic activities to improve your endurance as well as coordination and speed of movement.

Many changes in your health as you get older result from reduced activity levels. To prevent such changes as cardiovascular disease, decreased range of motion with arthritis, and decreased balance from changes in vision, flexibility, and muscle strength, you must find an exercise program you will adhere to. The program should include warm-up and cool-down sessions and stretching exercises. You need to hold your stretches longer, at least 15 to 30 sec, because your tissues are often less pliable and your decreased activity levels and increased sitting time produce tight muscles and **tendons**.

Fast walking is recommended in preference to jogging because it is less stressful on the joints. Monitor heart rate and rating of perceived exertion (RPE) consistently during aerobic activities so your intensity level does not exceed your level of training. Dehydration is common with exercise, so drink water before, during, and after exercise.

When exercise calls for changing position, be aware that **orthostatic hypotension**, a drop in blood pressure when assuming the upright position, is common when going from lying down to sitting and sitting to standing. Change positions slowly to avoid this and do some gentle, active range-of-motion exercises with your arms and legs before you stand. Changing positions to do a variety of exercises is important to give you good muscle balance and coordination.

Lifting weights for strength and conditioning is recommended. Concentrate on muscle endurance routines that take the weight through your full active range of motion. Do not perform the Valsalva maneuver (exhaling and "bearing down") while lifting weights, which can put undue pressure on your heart and raise your blood pressure. Inhale before you start, exhale with exertion, and remember to use slow, rhythmical breathing throughout the exercise.

Pay attention to your body and how it feels with exercise. Be knowledgeable about your "weak spots" in strength and flexibility training. Discuss with your doctor any exercise re-

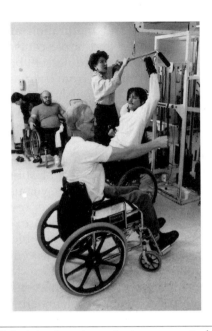

Strength training is an important component of fitness for all ages.

strictions stemming from osteoporosis, for example, and the effects that medication could have on exercise. Keep moving! Find exercises that you like to do, and will do, on a regular basis.

Equipment Availability

Before moving on to the last step of defining your exercise starting point or fitness baseline, you need to identify where you will work out. The equipment available to you, such as exercise machines, free weights, Theraband, and so on, will dictate your exercise modes. The typical resources and staff of the exercise facility can help with your preexercise fitness assessment. However, more in-depth assessments are possible using wheelchair accessible equipment or specialty equipment such as wheelchair rollers and arm crank ergometers, which are found typically in hospital-based programs and some community fitness centers (see Appendix A).

Because of the diversity of disabilities and lack of specialty equipment in community gyms, one standard assessment will not be entirely appropriate for each disability group. The baseline information you need to prescribe an exercise program will vary depending on your disability. Refer to the chapters about specific disabilities for recommended assessment areas for your disability.

Assessing Your Exercise Starting Point

Assessing your starting point for all fitness components (flexibility, strength, cardiovascular endurance, and body composition) is used to

- establish the fitness baseline for starting the exercise program at the appropriate intensity,
- identify strong and weak areas of the muscles needing work,
- set exercise goals, and
- customize the exercise program to fit your needs.

Different disability groups have different physical characteristics requiring special set-ups to meet specific physical needs in the exercise program. However, assessing flexibility, muscle strength, muscle endurance, cardiorespiratory endurance, and general body composition is appropriate for all disability groups.

Flexibility and Posture Assessment

To assess flexibility, identify both the areas of the body that are restricted in movement and the areas that show excessive movement. Restricted and unstable movements of joints can lead to inefficient muscular performance or injury. For example, if your chest and anterior shoulder muscles are tight and your posterior shoulder and upper back muscles are weak and stretched out, you may develop shoulder problems such as rotator cuff injuries, especially if you are a wheelchair user. Your exercise program should emphasize stretching your anterior shoulders and chest while strengthening your upper back. This manual uses general active range of motion (AROM) tests to determine the general areas that need to be stretched (see Table 1.2 on pp. 8 and 9). AROM tests can be performed at home or at any facility.

Posture is the end result of muscle balance or imbalance. To maintain an erect, upright posture, you need to use your strength and flexibility to keep a proper balance between opposing muscle groups: anterior muscles (flexors) must be in balance with posterior muscles (extensors), lateral muscles (abductors) must be in balance with medial muscles (adductors), and muscles that rotate extremities inward must be in balance with muscles that rotate extremities outward. Common muscle imbalances that you want to avoid include forward head and rounded back, rounded shoulders, and winged scapulae.

Forward Head and Rounded Back. If you spend a lot of time sitting in or pushing a wheelchair, gravity and activities in front of the body tend to pull body parts down and in. This tightens and strengthens the flexors. The result is the need to stretch the anterior neck and trunk musculature and strengthen the neck and back extensor muscles to promote muscle balance. The extensors of the neck and back are referred to as the antigravity muscles—they assist with upright posture. An upright posture, in turn, helps maintain a positive body image and can prevent problems with back pain.

Rounded Shoulders. Performing activities in front of the body and pushing a wheelchair often tighten and strengthen the adductors and internal rotators of the shoulder. The result is a need to stretch the tightened anterior muscles of the shoulder and strengthen the trapezius and rhomboids, which in turn may help prevent possible rotator cuff or shoulder impingement injuries.

Winged Scapulae. When use of the arms for overhead activity decreases, the postural result of winged scapulae often occurs, frequently accompanying round shoulders. It is important to recognize this postural weakness of the serratus anterior muscle and strengthen the muscle to prevent shoulder injuries. The serratus anterior and other scapular muscles must be strong before you work on strengthening movements above the shoulder level. Work on stabilizing the shoulder girdle musculature through free weight exercises before you progress to overhead strengthening.

Body alignment or the misalignment of extremities (e.g., arthritic hands or flat feet) needs to be monitored with repetitive activities or resistance training. Your physician should indicate the need for bracing or protective equipment on your preexercise medical form, or you should be aware of exercise restrictions you must observe to avoid injury. If you have a history of prior injuries or a muscle or skeletal disease (e.g., muscular dystrophy or osteogenesis imperfecta), you may require frequent training program modifications to avoid overstressing "weak links." Eliminating the weak links in your musculoskeletal system through proper training and biomechanical exercise techniques should be one of your goals to prevent injury. If you are a coach or instructor and you have questions

Table 1.2
Flexibility—General Active Range of Motion Tests

Joints	Movements	
Elbow	*Extension/flexion*—Hold arms straight out from the side of the body parallel to the floor. Flex elbows until the fingers touch the shoulders on the same side. (Fingers should touch shoulders with upper arm in any position.) *Limitations:* Elbow flexion and extension are usually not limited by nonpathological (without disease) muscle tightness; however, range of motion can be limited by spasticity (abnormal muscle tone) or orthopedic impairments.	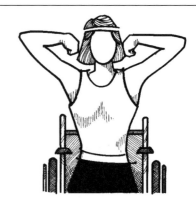
Shoulder	*Flexion*—Raise arms straight up in front of body with elbows extended. Arms should be approximately perpendicular to the floor with palms of hand facing forward. *Limitations:* Possible tightness in front or anterior shoulder (pectoralis major, anterior deltoid), back or posterior shoulder (posterior deltoid, latissimus dorsi, and teres major muscles).	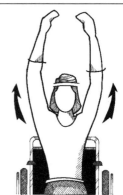
	Extension—Stand or sit in a tall erect posture. Grasp hands together behind back with elbows fully extended. Raise hands up maintaining elbow extension. Hands should reach chest level. *Limitations:* Possible tightness in anterior shoulder (pectoralis major, anterior deltoid).	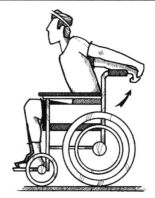
	Abduction—Raise arms straight out and up from sides with elbows extended until thumbs touch over the head or until arms are perpendicular to the floor. *Limitations:* Possible tightness in latissimus dorsi, front and back shoulder (anterior and posterior deltoid), and shoulder internal rotators.	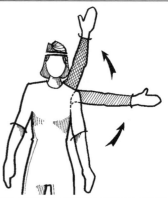

Joints	Movements

Shoulder *(cont.)*

External rotation (chicken wing)—Hold hands behind the head with elbows flexed in line or behind head.

Limitations: Possible tightness in anterior shoulder and chest (pectoralis major, anterior deltoid).

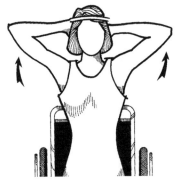

Ankle

Dorsiflexion—With leg straight curl foot up toward head. Foot and toes should at least be perpendicular to floor.

Limitations: Possible tightness in posterior calf muscles (gastrocnemius and soleus). Plantar flexion typically is not limited in range of motion.

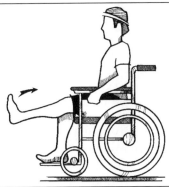

Knee

Extension—Sit erect on edge of chair or mat. Extend knee completely maintaining erect sitting posture. Low back should maintain a small curve; rounding of lower back indicates muscle tightness.

Limitations: Possible tightness in hamstrings, low back, or both.

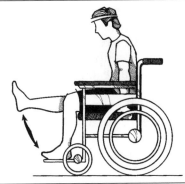

Straight leg raise—Lie on back, lift leg up as far as possible with knee extended. Leg should be able to move perpendicular to mat with knee fully extended. Inability to keep knee extended indicates muscle tightness.

Limitations: Possible tightness in hamstrings and low back.

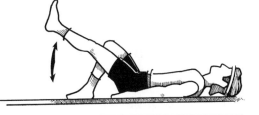

Hip

Flexion (knee to chest)—Lie on back. Raise knee up to chest as far as possible. Knee should be past the perpendicular toward head. Opposite leg should lie flat on mat.

Limitations: If difficult to raise knee to chest, possible muscle tightness in posterior hip muscles (gluteals) and/or low back. If difficulty with maintaining opposite leg flat on mat, possible tightness in anterior hip (hip flexors, iliopsoas).

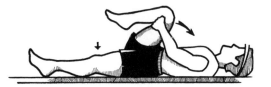

regarding an individual's alignment of extremities or joint laxity, consult the participant's physician or physical therapist.

Muscle Strength

People without the full use of their musculature require a specific assessment of the strength of their available working muscles. For example, if you have **quadriplegia**, you will show some muscle function loss in all four extremities. You need a strength assessment of all your working muscle groups to start an exercise program at the appropriate intensity for each one. The strength assessment also helps identify the proper mode of exercise and type of set-ups. For example, a weak triceps may not be able to extend the forearm up against gravity; however, if you bring the arm down to a table or a workout partner supports the upper arm, the weight of the arm is reduced, and you may be able to straighten the elbow. Your exercise program should then focus on the weak triceps.

Just as it is important to identify all your weak areas, it is also important to take a close look at all your proximal muscles. Proximal muscles are the muscles that surround the shoulder and pelvic girdles. For example, your smaller upper back muscles stabilize and position your scapula against your rib cage. Weakness in these muscles can position the shoulder improperly and cause impingement syndrome in your shoulder when you perform exercises above shoulder height, such as shoulder presses. If you are a wheelchair user, shoulder problems could make daily activities difficult. If you have shoulder problems, it is important to consult your physician.

Muscle Endurance, Tolerance to Aerobic Activities

Your exercise program should enable you to attain an appropriate level of strength and to maintain that strength over time or through a series of repeated muscular efforts such as wheelchair propulsion or transferring into and out of a wheelchair. Muscle endurance should not be confused with cardiorespiratory endurance. In individuals with an intact nervous system and no loss of muscle function, activities that promote cardiorespiratory endurance generally involve whole-body activities, such as running, whereas exercises to improve muscle endurance, such as

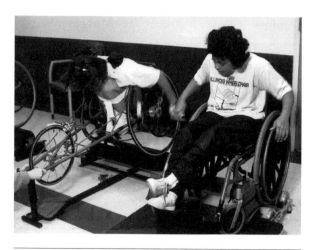

Performing short exercise time trials can assess your tolerance to aerobic activity.

strength training, are localized in a specific extremity or the trunk. People with intact nervous systems can use localized activities to improve muscle endurance and whole-body activities for cardiorespiratory fitness.

If you are a wheelchair user or have some degree of muscle loss, you will typically use localized activities for both long- and short-duration exercises. For example, you may use a wheelchair roller or an arm crank for long-duration, aerobic activities. These modes of exercise use the smaller muscle mass of the upper extremities, stressing primarily the peripheral system (the working muscles), as opposed to whole-body activities such as running, which use a larger muscle mass and stress both the peripheral (the working muscles) and the central (cardiovascular) systems. Decreased muscle strength and endurance can limit your ability to perform long-duration aerobic activities due to muscle fatigue. These limitations are even more prevalent with the loss of muscle function seen in people who have had a stroke or a **spinal cord** injury or who have been diagnosed with neuromuscular disease. Assessment of muscle endurance should focus on your ability to perform continuous aerobic activities.

Exercise Trials (Arm Crank, Wheelchair Rollers, Treadmill). Assess muscle endurance by performing a time trial on one of the above modes at low to moderate intensity, continuing for 5 min or until fatigued. People usually discontinue exercise due to muscle fatigue rather than cardiorespiratory factors. In addition, individuals with quadriplegia may experience exercise hypotension and may complain of dizziness or light-headedness (refer to p. 94 for specifics regarding exercise hypotension). Record your resting, exercise, and postexercise heart rate and blood pressure using the procedures that follow. Heart rate and blood pressure can be affected by your disability or medications. Refer to the assessment section of the chapter about your specific disability for information regarding the effects of medication on exercise.

Cardiorespiratory (Aerobic) Endurance

Cardiorespiratory or aerobic activities use large muscle masses continuously for a sustained period of time. The ability to perform exercise is limited by the delivery of oxygen to the muscles. Many devices and tests have been developed to assess cardiorespiratory fitness as indicated by maximum oxygen consumption ($\dot{V}O_2$max) and maximum aerobic power (both of which can be tested in exercise physiology laboratories). Exercise physiology tests and exercise stress tests are beyond the scope of this manual, and exercise technologists and elaborate testing equipment are generally not available in gyms and fitness centers. However, you can use a resting assessment of heart rate and blood pressure to prescribe aerobic exercise.

Resting Heart Rate. Palpation is the most practical way to assess the resting heart rate. The pulse can be palpated (felt) in one of the following areas:

- Radial artery—on anterolateral area of the wrist just above the base of the thumb
- Brachial artery—on the inside of the upper arm just above the elbow joint (antecubital space) and medial to the biceps tendon
- Carotid artery—on the neck just lateral to the larynx (Adam's apple), with caution if prone to syncope or slow heart rate. Be sure to palpate only one side at a time and do not press too hard or you could impede the blood flow.

To assess resting heart rate

1. Use the tip of the middle and index fingers to palpate the pulse. Do not use the thumb; it has a pulse of its own that can be misleading.

2. Start the stopwatch or second hand of wristwatch simultaneously with the pulse beat.

3. Count the first beat as zero, and continue counting for a designated time period (10, 15, 30, or 60 sec).

4. To obtain a count of beats per minute, multiply the beats registered for the designated time period times a multiplier that gives you a 60-sec count of beats per minute. For example you would multiply the number of beats counted in 10 sec by 6, in 15 sec by 4, and in 30 sec by 2.

5. Record the number in beats per minute.

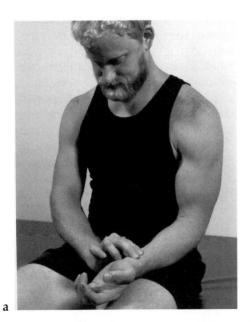
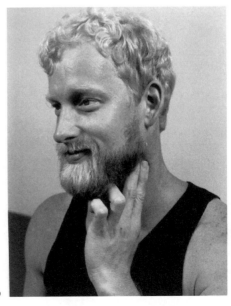

a   b

Taking (a) your radial pulse or (b) your carotid pulse is an easy method of measuring exercise intensity.

The heart rate varies due to anxiety, caffeine, smoking, body positions, and the like. Certain disabilities, such as quadriplegia from a spinal cord injury, and certain medications can also influence the heart rate. Refer to the disability-specific chapters for heart rate responses to exercise. The normal resting heart rate range is 60 to 100 beats per minute.

Blood Pressure.   Blood pressure is a measure of the pressure exerted on the arterial walls by the blood. It records two values, the systolic and diastolic pressures. Systolic blood pressure is the pressure when the heart contracts or pumps the blood out to the circulatory system. Systolic blood pressure normally ranges between 90 to 140 mmHg. Diastolic blood pressure is the pressure when the heart is filling up following a contraction. Diastolic blood pressure normally ranges between 60 and 90 mmHg.

Resting blood pressure can be measured indirectly with the use of a stethoscope and blood pressure cuff as follows:

1. Determine the proper cuff size. A cuff that is too large or too small can cause an inaccurate reading. Cuffs are available for children, adults, and people with particularly large arms.

2. With the subject seated and relaxed, wrap the cuff around the upper arm.

3. Place the bell of the stethoscope over the brachial artery located on the inside of the up-

per arm just above the elbow joint (antecubital space) and medial to the biceps tendon.

4. Inflate the cuff to 180 to 200 mmHg.

5. Slowly release the pressure of the cuff while watching the dial. Record the reading when you hear the first beat, or thud, which corresponds to the blood rushing through the open artery. This measure is your systolic blood pressure.

6. Continue to listen for the beats until they are muffled and disappear. Record this level as your diastolic pressure.

Blood pressure is recorded with systolic blood pressure on top and diastolic blood pressure on the bottom, for example 120/80 (systolic/diastolic).

Body Composition

Body composition refers to your percentage of total body fat. Excessive body fat can lead to obesity and may increase the risk of heart disease. In the past, body composition was estimated by recording measures of height and weight and consulting tables to determine the appropriate weight for the appropriate height. Height and weight tables have limitations, however, because they do not account for the body build and the proportion of bone, muscle, and fat.

Several techniques are available to assess percent body fat or percent of lean mass. Underwater weighing is a valid, reliable, and widely used laboratory technique for assessing body composition. The equipment necessary is not readily available in fitness centers and gyms, however. Skinfold measurement is another technique used for determining body composition, but it is invalid when assessing individuals with muscle loss (**atrophy**). Whatever the technique, all equations used in assessing body composition are considered population-specific. For accuracy, it is extremely important that the equation used to predict body composition matches the population. No standards to assess the percentage of body fat have been developed specifically for wheelchair users. Percent body fat is not a measure that is needed for exercise prescriptions. However, a general survey of body mass is necessary to direct the focus of the exercise program. If weight loss is the desired goal, program focus should be on long-duration aerobic activities (biking, running, wheelchair rolling, etc.) to burn calories.

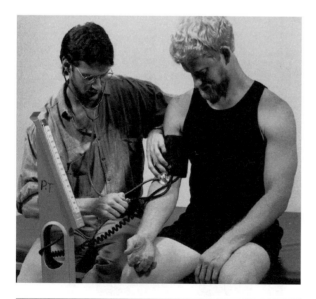

A baseline blood pressure measurement can be used as an indicator of aerobic fitness.

Athlete Medical Form

To be completed by the athlete

Date received by **facility name**: _____   Team affiliation: _____

Name _____   Phone (_____) _____

Address _____

City _____   State _____   Zip _____

Date of birth ____/ ____/ ____/   Health insurance _____   Policy # _____

Emergency contact _____   Relationship _____   Phone (_____) _____

Diagnosis _____

Cause: ___ Congenital (present at birth) or ___ acquired (if acquired, please complete the following)

   Date of onset/injury: _____

   ___ Head injury due to (type of accident): _____

   ___ Amputation level: _____   cause: _____

   ___ Stroke: cause: _____

   ___ Spinal cord injury: ___ complete   ___ incomplete, level ___   cause: _____

   ___ Other (specify disability and cause) _____

List all surgeries (procedure and date): _____

_____

Date of last tetanus shot: _____

Medication you are currently taking (prescription and over the counter): _____

_____

Allergies and specifics of reaction: _____

Medical history:

Seizures   No   Yes   Type _____

         Number in the past 12 months ____   Date of most recent seizure _____

Diabetes	No	Yes	
Insulin dependent	No	Yes	Explain _____
Hypertension (high blood pressure)	No	Yes	
Heart disease	No	Yes	Specify: _____
Lung disease/asthma	No	Yes	Specify: _____
Heat-related problems	No	Yes	Specify: _____
Injuries affecting sports participation	No	Yes	Specify: _____

Other (specify) _____

Are you currently involved in any outpatient therapies?   No   Yes   Explain _____

_____

Sports classification: track ___;   field ___;   swimming ___;   basketball ___;   quad rugby ___;   other ___

For the purpose of competitive/recreational participation in the following sports/activities: (check all that apply)

   ___ swimming   ___ boccie   ___ W/C basketball   ___ quad rugby   ___ amb. soccer   ___ field

___ target shooting   ___ W/C team handball   ___ equestrian   ___ bowling   ___ track   ___ archery   ___ slalom

   ___ cycling   ___ cross country   ___ table tennis   ___ powerlifting   ___ strength and conditioning   ___ tennis

Permission is given to **facility name,** _____ its representative, a representative of the local team, or local competition organizing committee to seek medical care in case of an emergency for the above person.

_____   _____
Signature of participant or parent/guardian if under 18   Date

(continued)

An athlete medical form should be completed before beginning an exercise program to detect the presence of disease, identify exercise restrictions, and help direct your program.

To Be Completed by Physician

Athlete's name: _____

Diagnosis (list all): _____

Impairments (e.g., hemiparesis, etc.): _____

_____

_____

Height: _____ Weight: _____ Pulse: _____ BP: _____ Sex: _____

Physical exam: Normal   Abnormal   Explanation of abnormalities

Head/neck   _____   _____   _____

Eyes/vision   _____   _____   _____

Ears/hearing _____   _____   _____

Heart/lungs   _____   _____   _____

GU   _____   _____   _____

CNS   _____   _____   _____

Skin   _____   _____   _____

Orthopedic exam:

   ROM loss/contractures: _____

   Joint laxity/instability: _____

   Other: _____

Dates of hospitalization over last 2 years with admitting diagnoses: _____

_____

_____

Significant "abnormal test" (EKG/X-ray/lab): _____

Approval for participation: ___ Yes   ___ No

Comments/restrictions: _____

_____

_____

_____

Physician's signature _____   Date _____

Print name _____   Phone (_____) _____

Address _____

City _____   State _____   Zip _____

Fax (_____) _____

Please return to: **program name and address**

(continued)

CHAPTER 2

Strength Training

Developing and starting a strength program is a rewarding experience. This chapter discusses the background information you'll need, including the factors you must consider if your strength program is to be safe and effective. We will also explain exactly how to design your own program.

Strength training is a general term used to apply to muscle development through the use of free weights, variable resistance, isokinetics, and isometrics. Strength training is used commonly in sports training, recreational fitness, and medical-related rehabilitation programs. There are many misconceptions about the use of strength

training and its potential for people with physical disabilities. However, it is clear that strength training can have many benefits in the presence of a disability, including enhanced sport performance, increased physical function, increased independence in daily living activities, and fewer medical complications.

Your Body's Response

The purpose of discussing the physiological effects of strength training is not to turn you into an

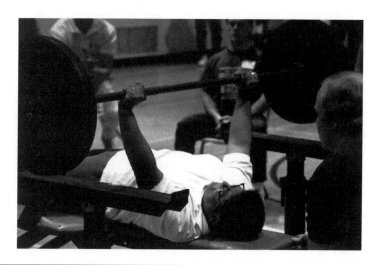

Strength training can show many benefits, including increased function with daily activities and increased self-esteem.

amateur exercise physiologist, but rather to give you a better understanding of how your body will react to the strength program that you design for yourself. Understanding cause and effect will allow you to better design and modify your exercise program to fit your needs and goals.

The human body has the remarkable ability to adapt according to the stresses placed on it. When the body is attacked by an infection, the immune system reacts by producing antibodies to counteract it. The musculoskeletal system functions similarly. When the muscles (muscle fibers) and the anaerobic energy system are stressed by weightlifting, they are modified. With appropriate rest and recuperation, the muscle can become larger (hypertrophy), stronger, or both as a positive adaptation to that stress.

True physiological changes in the muscle itself generally occur 4 to 6 weeks following the start of a strength training program. Initial gains in voluntary strength or the amount of resistance are possibly due to both the effects on the nervous system and direct effects on the muscles. The nervous system stimulates and controls the muscles. During the initial training phase, the nervous system controls learning the exercise movements, increasing stimulation of the muscles (prime movers), and improving coordination of movement by more efficient recruiting of muscle fibers. These initial, training-induced changes, without changes of the muscle such as muscle hypertrophy, are referred to as neural adaptations, and they occur prior to the physiological changes in the muscle. Most strength gains in individuals with neuromuscular diseases, such as muscular dystrophy, are attributed to these neural factors rather than to changes within the muscle.

Following the first few weeks of weight training, gains in strength or the amount of resistance tolerated will eventually taper off and become more modest as a result of physiological changes within the working muscles. Training-induced muscle changes include increased muscle cross-sectional area, attributed to muscle fiber **hypertrophy** (enlargement), and muscle fiber **hyperplasia** (increase in the number of muscle fibers) due to long-term effects of resistance training. Increases in strength are not always accompanied by muscle hypertrophy. Whereas in the early stages of muscular changes significant muscular hypertrophy can occur, after a certain improvement in strength, further increases occur with little or no gains in muscle size.

Generally, physiological changes in the muscle as a result of training do not differ for the physically disabled; the changes instead relate to the amount of active muscle mass used during exercise. The only exceptions are those conditions that directly involve the muscles, such as muscular dystrophy. In these situations, your goal is to increase strength through improving nervous system control rather than to affect the muscles directly. Table 2.1 summarizes the physiological effects of anaerobic strength training and how these effects improve the body's performance.

Muscle Soreness and Overwork Weakness

Muscle soreness 2 to 24 hours following strength training is a normal transitory response, usually as a result of muscle ischemia (decreased oxygen from the blood) and accumulation of metabolic wastes such as lactate. Delayed soreness 24 to 72 hours later may also occur. Muscle **spasms** are one theory about delayed muscle soreness. This theory states that pain from ischemia and build-up of waste products elicit reflex muscle spasms, which then produce more spasms and continue this cycle. Other research suggests that delayed muscle soreness is caused by the disruption in muscle connective tissue and its tendon attachments following eccentric contractions. Eccentric contractions produce a greater degree of delayed muscle soreness than concentric or isometric exercise, probably because fewer motor units are recruited during eccentric contractions compared to the same amount of work using concentric contractions.

You should not be alarmed about muscle soreness. You should recognize however, that soreness may be a sign of overtraining or overzealous progression of your exercise program. You can resume resistance training as muscle soreness declines. Recommended activities that can be used during recovery of muscle soreness include active rest (e.g., stretching), a reduction in the intensity or duration of the activity that initially caused the soreness, or use of an activity that utilizes different muscle groups (as in sport exercise routines and cross-training). If muscle soreness interferes with function—if, for example, it inhibits transfers or the ability to propel a wheelchair—you should not resume the exercise program until the soreness has completely stopped, and you should reevaluate the exercise program

Table 2.1
Physiological Effects of Resistance Training

System or organ	Effects of disuse (physiological)	Effects of exercise (physiological change)	Effects on performance
Cardiovascular system	• Higher resting heart rate • Lower cardiac output • Decreased circulation	• Increased absolute left ventricular wall thickness and left ventricular mass • Decreased resting heart rate • Greater absolute stroke volume • More efficient cardiac output and pulmonary ventilation • Increased oxygen extraction and delivery to muscles • Increased circulation	• Heart is more efficient (pumps same output with fewer beats)
Nervous system	• Suboptimal coordination • Decreased emotional state, possible depression, and lethargy	• Increased activation of motor units in prime movers • Increased EMG responses • Increased appropriate activation of synergists and antagonists	• Increased coordination and skill of movement • Increased accuracy, precision, and balance • Smooth, flowing movement • Improved self-esteem
Muscle	• Decreased muscle mass (atrophy) and strength • Early onset of fatigue	• Increased muscle mass (hypertrophy) • Increased muscle endurance • Improved ability to generate muscle tension (strength)	• Easier performance of daily activities • Increased ability for wheelchair propulsion on varied surfaces
Connective tissue/bone	• Bone demineralization (osteoporosis) • Decreased pliability of tendons and ligaments • Contractures • Pressure sores	• Increased bone density • Increased tensile strength in tendons and ligaments • Increased skin elasticity	• Decrease or elimination of pressure sores • Decreased incidence of injury from overuse activities • Stabilize and protect joints (ligaments)
Body composition	• Increased % body fat	• Decreased % body fat and increase in lean tissue	• Decreased risks of cardiovascular disease

Note. Adapted from Curtis (1981); Fleck (1983); Hakkinen (1989); Kraemer (1990b); Sale (1988); and Stone (1983, 1988).

design before restarting it. If you have prolonged bouts of muscle soreness without any recovery or relief after an exercise session, consult your physician.

Use extreme caution if you have a disease that affects muscle tissue directly, for example, muscular dystrophy or another neurological disease outside the **central nervous system** (brain and spinal cord), multiple sclerosis, polio, and numerous neuromuscular diseases. Progressive degenerative diseases result in gradual loss of muscle mass and strength. Muscle soreness with these conditions is an indication that the overload or intensity was excessive. This can result in *permanent* loss of strength. Researchers call this overwork weakness, and it is most commonly seen in people who have had polio or have some highly involved neuromuscular diseases.

Because of the possible deleterious effects, strength training is not appropriate for all populations. Research indicates that exercise training in people with neuromuscular diseases can be beneficial in maintaining strength and cardiorespiratory function if

- the degree of weakness is not severe—greater than 70% of residual muscle mass is available,
- the rate or progression of the disease is relatively slow,
- a survey of the individual's total daily activity level is considered in the program design, and
- the rate of increasing intensity is slow and supervised.

(Refer to pages 143-147 for more specifics about exercise for people with neuromuscular diseases.)

Muscle Contractions

Before discussing exercise principles and program design, we need to identify and clarify muscle contractions and types of training. This will give you a working vocabulary that can help you better understand this chapter. Categories of strength training can be based on the application of resistance. These categories include isotonic (both concentric and eccentric), isometric, isokinetic, and gravity-reduced exercise training.

Isotonic Training

Isotonic training consists of movements that contain both concentric and eccentric contractions. A concentric contraction refers to shortening a muscle during a muscular contraction, as in the up phase of a biceps curl. Performing "negatives" of an exercise refers to eccentric contractions.

Isotonic training generally emphasizes the concentric contraction; however, concentric versus eccentric contractions can only be completely isolated with physical assistance from a workout partner. The partner must place or lower the resistance (dumbbell) to allow you to perform only one type of contraction. For example, in order for you to perform only concentric biceps curls, your partner must lower the dumbbell each time. To perform eccentric biceps curls, your partner must place the dumbbell in your hand with your elbow flexed before each down phase. Isotonic training is considered a safe mode of resistance training during all phases of a training cycle.

Eccentric Training. Studies have confirmed that more muscle fibers are recruited during concentric contraction than eccentric contractions. Thus researchers have hypothesized that eccentric contractions are more efficient because they use fewer muscle fibers to lift the same load. Eccentric training is associated with muscle soreness—it produces a greater degree

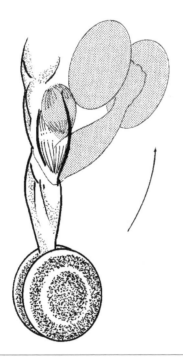

A concentric contraction.

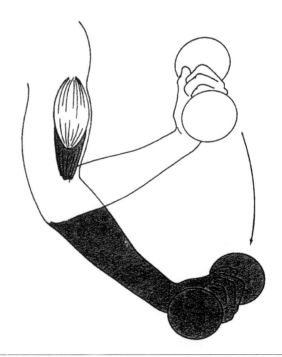

An eccentric contraction.

of muscle soreness than concentric or isometric training. This soreness has been attributed to muscle fiber connective tissue damage. Because eccentric exercise appears to produce the most trauma to the muscle fiber and the most muscle soreness, it should be reserved for use later in the training cycle or program. To avoid the potential of training-induced muscle damage in the neuromuscular diseases, eccentric training should not be a primary focus in the exercise program design. Remember that most strength gains in individuals with neuromuscular disease are attributed to neural factors, not muscle changes.

Isometric Training

Isometric contractions refer to a muscle contraction with no change in muscle length or without moving a joint, such as when pushing or pulling against a fixed object without movement. Strength improvements with isometric exercise occur at the specific muscle angle exercised; however, one source states that if you perform isometrics at different angles, it strengthens not only the specific muscle angle exercised but above and below that angle about 10 degrees in each direction. Isometric exercises are appropriate for individuals with arthritis when actual movement of the joint is limited due to pain. Isometric exercises can be performed anywhere without the use of equipment.

Isokinetic Training

Isokinetic exercise involves movement at a constant angular velocity. The velocity of the movement is controlled by the equipment and the tension is controlled by the participant. In this manner, torque can be measured and strength "quantified" so that different muscle groups on the right side of the body can be compared to the left side, and opposing muscle strengths can be measured. A few specialized machines deliver this type of training, but cost restricts their wide use. Isokinetic training is used commonly as an assessment tool in the sports medicine rehabilitation setting. One advantage of isokinetic training is the possibility of developing strength at speeds used during athletic or functional movements. Strength gains made in isokinetic training may be explained by a change in the recruitment patterns of the muscle fibers, suggesting that isokinetic

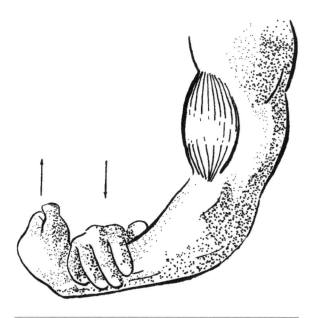

An isometric contraction.

training is velocity specific. Little or no muscle soreness occurs with isokinetic training, mostly because the muscle does not contract eccentrically.

Gravity-Reduced Exercise Training

This exercise training is performed in a position that reduces the effects of gravity and the weight of the exercising extremity. Gravity-reduced exercises are used for weaker muscle groups that have difficulty overcoming the weight of the extremity and gravity. For example, if you have very weak triceps, you may not be able to straighten your arm out over your head. However, if you bring your arm down onto a table at about shoulder level, you may be able to extend your elbow while it is supported on the table. This position would reduce the effects of gravity and the weight of your arm so your triceps could actually perform the movement. In some instances, gravity-reduced exercises can be performed until the muscle gains enough strength to perform the exercise in the antigravity position, giving you access to many more exercises. You may show great increases in function as you develop increased antigravity strength, such as the ability to perform independent transfers, to reach for objects, and so on. The amount of possible strength gains from performing gravity-reduced exercises with a very weak muscle depends upon external factors such as the amount of initial damage to the spinal cord with spinal cord injury or the amount of available working muscle fibers with multiple sclerosis. Gravity-reduced exercise training can be used for all disability groups.

Basic Training Principles and Considerations

Any safe, efficient exercise program follows the same basic principles of exercise. These principles—overload, progressive resistance, **symmetrical** muscle development, order of exercises, and specificity of training—apply to everyone, whether disabled or not. They may need to be modified, however, depending on your disability.

Overload Principle

The musculoskeletal system (muscle, tendon, ligament, bone) gains strength by being safely stressed or overloaded. This is called the overload principle. In conditions such as multiple sclerosis (MS) and neuromuscular diseases (NMD), however, the overload principle must be modified. Individuals with MS may show increased energy cost for walking and increased fatigue due to the effects of spasticity, ataxia, and weakness. Overworking the muscles in MS can contribute to excessive fatigue, which decreases the ability to perform daily functional skills such as dressing, walking, wheelchair propulsion, and the like. In the case of neuromuscular diseases and postpolio syndrome, overwork can possibly cause permanent loss of muscle fiber function.

Progressive Resistive Exercise (PRE)

As a muscle adapts to applied stresses, resistance must be increased for further positive changes to occur—thus the term *progressive resistive exercise*. Large increases in resistance should be avoided; if the muscle stress is too great, the muscle can react adversely and injury can result. If your increase in resistance results in poor technique, the increase was too great. How many times have we seen people arch their backs to perform a biceps curl with weights that are too heavy? Conditions such as MS and NMD require even slower progression. Often, the resistance exercise program goal when these con-

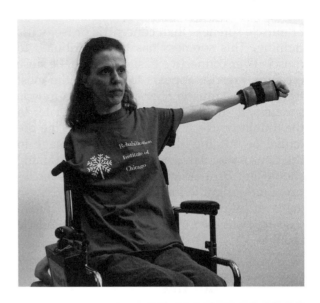

Performing a unilateral exercise allows the nonexercising arm to assist with balance.

ditions are involved is to maintain the present strength level, especially as the diseases progress. Because people with NMD apparently gain most increases in strength from resistance training due to neural factors rather than muscular changes (hypertrophy), large increases in exercise resistance (load) are not needed for strength maintenance or gains.

Symmetrical Muscle Development

Bilateral exercise—performing exercises with simultaneous use of the same extremity on both sides of the body—targets more proximal shoulder and pelvic girdle musculature and trunk strength than unilateral exercise—performing exercise with an extremity on only one side of the body. Bilateral exercise may be useful if you have minimal trunk coordination (**ataxia**) or balance impairments due to multiple sclerosis, closed head injuries, and similar conditions. Increases in proximal strength (in the trunk, shoulder, and pelvic girdle) may allow for improved coordination and movement of your extremities. But bilateral exercises are not appropriate for everyone. With bilateral exercises, a stronger extremity could compensate for a weaker extremity. If so, you would want to perform more unilateral exercises to allow your weaker extremity to catch up, thereby reducing the possibility of injury. If you have no use or limited use of one side of your body (for example with **hemiplegia** following a stroke), unilateral exercises are definitely appropriate. Unilateral exer-

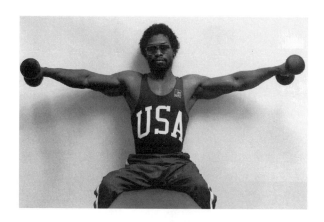

Bilateral shoulder raises force the trunk muscles to stabilize the body during arm movement.

cises may also be appropriate if you have significant coordination difficulties with your extremities or balance problems. Unilateral exercises may allow you to perform the desired exercise with better balance and proper technique. You may find it useful to hook your nonexercising arm around the push handle of your wheelchair or to hold on to your chair to help you keep your balance.

Order of Exercise

The order in which you perform exercises is important for maximizing the workout. Lifts working many muscle groups or multijoint exercises are the core exercises and should be performed before working individual muscles or single joints. Single-joint exercises before multijoint exercises may preexhaust the smaller

working muscles and limit the performance and safety of the multijoint exercises.

Your muscle groups need an appropriate amount of rest between sets for recuperation. This is easily achieved by working on one muscle group while another is resting to allow for full recovery. Work the opposing muscle group following exercise of the agonist. For example, follow the bench press with bent-over rows. Alternating an upper body exercise with a lower body exercise is another way to assure appropriate recovery time for each muscle group.

Specificity of Training

Specificity of training refers to choosing the exercises and program variables (sets, repetitions, loads, rest) used in selected activities. Specificity of movement in strength training may also include task-specific activation of motor units within a muscle and other **synergistic muscles**. This simply means working the muscles that you need to strengthen to perform a specific activity or sport. When selecting exercises for specific activities, you need to understand some basic biomechanics of movement or consult someone who does. Basically, you need to define the muscles that perform the activity and choose an exercise that works the specific muscle.

For example, if you wish to increase your strength to allow for independent transfers into and out of the wheelchair, you may perform dips or Rickshaw as your primary exercise. Dips focus on the triceps and shoulder depressors to allow

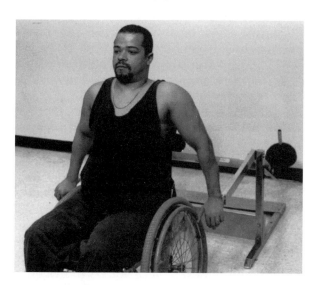

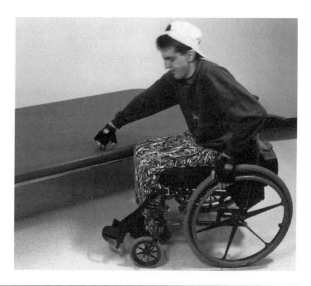

The Rickshaw exercise strengthens many muscle groups that are needed to perform wheelchair transfers.

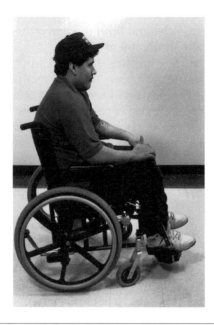

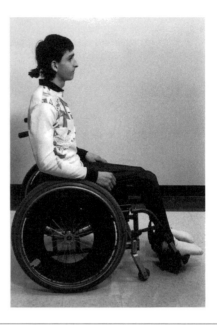

Poor posture (rounded shoulders) in stretched-out wheelchair back upholstery can set you up for a potential shoulder injury.

Good sitting posture exhibiting balanced front and back musculature is essential in avoiding injuries.

an individual to lift his or her body up to move from one surface to another. If you are interested in training for sport competition, you must analyze the movements needed for the specific activity and select appropriate exercises to strengthen the muscles used. An example would be using the seated shoulder press and the Rickshaw exercise to strengthen the drive phase of the track wheelchair forward push. A single-joint exercise could also be used for strengthening wrist extension to assist with the recovery phase of the wheelchair push.

Special Considerations and Concerns

Safety should always be the first concern when performing any activity. Most safety measures for exercise require a little knowledge and a lot of common sense. However, if you have a physical disability, you may have some special considerations or concerns unique to your disability. It is essential that you take responsibility for these safety issues, but you should not avoid exercise because of unfounded fears. Exercise is appropriate and safe for almost everyone. This section will spell out the special considerations for and concerns about exercise and instruct you on what to do about them.

Muscle Balance

Proper muscle balance is an important goal in all exercise routines because it is essential for maintaining good body alignment and avoiding injuries. Choosing balanced exercises for the muscles around each joint can help you avoid the sport- and exercise-related injuries associated with muscle imbalances, such as rotator cuff injuries in baseball pitchers and in wheelchair track athletes.

If you are a wheelchair user, you may exhibit very tight anterior musculature (tight pectoralis major and minor, anterior deltoid) and weak, overstretched back musculature. This imbalance is usually due to overuse of the anterior musculature in wheelchair propulsion and from performing most daily activities in front of the body. Poor posture (rounded shoulders) induced by old, stretched-out, ill-fitting wheelchair backs promotes this imbalance even further.

Over time, you may develop chronic shoulder problems that can greatly restrict your function or your only means of locomotion, wheelchair propulsion. When choosing your exercises, emphasize back and posterior shoulder musculature and not anterior musculature. Muscle balance can easily be achieved by using the push-pull routine. For example, if you perform a push exercise such as the bench press or triceps extensions, you should next perform a pull exercise that counters that motion, such as bent-over rows or biceps curls. This type of program will increase strength in all movements possible at a joint.

Spasticity can also contribute to muscle imbalance. Spasticity can be present in individuals with strokes, cerebral palsy, closed head injuries, and multiple sclerosis. Spasticity in certain muscle groups may habitually place an extremity in one position. Over time, this can cause muscle tightness and possibly muscle contractures (shortening of muscle and tendons). Resistance training to the muscles opposing the spastic muscles can possibly increase the range of motion of those joints. Be careful when using resistance training with spastic extremities, however, so as not to increase the abnormal muscle tone. Flexibility exercises are also recommended for individuals with spasticity. For more information, see chapter 4.

Single-Joint Versus Multijoint Exercises

Single-joint exercises such as triceps extensions isolate one muscle or muscle group by moving only one joint. Multijoint exercises such as the shoulder press involve more than one muscle group by moving many joints. Multijoint exercises may be preferred over single-joint exer-

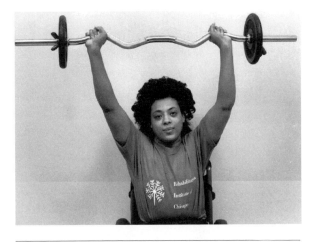

Multijoint exercises such as the shoulder press work both the shoulder and elbow joints simultaneously.

cises because they are more functional, movement specific, and time efficient. Many muscle groups are trained simultaneously during multijoint exercise, thus minimizing the chances of muscle imbalances. Use of single-joint exercises may be preferred when you are a beginner learning proper technique or when you have weaker areas that require special attention. If you have impaired coordination (common in cerebral palsy, closed head injury, stroke, and multiple sclerosis), you may require simple single-joint exercises to maintain balance and proper technique throughout the range of motion.

Free Weights Versus Machines

Machines allow movement only in a predetermined path, which balances the resistance to control extraneous movement throughout the exercise. The use of free weights, such as dumbbells, forces you to balance and control the weight throughout the exercise range of motion. One method is not better than the other. The choice of mode will be determined by your needs, availability of equipment, and the amount of neuromuscular control or coordination that you have.

If you display good trunk strength and stability, free weights may be the preferred mode. Free weights force the body or trunk to stabilize itself while the extremities are moving against a resistance. When using exercise machines such as the Universal shoulder press, the weight is balanced by the equipment, which minimizes the use of the small stabilizing muscles of the shoulder girdle. This can potentially set you up

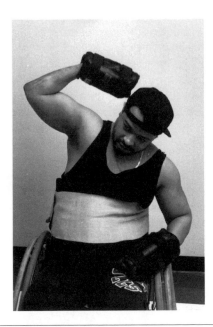

Athlete performs triceps extensions that isolate the elbow joint.

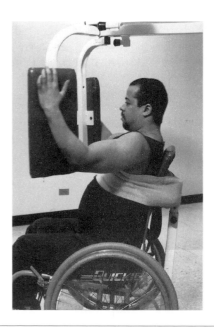

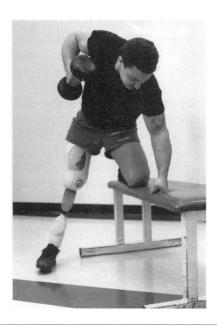

Exercise machines can aid in balance by controlling the exerciser's movement.

Free weight exercise forces you to balance and control the resistance through the exercise movement.

for a weak area or a muscle imbalance. With free weights, you must balance and control the resistance throughout the complete range of motion so that the nervous system is trained to learn the skill of the movement for that exercise. To assure safety, individuals performing free weight exercises may require spotting or supervision, especially during heavier lifts on the bench press and with squats. People with decreased upper extremity coordination and abnormal primitive **reflexes** may not find free weight exercises appropriate.

Damage to the motor areas of the brain may cause decreased coordination in the arms, legs, and trunk in the form of athetosis or ataxia, as in cerebral palsy, stroke, multiple sclerosis, and head injuries. For example, to assess your coordination during a free weight bench press with a partner spotting you, balance the bar with no weight. If you are capable of holding and maintaining the bar horizontally, perform one repetition. Notice the bar movement and your arm control. Be sure that you are positioned securely on the bench. Decreased balance on the bench can affect the control of the bar overhead. If you have only mild coordination deficits, you may be able to gain control of the bar during the exercise movement. If you have moderate to severe coordination difficulties, you may be unable to safely control the bar and you should use the machine bench press, which controls the exercise movement.

If you have moderate coordination difficulties, you may also exhibit abnormal primitive reflexes such as the tonic neck reflexes. If primitive reflexes are present, the free weight bench press is contraindicated. Refer to chapter 5, pages 68-69 for specifics on the primitive reflexes and the bench press. Individuals with spasticity may have an active "clasp-knife reflex." During the bench press, when enough tension develops in the golgi-tendon apparatus, this reflex, which immediately inhibits the extending muscles and causes the flexor muscles to pull the bar to your chest, can occur.

Machines are more appropriate if you do not have full trunk musculature or control, for example, for people with high-level spinal cord injuries who do not have active back and abdominal muscles. As mentioned earlier, if you have full use of trunk musculature but decreased control (which may be seen with multiple sclerosis, closed head injuries and cerebral palsy), you may benefit more from the use of exercise machines, which allow you to balance and control the resistance so you can complete through the full range of motion safely without loss of balance. When you don't have to balance the resistance yourself you can better isolate the prime movers—the muscles needed to perform the exercise—and concentrate on achieving proper technique. In variable resistance exercise machines, the resistance level changes to coincide with the biomechanical movements of the body, allowing full range of motion and the ability to exercise eccentrically.

Should I Exercise With Spasticity?

Spasticity is defined as hypertonus, or too much muscle tone, which may result in decreased range of motion, overactive tonic reflex activity, and stiff, awkward movements. Basically, your muscles have a mind of their own and may contract independent of your conscious efforts. The distribution and quality of spasticity is thought to be related to the site and extent of the brain or spinal cord damage.

Spasticity may exist at birth or develop in the postnatal period, as in cerebral palsy. Over time, some individuals with progressive neurological disorders, such as multiple sclerosis, may develop spasticity. Damage to the brain from a stroke or head injury may also produce spasticity following a period of hypotonia or low muscle tone.

The presence of spasticity may limit or totally restrict purposeful movement. Be careful when exercising a spastic extremity not to set off or increase abnormal muscle tone. You should have control of a movement before using resistance training to strengthen that movement. If movements are not functional due to spasticity in that muscle group, the exercise program should focus on the movement and muscles opposing the spastic muscle groups. For example, if you cannot extend the elbow due to strong flexor tone (spasticity) in the biceps, the use of resistance exercise for the biceps is not appropriate. However, if you can extend the elbow in the presence of biceps flexor tone (spasticity), resistance training may be indicated to strengthen the triceps. Exercising the triceps may help decrease or normalize the abnormal tone of the biceps through a mechanism called **reciprocal inhibition**. Decreased spasticity in the biceps and increased strength in the triceps may give you greater control and function in your arm.

There may be some cases, however, in which strengthening spastic muscles is appropriate. A spastic muscle is not necessarily a strong muscle. If you have full isolated control of all movements in an extremity or muscle with minimal spasticity, resistance training may be indicated to strengthen the spastic extremity to increase use or function in it. However, any exercise or activity that limits function or motor control (coordination) of the extremity should be stopped.

Spasticity may temporarily increase in the involved extremity with increasing muscle effort on the noninvolved side; however, it should subside shortly after exercise. If spasms occur, they do not typically have a detrimental impact on your function or daily activities. Remember, spasticity is a dynamic condition and may differ with each individual. When in doubt, consult your physician, physical therapist, or appropriate medical professional.

Exercising From Your Wheelchair

Most techniques and exercise principles also apply to the wheelchair user; however, the wheelchair itself offers some unique challenges. Like people, wheelchairs come in many different dimensions and offer a variety of features. To allow for safety, you should be aware of the limits of your wheelchair. In particular, you should be aware of your wheelchair stability and center of gravity (COG) and its back height.

Wheelchair Stability and Center of Gravity. When exercising from the wheelchair, the first concern is that it is immobilized. It is not uncommon that wheelchair brakes do not hold, and many athletic wheelchairs do not even have brakes. If this is your case, you may not have any difficulty performing exercises down at your sides and close to your body, such as a biceps curl, but you may have some trouble with over-the-head exercises like the shoulder press.

A second concern that affects the stability of your wheelchair is its center of gravity. Some of the athletic wheelchairs move the center of gravity toward the front of the chair by simply moving the axle plate forward. This allows for faster turning and speed, but it also reduces the force needed to flip the chair backward. If your axle plate or COG is forward, you need to make sure your chair is adequately stabilized before performing over-the-head exercises.

You can immobilize your wheelchair in several ways:

- Weigh down the front end of your wheelchair with sand weights. You can also place sand weights behind the wheels to further prevent any forward or backward shifting or tipping.
- Position your wheelchair back against a wall. Be sure to place sand weights in front and behind the wheels in this technique as well.
- Hook the push handles over a high/low table if one is available. A high/low table will probably not be available in a community fitness setting, but most rehabilitation centers will have one.

- Have your workout partner stabilize your chair. This technique is probably the least desirable because it does not allow you total independence.

Back Height. Back height should be determined by personal preference based on your level of injury, sensation, and balance. With spinal cord injuries, the general rule of thumb is that the higher the level of injury, the higher the backrest, because of the need for balance and stability.

Some of you, wheelchair athletes in particular, may have a low backrest. This increases your mobility but the trade-off is comfort and stability. With a low back height, you may have difficulty with over-the-head exercises. Even with a strong trunk, including abdominal and back muscles, over-the-head exercises may be difficult without stabilization from your legs. You have some of the same options as you did for immobilizing your wheelchair. Try these suggestions:

- Back your wheelchair against a wall for support.
- Have your workout partner spot you for all over-the-head exercises.
- Perform unilateral over-the-head exercises and use the nonexercising arm for balance.
- Transfer into a chair with a higher back to perform your over-the-head exercises.

- Perform your over-the-head exercises with exercise machines rather than free weights. Without having to balance the weight, you may be able to safely and independently perform your exercise program.

Positioning and Strapping

An aligned, secure, and stabilized position is a necessity for you to perform exercises with your extremities. Your position or posture can also greatly influence your muscle tone and set off or prevent primitive reflexes if you have a head injury or cerebral palsy. Posture and trunk stability during exercise also affects your balance, no matter what your disability. General guidelines for positioning and strapping follow.

Head. To avoid the influences of primitive reflexes, your head and neck should be maintained in a neutral position during upper and lower extremity exercises. Refer to Table 5.3 on page 69.

Trunk. The trunk or body position should be erect, stabilized, and secure during upper and lower extremity exercises to avoid substitution of muscles. An elastic binder or belt can be wrapped around you and the wheelchair to stabilize the trunk and maintain balance. We recommend an elastic binder for anyone with mild to moderate balance deficits in the trunk. The elasticity of the

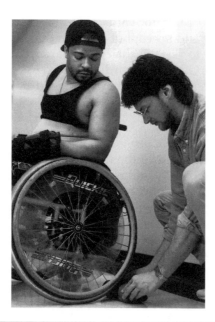

Sand weights under the wheels can help prevent your wheelchair from tipping.

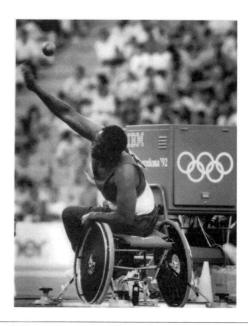

Immobilizing your wheelchair allows you to perform physical activity safely.

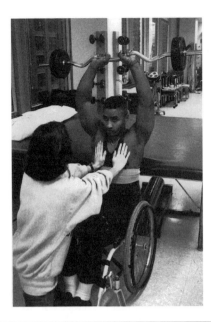

Performing over-the-head activities in low-back wheelchairs requires help with trunk balance.

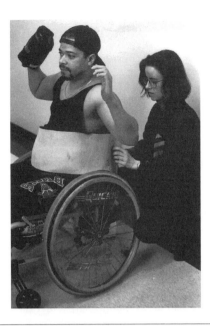

The use of an elastic binder around you and your chair can assist your balance in the absence of upper trunk muscles.

binder allows some degree of control and enables the trunk musculature to contract for balance and stability during upper and lower extremity exercise. The more trunk control you possess, the looser the binder should be. People with moderate to severe trunk balance difficulty can use nonelastic belts or wraps. For example, if you do not have any trunk muscles (abdominal or back), you would benefit from a nonelastic strap that stabilizes your body against your chair while you exercise with your arms. If you have good trunk control, you may want to remove arm rests to allow more freedom of movement.

Upper Extremities. Some individuals with head injuries, stroke, or cerebral palsy may have one upper extremity that is more severely involved than the other. In many cases the more involved extremity can interfere while the opposite side is being exercised. Strapping your nonexercising extremity in a neutral position to the armrest of the wheelchair is often helpful. You could also secure the arm under your wheelchair seat belt.

Lower Extremities. People with conditions such as cerebral palsy, multiple sclerosis, head injuries, and spinal cord injuries often exhibit an extensor pattern or posture characterized by trunk, hip, and knee extension, hip adduction and internal rotation, and ankle plantarflexion (toes pointing down).

If spasticity creates a positioning problem, your lower extremities should be positioned securely

in full flexion when performing upper extremity exercise. The full flexion position can break up the lower extremity extension tone and securely position the buttocks and trunk to the back of the wheelchair seat and back. A strap or seat belt coming from underneath the wheelchair and crossing over the proximal (upper) hips can secure you in the wheelchair.

The ideal 90/90-degree hip and knee angle may need to be modified by increasing the hip

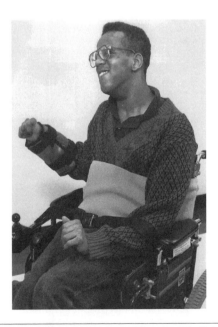

The nonexercising arm is secured by a seat belt to avoid interference when exercising.

Positioning and strapping the lower extremities

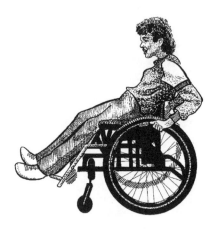

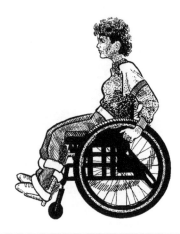

Without proper positioning, exercise may elicit an extensor thrust that would interfere with exercise performance.

The use of proper positioning and strapping with a waist belt secured to the frame can aid in trunk stability during exercise, diminishing an extensor response.

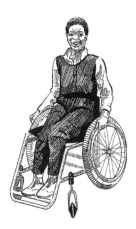

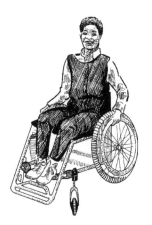

A strap placed above the footrests can allow for increased hip and knee flexion, decreasing the potential of an extensor response during exercise.

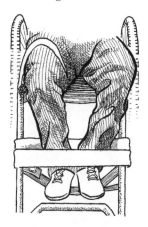

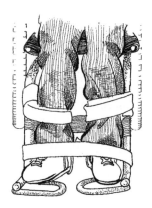

A single strap tightened around the right hip and wheelchair frame maintains proper alignment in the presence of right adductor spasticity. The anterior and posterior straps secure the lower extremities and can prevent involuntary knee extension during exercise.

Strapping below the knees controls bilateral adductor spasticity.

flexion if your hips continue to extend. Raising the footrests can also increase hip flexion. If footrests cannot be raised, use a strap above the footrests to allow more flexion at the hips and knees.

Straps can also be applied around the front of the footrests to prevent knee extension and hip adduction with upper extremity exercise.

General Precautions With Strapping

When using straps, it is important to be aware of any areas of decreased sensation, typically seen with spinal cord injuries, strokes, head injuries, and multiple sclerosis. These areas of the body are prone to skin breakdowns. All areas that are strapped should be checked for redness. Straps should be at least 2 in. wide to increase the area of contact with the skin. Thinner straps may cause a tourniquet effect by applying too much pressure over one area. Be on the alert for skin color changes or swelling following strapping. If you feel some unusual sensations such as a "pins and needles" feeling, it is time to loosen and adjust your straps because the strap may have been placed over a major nerve or blood vessel. As a general rule, all straps should be loosened between sets.

If your legs are strapped to a bench to perform exercise such as the bench press, stretch your legs before strapping to decrease the possibility of setting off spasms in your legs.

Anyone with a history of hip pain, hip dislocations, and total hip replacements must be especially careful because strapping the lower extremities with the legs extended against spasticity can aggravate the hip condition.

The lower extremities should be positioned with some degree of hip and knee flexion to allow for muscle slack and to avoid setting off a muscle spasm. Place rolled-up pillows, towels, or a bolster under the knees. If strapping is still needed for balance, place the straps above the hips to allow good stability on the bench without putting extra stress on the hips if spasms do occur.

Spotting

Another factor to monitor for a safe exercise program is spotting. Spotting is not always needed, but it is required for safety in the following situations:

- To teach proper technique or posture for an exercise

- When using heavy squat and bench press exercises
- Whenever safety may be a concern

Spotters need to be alert to avoid unexpectedly giving way if inexperienced with free weights or in the presence of spasticity.

Bench Press.   Position the primary spotter behind you to assist as needed. Two auxiliary spotters can be used at each end of the bar during heavy lifts. The primary spotter helps you during the exercise if you have trouble or require assistance to keep the weight moving (sticking point). The auxiliary spotters should not touch the bar unless the primary spotter calls for assistance or unless you cannot complete the range of motion of the exercise. Auxiliary spotters should always be used if you exhibit decreased motor control and coordination during free weight bench press and squats.

Squats.   Position the primary spotter behind you with hands on your waist. Two auxiliary spotters can be used at each end of the bar during very heavy lifts if a barbell is used. The primary spotter helps you during the exercise if you require assistance to keep the weight moving by pulling or guiding your hips upward. The auxiliary spotters should not touch the bar unless the primary spotter calls for assistance.

Choosing the Appropriate Exercises

You should now have the background knowledge you need to select appropriate exercises to

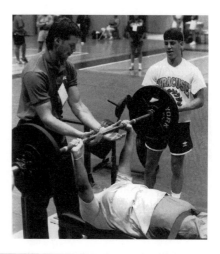

The primary spotter assists with an even lift-off.

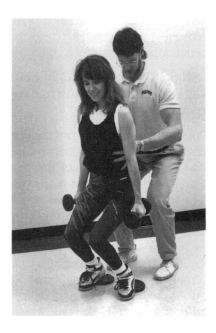

The spotter can assist in continuing movement and can also aid in maintaining proper exercise posture and technique.

meet your needs. In the disability-specific chapters, you will also find more tips about modifying exercises for your disability.

Based on your new knowledge, you now know to ask yourself the following questions before selecting your exercises:

- Which muscle groups are my weak areas?
- Do I have adequate muscle balance around my joints?
- What kind of exercise equipment is available to me?
- Which exercise modes are most appropriate based on my coordination, strength, and balance?

The last step for selecting your exercises is to have a general knowledge of anatomy so you know which exercises work each muscle. For example, following your strength assessment, you discover that your right triceps are significantly weaker than your left. Before choosing the appropriate exercise for the triceps, you need to know where the muscle group is and the type of action it performs. Table 2.2 will assist you in your exercise selection. The following, "Movement Terminology," provides you with a working vocabulary to understand the actions your muscles perform. Table 2.2 shows detailed drawings of the muscles of the body followed by a description of the action each muscle performs. It also gives a list of appropriate exer-

cises to work each muscle. After finding triceps on the muscle chart, look at the exercise column for some exercise suggestions. For example, if you decide that you need to perform a unilateral single-joint exercise to focus on weak triceps, you then select the dumbbell triceps extensions exercise.

Movement Terminology

Flexion—Movement of a body part that results in a decrease in the angle of the articulating bones (bending of a joint).

Extension—Movement of a body part that results in an increase in the angle of the articulating bones (straightening of a joint).

Rotation—Movement of a bone or body part around its own axis.

Abduction—Movement of a body part away from the center of the body.

Adduction—Movement of a body part toward the center of the body.

Circumduction—Movement of a body part combining flexion, extension, abduction and adduction, resulting in a cone-shaped path (the shoulder, hip, and trunk can circumduct).

Inversion—Movement of the foot, resulting in turning the sole inward.

Eversion—Movement of the foot, resulting in turning the sole outward.

Supination—Outward rotation of the forearm (movement to palm up position).

Pronation—Inward rotation of the forearm (movement to palm down position).

Dorsiflexion—Ankle movement resulting in the toes moving toward the shin.

Plantarflexion—Movement of the foot away from the shin, downward movement of the foot with toes pointing toward the floor.

Horizontal adduction—Moving the shoulder joint in toward the front of the body with arm parallel to the floor.

Horizontal abduction—Moving the shoulder joint away from the front of the body and toward the back with arm parallel to the floor.

Scapular adduction—Moving the scapula toward the spine.

Scapular abduction—Moving the scapula around the trunk away from the spine.

Scapular upward rotation—Movement of the shoulder joint pointing it more upward.

Scapular downward rotation—Movement of the shoulder joint pointing it more downward.

Table 2.2
Anatomical Muscle Chart (Anterior)

Muscles	Action	Exercise
Abdominals External obliques Internal obliques Rectus abdominus Transversalis	Flexion of the spine (trunk), supports and compresses abdominal viscera, lateral flexion of the spine, rotation of the trunk	Pelvic tilts, crunches, lateral crunches, bent knee sit-ups, leg lift progression, medicine ball toss
Biceps brachii Brachialis	Flexes elbow	Biceps curls with palm up, upright rows, lat pull-downs, back rows
Brachioradialis	Strong elbow flexor with forearm pronated or partially pronated	Biceps curls with palm down, upright rows, lat pull-downs, back rows
Deltoid	*Anterior:* Horizontal adduction, shoulder flexion, internal rotation of shoulder	Front raise, chest flys, bench press, shoulder internal rotations
	Middle: abducts the shoulder	Side raise, upright rows, shoulder press, back rows
	Posterior: Extends the shoulder, externally rotates shoulder	Back raise, shoulder external rotations,
Gluteus medius	Abducts the hip joint	Side leg raises
Hip adductors	Adduct the hip joint	
Iliopsoas	Flexes hip	Knee to chest, lunges, leg lift progression, straight leg raise
Pectoralis major	Horizontal adduction, shoulder flexion, internal rotation of shoulder	Chest flys, bench press, front raise, shoulder internal rotations
Pronator teres	Pronates forearm, assists in flexing elbow	Biceps curls, upper pulley diagonal cross to open, slow rotation of forearm holding dumbbell and turning hand palm down
Quadriceps muscle group Rectus femoris Vastus lateralis Vastus medialis Vastus intermedius	Extends knee (rectus femoris portion of the hip joint)	Leg extension, lunges, squats
Sartorius	Flexes, laterally rotates, and abducts the hip joint. Flexes and assists in medial rotation of knee joint.	Marching in sitting or standing position, knee to chest
Serratus anterior	Abducts and upwardly rotates scapula, holds medial border of scapula to thorax	Bench press, serratus punches
Supinator	Supination of forearm	Lower pulley diagonal open to cross, slow rotation of forearm holding dumbbell and turning hand palm up
Tibialis anterior	Dorsiflexes the ankle joint and assists in inversion of the foot	Dorsiflexors
Wrist flexors Flexor carpi ulnaris Flexor carpi radialis Palmaris longus	Flexes wrist toward palm	Wrist curls with barbell/dumbbell, wrist rollers (clockwise)

(continued)

Table 2.2   *(continued)*

Anterior Muscles

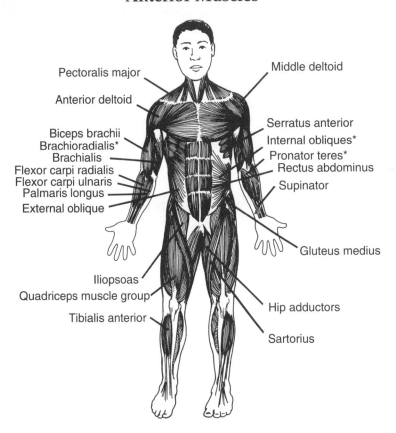

Pectoralis major
Anterior deltoid
Biceps brachii
Brachioradialis*
Brachialis
Flexor carpi radialis
Flexor carpi ulnaris
Palmaris longus
External oblique
Iliopsoas
Quadriceps muscle group
Tibialis anterior

Middle deltoid
Serratus anterior
Internal obliques*
Pronator teres*
Rectus abdominus
Supinator
Gluteus medius
Hip adductors
Sartorius

Posterior Muscles

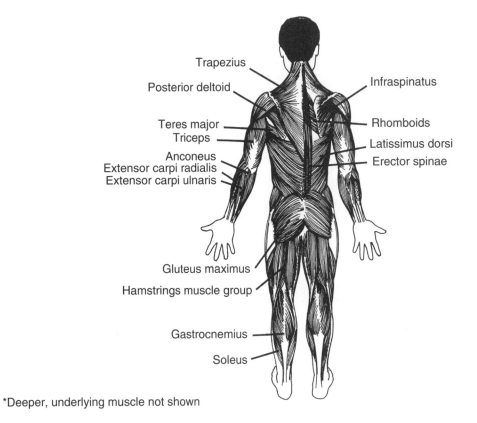

Trapezius
Posterior deltoid
Teres major
Triceps
Anconeus
Extensor carpi radialis
Extensor carpi ulnaris
Gluteus maximus
Hamstrings muscle group
Gastrocnemius
Soleus

Infraspinatus
Rhomboids
Latissimus dorsi
Erector spinae

*Deeper, underlying muscle not shown

Table 2.2 *(continued)*
Anatomical Muscle Chart (Posterior)

Muscles	Action	Exercise
Erector spinae	Extends spine, rotates spine	Back extension, trunk rotations
Gastrocnemius Soleus	Plantar flexion of ankle Gastrocnemius assists with flexion of the knee	Toe raises
Gluteus maximus	Extends the hip, assists in internal rotation of the hip	Lunges, squats, back leg raise
Hamstrings/knee flexors Semitendinosus Semimembranosus Biceps femoris	Flexes knee, internally rotates the knee joint (semitendinosus and semimembranosus). Flexes knee, extends and assists in external rotation of hip joint	Leg curls, lunges
Latissimus dorsi	Shoulder internal rotation, draws shoulder down and back (extends shoulder)	Lat pull-downs, bent-over rows, chin-ups
Rhomboids	Adducts and elevates scapula, rotates scapula downward	Back rows
Teres major	Internal shoulder rotation	Upper and lower diagonals, dips, bent-over rows, lat pull-downs, back shoulder raise, shoulder depressors, shoulder rotations
Trapezius	*Upper:* upward rotation of scapula, elevates the scapula, extends, laterally flexes, and rotates head when acting on one side. Acting bilaterally, extends head. *Middle:* adduction of the scapula *Lower:* upward rotation of scapula, depression of the scapula	Shoulder shrugs

Bent-over rows Dips, shoulder depressors |
| Triceps Anconeus | Extends elbow | Triceps extensions, dips, shoulder press, bench press |
| *Wrist extensors* Extensor carpi radialis Extensor carpi ulnaris | Extends wrist away from palm | Wrist extension (reverse curls), wrist rollers (counterclockwise) |

Maintaining an Exercise Log

Maintaining an exercise log (see page 35) is an important part of your exercise program. Keeping track of your exercises and the resistance used can help you increase the demands of your program. Improvements in duration and resistance can also serve as positive reinforcement to further motivate you and to set new exercise goals. A good exercise diary can also provide your physician with helpful data. We suggest that you photocopy the blank exercise logs and later fill them in after your workout sessions.

During your first few weeks, it may be useful to fill in your exercise log with each training session. It is typical to change your resistance frequently as you find the starting point appropriate for you. Following the first 4 weeks, you can update your log weekly for strength exercises, but you should continue to chart your aerobic exercise following every session.

The following case study will show you how to use the exercise logs most effectively.

CASE STUDY:

You are a 30-year-old individual who has just completed your rehabilitation following a spinal cord injury. You no longer have use of your upper trunk and leg muscles. You have also lost use of your hand muscles. Your triceps on your right side has normal function; however, your triceps on your left side is too weak to extend your elbow straight up against gravity with use of any weights or resistance.

Basic Variables of Exercise Program Design

Now that you have selected your exercises, you are ready to customize or design your own program. Four basic variables—training load, sets and repetitions, rest periods, and frequency of exercise sessions—determine the amount of work (exercise volume) in an exercise program. These variables dictate exercise program outcome and can be manipulated to develop muscle endurance, muscle strength, and muscle power.

Training Load

The appropriate training load (amount of resistance used) relates to your fitness level. If you have been very inactive and are deconditioned, you will benefit from training at a very low workload. Low workloads are recommended for all beginners to prepare the body for greater stress as the program progresses. Starting with a low workload also gives you an opportunity to learn proper and safe exercise technique. Health and fitness professionals now know that the popular "no pain, no gain" motto is insane! Trying to lift too much weight can promote poor exercise technique and possible injury. It is important that you start out slow and work within your own physical limits. Listen to your body. Pain is a sign of possible trauma to your tissues.

Remember, to avoid injury, not only the muscles but also the tendons and ligaments need to be strengthened before using high-load exercise. One criteria for determining proper workload is the subjective feeling of being minimally out of breath during the training. The training load is only one variable of the total exercise program. The load should strictly follow the designated sets and repetitions to achieve outlined goals. The term *repetition maximum* (RM) refers to the maximal resistance that can be lifted for a certain number of repetitions. For example, if you are performing 3 sets of 6 repetitions, the load should be high enough to challenge you but low enough so you can complete the designated number of sets and repetitions.

Forced repetitions mean performing an exercise to exhaustion and requiring assistance from a partner to finish the last few repetitions. Forced repetitions should not be used on a daily basis because they can promote overtraining and injury. People with multiple sclerosis or neuromuscular diseases should avoid forced repetitions completely due to the possible effects of overwork weakness.

Sample Exercise Log

Notes	Exercises	Sets/reps	Weight				
			Date 4-1	4-8	4-15	4-22	
—Need an elastic binder around trunk and chair for all shoulder exercises	Rickshaw	3/10	40#	45#	45#	50#	
—Straight-arm back raise performed bent-over knees in chair	Lat pull-downs	3/10	50#	50#	55#	55#	
4/1/93 Lightheaded following arm crank	Shoulder front raise	3/10	5#	5#	7#	7#	
4/15/93 Not lightheaded following arm crank (4 mins)	Shoulder back raise	3/10	5#	5#	7#	7#	
—Arm crank performed by using velcro gloves	Straight-arm back raise	3/10	3#	3#	3#	5#	
—Shoulder exercises with one arm at a time	Right triceps extension	3/10	20#	25#	25#	30#	
	Left triceps extension	2-3/10	0#	0#	0#	1-2#	
	Biceps curls	3/10	15#	20#	25#	25#	
	Arm crank	3/10	2 min	2 min	4 min	6 min	

Sets and Repetitions

With use of the appropriate training load, the number of sets and repetitions govern the goal and outcome of the exercise program. Sets and repetitions can be set up for muscle endurance, basic muscle strength, and muscle power routines (see Table 2.3).

Muscle Endurance. This term refers to the ability to repeatedly perform submaximal muscle contractions. Muscle endurance routines are high-repetition programs with a lower load or resistance. Lower intensities or loads are required when training for repetitive continuous contractions over time. Continued muscle exertions include walking, wheelchair propulsion, and many other activities of daily living. The higher number of repetitions with lower resistance allows you to safely learn the skill and technique of each exercise. Such routines allow for positive changes or adaptations with less risk of overstressing the neuromuscular system. The recommended program design for muscle endurance includes 3 to 5 sets of 8 to 20 repetitions. One author recommends a minimum of 8 repetitions per set for the first year of training before progressing to higher workloads. This allows the body to "build a base" or make early changes to allow for further stresses. With all routines the overload principle must be followed or there will be minimal to no gains in muscle endurance, strength, or power.

Muscle endurance routines are recommended for all beginners and are the most appropriate routines for people with neuromuscular diseases. With multiple sclerosis, postpolio syndrome, or a neuromuscular disease, you may have to lower the number of repetitions and the load according to your physical fitness level and tolerance. You will still require a **submaximal workload** (lower weight) to avoid the risk of overstressing the neuromuscular system.

Muscle Strength. This term refers to the force a muscle can exert against its maximal resistance in a single effort. Muscle strength activities are of short duration and are most frequently used in sports and in daily activities such as transferring into and out of a wheelchair. Muscle strength routines can increase your ability to move your own body, allowing for easier, more independent pressure reliefs and transfers. If you have a high-level spinal cord injury or are a wheelchair user, an increase in muscle strength will make propel-

Table 2.3 Exercise Program Design—Muscle Capabilities		
	Volume (reps/sets)	Intensity (load)
Muscle endurance	8-20/3-5	Low to medium
Stength	3-9/3-5	Medium to high
Strength-power	1-3/3-5	Very high
	8-10/1-2	Low to medium

Note. Adapted from Pauletto (1986); Poliquen (1984); and Stone et al. (1982).

ling a manual wheelchair outdoors on uneven surfaces easier. These routines are also appropriate for short-distance walkers, including people with cerebral palsy, multiple sclerosis, stroke, closed head injury, and spinal cord injury.

A basic strength routine is a progression from the muscle endurance routine and is appropriate for most populations, especially athletes. Research has reported that routines of three to nine repetitions produce the highest increase in strength. Muscle strength can also increase muscle endurance. The stronger the muscle fibers, the fewer fibers are needed to perform an activity. This leaves more fibers to maintain the activity for longer time periods.

Muscle Power. This term refers to a progression from muscle strength routines and is an important but often unemphasized area of strength training. The definition of **power** is force x distance ÷ time. Strength training typically emphasizes the force component of exercise and sport but not the speed or acceleration component. Power routines should reflect both the force and speed components. The force component is emphasized by performing fewer exercises with heavier workloads, fewer repetitions, and longer recovery intervals; for example, performing one to three repetitions of your determined weight resistance with three to five sets and a 4-min rest period between each set. You should also perform higher repetitions at relatively low workloads emphasizing speed and explosiveness.

Rest Periods

Your muscle groups need an appropriate amount of rest between exercise sets for recuperation. This rest will allow your working muscles to replenish their energy to perform the next set. For general strength training, 2 to 4-min rest periods are recommended. Adhering to recommended rest periods is necessary to show any positive training effects. Rest periods that are too long do not stress the system enough to allow for significant training effects, whereas rest periods that are too short can promote muscle fatigue because they don't allow for energy replenishment. Muscles need these energy sources to maintain exercise at high intensities. Shorter rest periods of 2 min or less can be used to train for muscle endurance activities like wheelchair road races, swimming, and long-distance walking. People with multiple sclerosis, postpolio syndrome, and the neuromuscular diseases should use rest periods judiciously to avoid fatigue. If you have a limited available working muscle mass, it is also very important that you allow for adequate rest between sets to prevent overtraining injuries. With a decreased muscle mass, you may be limited in alternating muscle groups with your routine.

Frequency of Exercise Sessions

The frequency of exercise depends in part on the duration and intensity of the exercise sessions. The frequency can vary from three to seven periods a week depending on your needs, interests, and functional abilities. Alternate a day of exercise with a day of rest. This is imperative if you have limited active muscle mass. Working the same muscles on consecutive days can cause overuse injuries. Once you have achieved the initial positive training responses including an increased strength in muscles, **ligaments**, and tendons, you can achieve a greater conditioning response on a daily basis if you can alternate your muscle groups. For example, work your chest and arms on Monday and Wednesday and work your shoulders and back on Tuesday and Thursday. This is referred to as a split routine.

With progressive disorders such as multiple sclerosis and the muscular dystrophies, you should stop or lower your frequency during periods of **exacerbations**. During **remission** when you are showing progressive return of strength and function, you may gradually increase frequency as tolerated; however, medical clearance is highly recommended before restarting the exercise program.

Maintenance of Strength Gains. Muscle strength and endurance are not compromised easily once you stop resistance exercise. When training goals have been achieved, you can maintain strength with as little as one training session per month, according to one source.

Program Progression

Your initial exercise program should include an orientation to exercise and education about it. Take your time to familiarize yourself with all the exercises you are going to perform. Do not rush yourself—it is important to develop good technique with your exercises. Remember, your base program should prepare you for higher intensity work. Your base program should generally last 4 to 6 weeks, depending on your starting physical condition.

The progression of your exercise program depends on your functional capacity, health status, age, needs, and goals. Progression of program design must be individualized, especially if you have a dynamic or progressive disability. Nonprogressive disorders typically progress gradually when you follow an exercise program of appropriate design. But exercise with progressive disorders such as multiple sclerosis and the neuromuscular diseases should be governed by the condition's severity and rate of progression. People with these disorders may show gradual increases or maintenance of strength during periods of disease inactivity. However, when the disease is in an active state, they should stop their exercise programs or adjust them according to health and ability. A physician's clearance to restart the exercise program is sometimes indicated with complicated dynamic disorders. If you have any doubt about exercise program progression, consult your physician.

Your program should be upgraded and evaluated weekly. The strength training variables need to be progressing toward the training goals so you can maintain stimulus. You also need to upgrade your exercise program to keep it interesting and to avoid overtraining and injury.

Upgrading your program for a specific sport season requires proper timing of program development. Chronic program variables have been established and the concept of periodization proposed to give a theoretical basis for changing workouts (see Table 2.4). This theoretical model is for strength-power training; it deals with the variables of volume (total number of repetitions) and intensity (amount of resistance used). The

Table 2.4
The Four Phases of Periodization

	Volume (reps/sets)	Intensity (load)	Rest (minutes)	Frequency (days/week)
Muscle endurance (hypertrophy)	10+/3-5 High	Low	0-2	3-4
Strength	5/3-5 Moderate	High	3-4	3-5
Strength-power	2-3/3-5	Very high	3-4	4-6
Peaking-maintenance	2-3/1-3	Very high	3-4	1-5
Active rest (3-4 weeks after peaking)	Low	Very low		2-4 days off

Note. Adapted from Kraemer (1984/1985, 1990a) and Stone et al. (1982).

chronic variables are part of a four-phase model that aims to avoid overtraining and is planned so you reach optimal performance at a specific time (peaking at the time of athletic event).

Preventing Overtraining

Being able to recognize overtraining is important to prevent overuse injuries. Overtraining is a plateau or decrease in your performance that results from the inability to tolerate or adapt to your training load. There are two types of overtraining, monotonous and chronic overwork.

Monotonous Program Overtraining. This occurs when you consistently and unvaryingly use the same type of exercise. This type of overtraining does not result from overwork or excessive fatigue; it is thought to be due to an adaptation of the central nervous system (brain and spinal cord) to unvarying training routines.

Chronic Overwork Overtraining. This type of overwork is more severe. It involves excess fatigue or exhaustion from overwork that has been sustained too long or repeated too frequently. You will no longer obtain positive changes in response to the training stimuli because your body's defense systems are overwhelmed and cannot adapt. Chronic overwork can be seen in all

sports, but it occurs most often in anaerobic sports where speed, strength, and skill are emphasized.

To avoid overtraining, review the following principles:

- Use appropriate training variables (e.g., periodization) and be alert for the symptoms of overtraining. Symptoms include lack of motivation, anxiety, depression, irritability, lack of self-confidence, fatigue, the inability to concentrate, decreases in weight, and increases in resting heart rate, blood pressure, or both.
- Monitor your body for signs of impending injury, such as fatigue and lack of enthusiasm for training. These signs may indicate that exercise has been too intense or that rest and recovery have not been adequate.
- Pain usually indicates that a body part is or has been overstressed, and discomfort that causes changes in your daily activities (e.g., difficulty transferring out of wheelchair) requires toning down and varying your exercise program.
- Appropriate use of warm-up, stretching, and cool-down periods prevents injury and improves performance.
- A well-balanced exercise program must include strengthening all major muscle groups and monitoring muscle balance so you will be less susceptible to injury.

CHAPTER 3

Aerobic Training

Aerobic exercise is an essential component of fitness and is important in achieving a healthier, more active lifestyle. In this chapter, we will discuss how your body responds to regular aerobic activity. We will give you the tools and knowledge to select the appropriate modes of exercise and show you how to monitor your exercise intensity.

Regular aerobic exercise has powerful implications for positive changes physically and mentally. Regular aerobic exercise is even more important if you are deconditioned and want to avoid health risks that result from a sedentary lifestyle, such as cardiovascular disease. Studies have shown that people who participate in wheelchair sports and fitness programs show decreased medical complications and hospital admissions.

Aerobic exercise and activities are commonly called endurance training because they involve elevating the heart rate over a prolonged period of time. In order to do this, aerobic training requires a continuous, long-duration activity that works large muscle groups, typically the large muscles of the torso and legs that are used in jogging. Aerobic training is also referred to as *cardiorespiratory endurance* because it relies on oxygen to provide energy. When the cardiorespiratory system is stressed, positive central changes occur, resulting in a more efficient heart and lungs.

Your Body's Response

Cardiorespiratory endurance relies on the strength of the heart muscle and performance of the lungs to withstand the increased load that aerobic exercise requires. As with other muscles, the heart and lungs need to be stressed to produce positive training changes. For the cardiorespiratory system, exercise must be appropriately intense to force the aerobic energy system to use

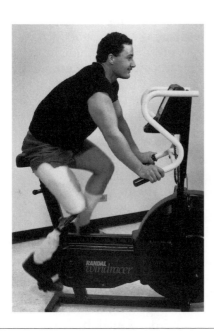

Aerobic exercise promotes an active lifestyle and decreases health risks that result from being sedentary.

39

oxygen as a source for its energy metabolism. Aerobic exercise allows no rest periods during the activity, because with rest the energy system would not be forced to use oxygen and would turn to **anaerobic** (without oxygen) energy sources. Anaerobic energy sources are what you use for strength training.

The primary stimulus for a more efficient heart is an increased load on the heart that is proportional to the size of the muscle mass active during training. As mentioned earlier, typical activities that train the heart muscle usually involve the use of large muscle groups. Hence jogging stresses the cardiovascular system more than wheelchair rolling because jogging uses larger muscle groups. Cardiovascular training produces an increased ability to circulate blood from the heart and to obtain a lower resting heart rate. Basically the heart muscle becomes stronger and more efficient by being able to beat less and pump out more blood for circulation to the lungs and all other body systems. People with some conditions, such as quadriplegia, may not be able to recruit, or may not have, a sufficient active muscle mass to create an adequate volume load on the heart during aerobic exercise. Often muscular fatigue of the arms or legs sets in before target heart rates can be achieved. As a result, central cardiovascular training changes may not occur, but other significant and beneficial peripheral changes do, including increased exercise tolerance, improved muscle endurance due to muscle fiber growth in size (hypertrophy) and their improved ability to extract oxygen from the blood, increased good cholesterol (HDL-C) with a decreased risk of cardiovascular disease, increased peripheral circulation, and strength gains that may allow increased cardiorespiratory endurance. These peripheral changes help people perform the activities of daily living, such as wheelchair propulsion, that require muscle endurance. Table 3.1 summarizes the physiological effects of aerobic training and how these effects improve the body's performance.

Blood Pressure and Heart Rate Changes

Before moving on to a discussion of training modes and exercise intensity, it is important to have a basic understanding of how your heart and circulation system actually work. This is especially important because you will monitor exercise intensity and progress through blood pressure and heart rate.

The heart consists of two pumps, the right and left ventricles. The right ventricle pumps blood to the lungs, creating pulmonary circulation. The left ventricle pumps blood to all other body systems, creating systemic circulation. Systemic circulation is accomplished through arteries that carry blood away from the heart and veins that return blood to the heart.

Blood pressure, or peripheral arterial pressure, measures two separate components, systolic, the lateral pressure of the blood against the walls of the arteries associated with the pumping of blood from the heart, and diastolic, the arterial pressure during the relaxation phase of the heart cycle as the heart refills with blood that holds the arteries open. Diastolic pressure is normally lower than the systolic pressure. Systolic blood pressure increases during aerobic (endurance) exercise, whereas diastolic blood pressure should remain stable or increase only slightly. The average normal blood pressure for a young adult is 120/80. The top number represents the systolic blood pressure and the bottom number represents the diastolic blood pressure.

The heart is able to vary how much blood is actually pumped out to allow it to adjust to different stresses or demands such as exercise. The amount of blood that the heart pumps out to your circulation is referred to as cardiac output. **Cardiac output** is defined as the product of stroke volume and heart rate: Cardiac output = stroke volume (SV) x heart rate (HR).

Stroke volume is the amount of blood that is ejected with each heart contraction. The more full the heart is before a contraction the more blood is pumped to the circulatory system (stroke volume). Of course, the more blood that is pumped out with each heart contraction, the more blood can reach your exercising muscles. The amount of blood that is returned to the heart can be affected by pooling of blood in inactive extremities, as in people with paraplegia or quadriplegia and some people with hemiparesis following a stroke. This decrease in stroke volume decreases cardiac output as well as the overall effectiveness of your heart during exercise.

During exercise, heart rate is also an important factor for increasing cardiac output. Regulation of heart rate is under the control of the **autonomic nervous system**, a regulatory control system that governs involuntary organs (visceral) or internal function. It consists of two branches, the **parasympathetic** and **sympathetic**,

	Table 3.1 Physiological Effects of Aerobic Training		
System or organ	**Effects of disuse (physiological)**	**Effects of exercise (physiological change)**	**Effects on performance**
Cardiovascular system	• Higher resting heart rate • Higher resting blood pressure • Lower cardiac output • Decreased circulation	• Decreased resting heart rate • Decreased resting blood pressure • Greater absolute stroke volume • More efficient cardiac output and pulmonary ventilation • Increased oxygen extraction and delivery to muscles • Increased circulation	• Heart is more efficient (pumps same output with fewer beats) • Increased endurance • Decreased risk of cardiovascular disease
Nervous system	• Suboptimal coordination • Decreased emotional state, possible depression and lethargy	• Increased activation of motor units in prime movers • Increased EMG responses • Increased appropriate activation of synergists and antagonists	• Increased coordination and skill of movement • Increased accuracy, precision, and balance • Improved self-esteem
Muscle	• Decreased muscle mass (atrophy) and strength • Early onset of fatigue	• Increased muscle endurance	• Easier performance of daily activities • Increased ability for wheelchair propulsion on uneven outdoor surfaces
Connective tissue/bone	• Bone demineralization (osteoporosis) • Decreased pliability of tendons and ligaments • Contractures • Pressure sores	• Increased bone density and mass • Increased tensile strength in tendons and ligaments • Increased skin elasticity	• Decrease or elimination of pressure sores • Decreased incidence of injury from overuse activities
Body composition	• Increased % body fat	• Decreased % body fat and increase in lean tissue	• Decreased risks of cardiovascular disease

which normally act in a balanced reciprocal fashion. Stimulation of the parasympathetic system promotes relaxing and vegetative (resting) functions of the body, maintaining a lower heart rate. Stimulation of the sympathetic system prepares the body for movement and emergency situations by alerting the body's organs as needed, elevating the heart rate. At rest, the parasympathetic branch dominates, and during exercise, the sympathetic branch dominates. Disruption of the sympathetic system, possibly seen following a spinal cord injury, shifts control of involuntary organs and glands to the parasympathetic system, which modifies the organs'

physiological responses and adaptations to exercise by restricting the maximum heart rate. This limited, or lower, heart rate also decreases the overall cardiac output (see Table 3.2). Refer to page 96 for more information about the effects of exercise following autonomic nervous system dysfunction.

Modes of Aerobic Training

Your mode of aerobic training depends on your available muscles. If you can walk, you have the same options as the nondisabled population, with modifications for balance and bracing as needed. If you are a wheelchair user, you can participate in modified wheelchair aerobics; upper body **ergometry**, which is bicycle pedaling with the upper extremity (arm cranking); or wheelchair ergometry, which is pushing a wheelchair on a treadmill or stationary rollers.

The main advantage of wheelchair ergometry as compared to forearm cycle ergometry is its training specificity for wheelchair users and wheelchair sports. The disadvantage of wheelchair ergometry is that its net mechanical efficiency is lower than that of forearm cycle ergometry. Wheelchair ergometry may require more energy than forearm cycle ergometry because neural pathways tend to favor asynchronous over synchronous arm movements, greater isometric muscle activity may be required to stabilize the trunk during application of force to the hand rims, and transmission of forces by a handle is more efficient than by rim pressure. Consider these differences when starting an aerobic exercise program. If you have quadriplegia and limited trunk balance or if you have been diagnosed with multiple sclerosis and mechanical efficiency and ease of movement is more important than task-specific wheelchair propulsion, upper body ergometry is an appropriate choice; the proper mode is based on whether you are training for general fitness (upper body ergometry) or sport (wheelchair ergometry).

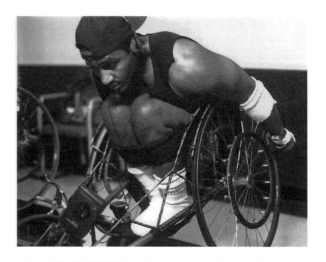

Wheelchair ergometry allows you to perform sport-specific aerobic exercise.

Monitoring Your Exercise Intensity

Target heart rate range and rating of perceived exertion (RPE) are two ways to monitor your aerobic exercise intensity. They appear to be the most accurate and easy to use measures of exercise intensity for strength and conditioning at home or in a group exercise setting. Heart rate and RPE are individually specific, and after instruction and guidance in their use you can monitor either indicator independently. Based on your monitoring, you can control the aerobic

Table 3.2 Autonomic Nervous System Responses		
Organ	**Parasympathetic**	**Sympathetic**
Sweat glands (thermoregulation)	No connections	Secretion
Smooth muscle in skin	No connections	Constriction
Blood vessels in skin	No connections	Constriction
Blood vessels in skeletal muscle of arms	No connections	Relaxation
Blood vessels of abdomen	Vasodilation (increases blood flow)	Vasoconstriction (decreases blood flow)
Colon wall	Peristaltic contraction	Relaxation
Bladder	Contraction (emptying)	Relaxation
Sphincter muscles	Relaxation (emptying)	Contraction
Heart	Slows heart rate and decreases metabolism	Increases heart rate, vigor of contraction and metabolism

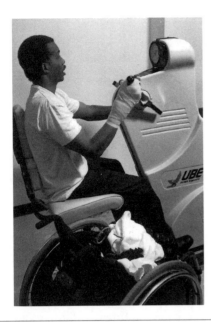

An upper body ergometry hand grip can be assisted with the use of an ace wrap to allow for aerobic exercise.

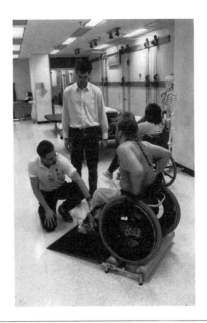

Wheelchair ergometry is more specific for everyday activities and sport-related training.

intensity of an activity by changing the speed of movement and the amount of resistance. Table 3.3 relates exercise levels to common physical activities, starting at resting levels and progressing to athletic levels of aerobic conditioning.

Target Heart Rate Range

An easy way to monitor aerobic exercise intensity is to take your heart rate during or immediately after exercise (refer to chapter 1, p. 11). As you become more fit, the same speed of movement will elicit a lower heart rate. This is why it is important to know your target training heart rate range. This range indicates a progressive adjustment of activity level as you get stronger so you can train your heart safely. Three methods can be used to monitor heart rate: age-adjusted maximal heart rate, actual tested exercise heart rate, and the Karvonen formula.

Age-Adjusted Maximal Heart Rate. Your target heart rate is found by taking a percentage of your maximum heart rate according to your fitness level. Maximum heart rate (max HR) decreases with age and is different for each individual, but it can be approximated by subtracting your age from 220. However, if you are a beginner in an exercise program doing only arm work from a wheelchair, one source recommends using 200 as a starting point instead of 220. Maximum heart rate for individuals with high-level

spinal cord injuries (Class 1A, B, C) is an average 20 to 40 beats lower, so people with these injuries should subtract their age from 190.

Ideally, you should reach 60% of maximum heart rate when you begin aerobic exercise, the lowest point that will adequately stimulate the heart and lungs. But remember, if you are deconditioned or unable to achieve an elevated heart rate level with starting aerobic exercise (e.g., secondary to medication or muscle fatigue), you will still benefit from the peripheral changes of aerobic activities. Achieving 75% of the maximum heart rate may require too strenuous aerobic exercise unless you train regularly and are close to your ultimate fitness level. According to the American Heart Association then, your target heart rate range should be 60% to 75% of your maximum heart rate, and after 6 months or more of regular exercise training you can work up to 85% of your maximum heart rate if you have no heart rate restrictions.

Actual Tested Maximal Heart Rate. The age-adjusted estimate of maximum heart rate above varies by plus or minus 10 to 15 beats per minute according to two different sources. A second method for determining target heart rate range takes a fixed percent (60%-85%) of the actual tested maximal heart rate. This fixed percent depends on your desired intensity and training level. It is measured by a maximal heart rate test running or pushing on a treadmill or riding or pushing a bicycle ergometer. Most fitness centers

Table 3.3
Exercise Levels Related to Common Activities

Recreation	Activity
Standing Walking (1-2 mph) Bed exercise	Shaving, dressing, showering, desk work, automobile driving, dusting, light housework
Walking (2-3 mph) Cycling (5 mph) Canoeing (2.5 mph)	Car washing, manual typing, using hand tools, auto repairs, cleaning, scrubbing, waxing
Calisthenics (light) Softball (noncompetitive) Volleyball (6-person noncompetitive) Walking (3-3.5 mph) Cycling (6 mph)	Janitorial work, raking leaves, window cleaning, light lawn mower pushing, mopping, hanging wash
Dancing (social) Calisthenics (moderate) Swimming (light) Baseball (noncompetitive) Walking (5 mph) Cycling (6.5-8 mph) Canoeing (3 mph)	Stair climbing (slow), heavy machine repair, pushing a power mower, carrying trays, walking room to room, lifting and carrying 20-44 lb
Softball (competitive) Soccer (noncompetitive) Walking (4 mph) Cycling (8.5 mph) Canoeing (4 mph)	Stair climbing (moderate), construction, garden digging
Dancing (rumba, square) Calisthenics (heavy) Walking (5 mph) Cross-country hiking Swimming (moderate)	Shoveling 10-lb loads 10 times/min, hand lawn mowing, splitting wood, lifting and carrying 46-64 lb
Basketball (nongame) Jogging (5 mph) Walking (6 mph) Cycling (12 mph) Canoeing (5 mph) Mountain climbing Swimming (fast)	Stair climbing (fast), ditch digging, hand saw, lifting and carrying 65-84 lb, carrying 20 lb up stairs
Basketball (vigorous) Soccer (competitive) Running (5.5 mph) Cycling (13 mph)	Shoveling 14-lb loads 10 times/min, climbing a ladder, lifting and carrying 85-100 lb
Basketball (competitive) Running (6 mph, 7 mph, 8 mph, 9 mph, 10 mph) Cycling (14 mph, 15 mph, 16 mph) Swimming (crawl) 850 yd/18-20 min 950 yd/20-22 min 1,000 yd/20-22 min Gymnastics Judo Wrestling	Shoveling 16-lb loads 10 times/min

Note. Adapted from American College of Sports Medicine (1991); Richard and Birrer (1988); and Skerker (1991).

and gyms do not have the equipment to perform maximal exercise testing. Although it is the most accurate method to base aerobic training on, it is costly and is typically only available in exercise physiology laboratories or research centers.

Karvonen Formula.   A more aggressive method, which is 15% more intense than the age-adjusted heart rate or the actual maximal heart rate calculation, is the Karvonen formula. This formula takes into account your maximum heart rate and resting heart rate, thus incorporating your aerobic fitness level as you improve with training. First your heart rate range or reserve (HRR) must be calculated by subtracting the resting heart rate (rest HR), which is taken in the morning before any activity has been performed, from the max HR, which is taken from an observed exercise test or estimated from the age-adjusted equation. The heart rate range is then used to calculate the desired percentage of target heart rate (THR):

$$HRR = max\ HR - rest\ HR$$
$$\%\ THR = (\% \times HRR) + rest\ HR$$

This aggressive method of heart rate training can only be used if you have no heart rate restrictions and are training at a consistent level.

The heart rate ranges in Table 3.4 clearly show the importance of adjusting the conditioning intensity to your fitness level and health status. This individual should follow the method where the maximal heart rate is actually tested because the age-adjusted and Karvonen formula produce ranges that exceed the actual tested maximal heart rate. But, realistically, you are not always able to be safely tested and monitored for max HR in the gym or group setting, and the age-adjusted method is often used. The Karvonen formula may be best if you are an advanced athlete who would like to be more aggressive and progressive as your resting heart rate decreases. However, the Karvonen formula will be too aggressive if you have sympathetic nervous system involvement and are not able to achieve the maximum heart rates predicted for your age, for example, if you have a complete spinal cord injury above T6 or if you have had a stroke. If you have a chronic disability such as postpolio syndrome, MS, or a progressive neuromuscular disorder, you may not be able to achieve maximal heart rates because of muscular fatigue. In this case, an interval approach is recommended with 2 to 3 min of aerobic activity followed by a 1-min rest. You can monitor your exercise by using RPE.

RPE—Rating of Perceived Exertion

If you are not able to meet the target heart rate ranges because of muscle fatigue, if your pulse is difficult to monitor, or if cardiac medication restricts your true heart rate reading (e.g., beta-blockers), then you can modify your exercise intensity by the perceived exertion scale. Please note that the American College of Sports Medicine (ACSM) recommends blood pressure monitoring for those with fixed heart rates secondary to medication or use of a pacemaker.

Rating of perceived exertion (RPE) is a technique developed by Borg (1982) to quantify subjective exercise intensity as it relates to the degree of physical strain. To use the Borg or RPE scale, you select numbers that correspond with your perception of how intense the exercise feels (Table 3.5). On a scale from 6 to 20, the number 6 is the baseline, which is no exertion. The top of the scale, number 20, is maximal exertion, the most exhausted you can feel for the exercise being performed. The scale values correlate to heart rates ranging from 60 to 200 beats per minute for subjects 30 to 50 years old.

Using RPE, heart rate increases parallel to aerobic exercise ($\dot{V}O_2$). On the original scale by Borg, the numbers 12 to 13 correspond to

Table 3.4 Target Heart Rate Range		
	Lower limit	Upper limit
Age-adjusted maximal heart rate		
Max HR (190 – 25)	165	165
Conditioning intensity	x.65	x.75
Target heart rate	**107**	**124**
Actual tested maximal heart rate		
Max HR	120	120
Conditioning intensity	x.70	x.85
Target heart rate	**84**	**102**
Karvonen formula		
Max HR (190 – 25)	165	165
Resting HR	– 85	– 85
HRR	80	80
Conditioning intensity	x.60	x.80
(60%-80% of HR range)	48	64
Resting HR	+85	+85
Target heart rate	**133**	**149**

approximately 60% of the max HR, whereas a number rating of 16 corresponds to approximately 85% of the max HR. On an updated ratio scale, 4 to 6 corresponds to approximately 60% to 85% of the heart rate range. If your RPE is in this range, exercise intensity should not exceed the intensity at which you are working.

According to Borg, the original RPE scale is the best one for exercise testing and for prescribing exercise intensity in sports and medical rehabilitation. The Borg scale is considered in exercise prescription because it is related to heart rate and integrates other important strain variables. The new category scale with ratio properties is most often used for determining other subjective symptoms, such as breathing difficulties, aches, and pain.

Studies have shown that practice with the Borg scale can help you learn the relationship between heart rate and RPE, allowing less frequent monitoring of heart rate and independent use of RPE.

RPE is a valid and reliable indicator of exercise intensity for the general population, but caution should be used when applying these scales to specific disability populations because they have not been validated with all these groups.

Table 3.5
Rating of Perceived Exertion (RPE) Scales

Borg scale	Updated ratio scale	
6	0	Nothing at all
7 Very, very light	0.5	Very, very weak (just noticeable)
8	1	Very weak
9 Very light	2	Weak (light)
10	3	Moderate
11 Fairly light	4	Somewhat strong
12	5	Strong (heavy)
13 Somewhat hard	6	
14	7	Very strong
15 Hard	8	
16	9	
17 Very hard	10	Very, very strong (almost max)
18	*Maximal	
19 Very, very hard		
20		

Note. Reprinted by permission from Borg (1982).

However, the RPE scale can be used as a guide to safely adjust exercise intensity to your own tolerance.

Aerobic Exercise Program Design

Intensity is just one of the variables to control when starting an aerobic exercise program. The other variables are duration and frequency.

Duration

The recommended aerobic exercise duration is 15 to 60 min of continuous activity or a series of work/rest period intervals in which the work time equals 15 to 60 min of exercise.

To significantly increase your aerobic fitness you should exercise a minimum of 20 min at your target heart rate. However, inactive and untrained individuals should not maintain exercise target heart rates for the entire 20 min when starting an aerobic program. In the presence of chronic diseases, 20 min at the target heart rate may be even more difficult or unsafe to achieve. Your initial aerobic exercise duration should be within your tolerance, whether it be 5 min or 50 min. If you have difficulty maintaining continuous activities, decreased strength may be a major factor, and you should start out with low intervals, for example, 1 min of exercise and 1 or 2 min of rest.

Frequency

The recommended exercise frequency also depends on your starting fitness level, including muscular strength, cardiorespiratory endurance, and how easily you become fatigued. Three to five exercise periods a week is a common recommendation. If you are significantly deconditioned, you can benefit from short daily sessions until you can tolerate longer exercise periods. For example, you could perform three 10-min exercise bouts throughout the day and gradually increase your exercise time to 30 min three times a week if tolerated. Once again, it is important to work within your limits. It is desirable to alternate a day of exercise with a day of rest, especially if you are easily fatigued.

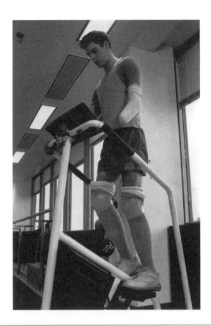

Your aerobic activity should be something that you like to do and that fits into your schedule.

Rate of Progression

Each of you will progress at a different rate depending on your starting fitness level and how your disabling condition affects you. The ACSM breaks the exercise rate of progression into three stages of varying intensity or duration that you can easily modify to fit your needs: the initial conditioning stage, the improvement conditioning stage, and the maintenance conditioning stage.

Initial Conditioning Stage

This is your beginning exercise program. This stage includes selecting an appropriate exercise mode, whether it be swimming, walking, or wheelchair rolling. Your program should include light calisthenics and low-level aerobic activities within your exercise tolerance. Your aerobic activities can last up to 10 to 15 min; however, you may use shorter durations if you have a low tolerance to exercise. If you are easily fatigued, you may benefit from performing a series of work/rest intervals initially and gradually building yourself up by increasing your exercise time period and keeping your rest period the same. If you have multiple sclerosis or if you are working with a very limited muscle mass, as can be seen in the muscular dystrophies, the interval approach may allow you to

exercise while avoiding fatigue and overtraining. Your base program should last 4 to 7 weeks before you progress to the next stage.

Improvement Conditioning Stage

The goal of this stage is to progress from short-duration exercise bouts and discontinuous exercise to continuous aerobic exercise lasting 20 to 30 min. Once again, you need to work within your tolerance. By this stage, you will have found the exercise mode that best fits your lifestyle and needs. If overheating or early onset of fatigue is still a factor, you should continue the interval approach but advance by increasing the total duration of your work/rest exercise bouts. For example, you may perform 5-min walks with a 1-min rest period for a total of 30 min and gradually increase your total exercise duration time.

Maintenance Conditioning Stage

This is your long-term training stage. This stage begins after the first 6 months of training. By this time, you will have made significant gains in your cardiorespiratory endurance. Unlike muscular strength, you can lose cardiorespiratory endurance rather rapidly—a few weeks of inactivity can set you back to your starting stages. So it is important to remain active by performing some type of aerobic activity two or three times a week. Cross-training may allow you to keep

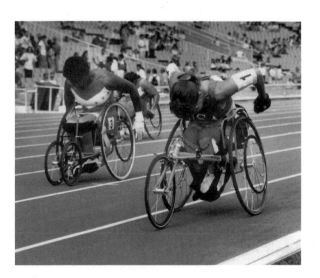

Proper positioning along with protective taping and gloves can assist with your aerobic performance as well as safety.

active without boredom from performing the same activity. Remember, it is much easier to maintain your fitness level than to start over to regain it.

For more specific modifications for aerobic exercise, turn to the disability-specific chapter that relates to you.

CHAPTER 4

Flexibility Training

Flexibility is a very important, but often neglected, fitness component. How many times have you jogged, wheeled, or performed a workout without taking the time to stretch? You must remember that balanced muscle length and unrestricted movement around your joints are necessary to avoid injuries.

Flexibility is the maximum ability to move a joint or a combination of joints through a range of motion. Many factors can influence your flexibility, including muscle temperature and elasticity, the distensibility of the joint capsule, and the extensibility of your ligaments and tendons. Not everyone has the same available movement— flexibility is related to your age, gender, and physical activity. Evidence suggests that girls are more flexible than boys and that exercise improves flexibility. Weight training has been found to increase flexibility if the exercises are performed using a full range of motion in the same plane of motion as the one in which flexibility is measured.

Not only do people have different degrees of flexibility, but flexibility can vary in different areas of the same body, for example, the hamstring muscle group is often tighter than the quadriceps muscle group. Repetitive movement patterns using the same muscle groups (e.g., wheelchair propulsion) and habitual postures (e.g., sitting in a chair with rounded shoulders) can promote muscle tightness or decrease flexibility. This decrease in flexibility can then cause

improper or inefficient movement. Also, when a muscle is tight, it tends to lose sensation. This sequence of muscle tightness causing altered movement patterns and decreased sensation shows how lack of flexibility in one area can cause injuries in another.

It is possible to improve flexibility at any age with appropriate training. Both muscle and joint flexibility is best improved by regular stretching

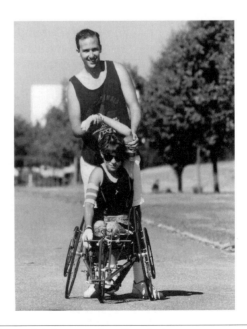

Active assisted range of motion during warm-up can help prepare you for an athletic event and prevent musculoskeletal injuries.

routines, so flexibility training requires a knowledge of joint range of motion and muscle reactions to stretching. Stretching exercises can be used to

- increase range of motion,
- maintain available range of motion,
- improve posture,
- reduce muscle soreness,
- prevent musculoskeletal injuries,
- provide relaxation and relieve neuromuscular tension, and
- control spasticity.

These benefits illustrate the importance of including stretching for flexibility in an exercise routine. Optimizing your flexibility can allow for more efficient movement that will enhance mobility and sports skills as well as prevent injuries.

When Should I Stretch?

Stretching should always be included as part of your warm-up; however, you should not just jump in and start stretching your cold muscles. Like an old car in the winter, your muscles require some time to warm up. The ability to perform physical work tends to be improved at elevated body temperatures. Gentle physical activity allows the blood to circulate to the muscles and tendons, which warms them up and makes them more pliable. This will reduce the potential risk of stretching-induced injuries. Simple warm-up activities can include rolling your shoulders forward and backward and slow wheelchair propulsion. Arm circles, clockwise and counterclockwise, are also excellent general activities to warm up the whole arm. If you are going to perform leg exercises, walking or a slow jog may be useful to increase the circulation to the working muscles of your legs. Gentle riding on a stationary bicycle for 3 to 5 min is also a good activity. Once you have increased the circulation to your working muscles, you can perform gentle static stretches to prepare your muscles for your workout. The static stretches should concentrate on the muscles and movements specific to the activity or exercise that you are going to perform, for example, arm stretches for wheelchair basketball and leg stretches for resistance exercise with the legs. Again, a warm and stretched muscle is less likely to be injured during your workout.

The cool-down phase of your workout should also include stretching. In your cool-down you again want to exercise at a submaximal level for 5 to 10 min to prevent muscle cramps and allow your heart rate and circulation to return to their preworkout levels. You then should perform your warm-up stretching routine again. At this point in your exercise program the muscles are warm and most pliable so additional flexibility can often be achieved, making this a good time to work on problem spots or tight areas. Stretching during cool-down also helps decrease the muscle soreness that tends to occur 24 to 48 hours after strenuous activity.

Principles of Stretching

Before we address exactly how to stretch and identify some techniques, we need to discuss the principles of safe, effective stretching. The three main principles of stretching, as with aerobic exercise, are frequency, intensity, and duration. Monitor and adjust all three according to your specific functional range of motion limitations.

Frequency

Stretching exercises need to be performed at least three times a week to maintain flexibility. You can progress to daily stretching routines, especially if spasticity is present and functional range of motion is essential to perform your daily activities. Whole-body stretching is necessary to maintain functional range of motion so you can perform the activities of daily living, even if you are nonambulatory. For example, if you use a wheelchair for locomotion, stretching your legs may not relate to wheelchair propulsion but it can assist with proper positioning in your wheelchair and with the ability to get the lower half of your body dressed.

Stretches should be done in the warm-up and cool-down phases of your exercise program. They can also be done while you are resting between sets of exercises. You should perform 1 to 3 repetitions of each stretch, but you can increase the number of repetitions if the goal is to increase range of motion in a particular area. For example, if you have tight heel cords and want to work on fast walking on the treadmill, it would be beneficial to stretch your heel cords and other leg muscles after a 3- to 5-min warm-up of walking. However, you would want to concentrate on performing at least two static stretches of both heel cords for 30 to 60 sec before and after the exercise; the other leg muscles may only require one static 30-sec stretch before and after the exercise.

Intensity

In regard to stretching, intensity refers to how much tension is produced by the stretch. The degree of stretch can be increased or decreased by the amount of time the stretch is held and the amount of external force applied to produce the stretch. The tension produced should not cause pain—pain means you have pushed too far. Begin high-intensity stretching to gain range of motion with proper medical instruction. To avoid damage to the joints and muscles, never stretch a multijoint muscle maximally over more than one joint at any time. For example, the quadriceps muscle group stretches across the front of the knee and hip. You should stretch this muscle group by lying on your stomach and grasping one leg above the ankle with a flexed knee. Do not maximally force the knee to flex or you could damage the knee joint, the quadriceps muscles, or both.

Again, there should be no pain when you stretch; you should feel only slight tension that slowly diminishes with the stretch. Apply stretches gradually, building to a maximum as the tissues release, and then remove the stretch gradually to prevent rebound or tightening of the muscle. When stretching after a workout to gain range of motion, apply slightly more tension than when stretching before a workout.

Duration

How long you hold a stretch contributes to the intensity. Static stretches should be maintained for 10 to 60 sec. Use a variety of moderate-intensity 10-sec stretches to warm up for an activity. A 60-sec moderate-intensity stretch may be used with spasticity (e.g., multiple sclerosis, cerebral palsy, spinal cord injury) or coordination problems (e.g., head injury, stroke) to stretch and relax a specific muscle group. Begin general stretching for 10 sec and then increase the time and intensity according to the tightness of the muscle group. Stretch for longer periods after workouts (during cool-down) to increase range of motion and decrease muscle soreness.

BASIC STRETCHING RULES

- **No bouncing.** Hold static stretching to build up soft tissue tension so change can occur in tissue length. Bouncing can tear tissues or cause injuries in other affected areas.
- **No pain.** Stretching should cause a sensation of discomfort or tension; pain indicates that you have pushed too far.
- **Do not hold your breath.** Exhale with short-duration stretches and breathe slowly and rhythmically with longer duration stretches so you are relaxed and focused on the muscles you are stretching.
- **Know what you are stretching and why.** Each individual and sport has different flexibility requirements; individual assessments are required to recognize tight and unstable areas.
- **Watch for muscle substitution and make sure the proper group is being stretched.**

Precautions With Stretching

If you have any of the following conditions, check with a physician or physical therapist before implementing a flexibility routine. You need to be knowledgeable about the structural stability of your bones, joints, and muscles and understand restrictions or precautions that you may have to follow both with stretching and with exercise. For example, if you have a history of joint laxity at the knee, you may have to wear a knee brace to help control this laxity during stretching and exercise. These conditions require professional clearance:

1. Severe spasticity with resultant joint contractures; the presence of a joint contracture or deformity
2. The diagnosis of osteoporosis or heterotopic ossification
3. A history of joint laxity (hypermobility), joint subluxation (partial dislocation), or joint dislocation
4. A surgical history with resulting scar tissue, tissue adhesions, joint fusions, or placement of instrumentation to stabilize a fracture
5. Pain that limits movement or that has not yet been evaluated by a physician or physical therapist

Contraindications With Stretching

The following existing conditions indicate that a stretching routine should not be performed at all or only by a medical professional. These conditions need to be evaluated and monitored by a medical professional to prevent injury:

1. An infection in an extremity or joint
2. Excessive swelling in a joint
3. Severe, painful joint crepitus
4. An open wound in the area you want to stretch
5. The onset of pain in an extremity
6. New joint instability or laxity that has not yet been evaluated by a physician or physical therapist

Stretching Techniques for Developing Flexibility

Review the following techniques of stretching so you are aware of the most appropriate way to stretch based on your physical disability as well as your strength and muscular control.

Passive Range of Motion (PROM)

Use this type of range of motion when you require assistance from a partner or when one body part is stabilized to stretch another part. *Passive* means there is no active muscle contraction while the joint is being moved through its range of motion. Slow, rotational passive range of motion can be used to decrease tight muscles around a joint for people who lack or have inadequate muscle control, the presence of spasticity, or both, as with spinal cord injury, cerebral palsy, and multiple sclerosis. However, when sensation is lacking, such as in complete spinal cord injury or stroke, PROM should be performed only by medically trained personnel to prevent stretch-induced injuries.

Active-Assisted Range of Motion (AAROM)

If you can perform an active muscle contraction but are too weak to perform the entire motion, after a stroke, for example, or if you have a neuromuscular disease, you will require a partner's assistance to stretch through the complete range of motion. When someone is assisting you with range of motion, you must know your functional range of motion, or your own limits, so stretch-induced injuries do not occur. AAROM can also be used to enhance the warm-up and cool-down phases of exercise and athletic events.

Active Range of Motion (AROM)

This type of range of motion is done with no assistance. It requires an active muscle contraction and joint movement to elongate the opposing muscle group. Active range of motion is often used for general whole-body warm-up and stretching. AROM does not develop as much range of motion as passive or active-assisted range of motion.

Static Stretching

Static stretching is the preferred mode of stretching for most individuals because if done properly there is little risk of injury. *Static* means that the stretch is held constant for a certain range of motion around one or a sequence of joints.

Dynamic Stretching

Dynamic stretching is a more specific mode of stretching for sport-specific movements. Sometimes referred to as ballistic stretching, it involves resistance in a joint to movement. Dynamic stretching often involves quick motions that are generally recommended only for highly conditioned athletes. Dynamic stretching should never be performed if you have spastic muscles. This type of stretching may increase your abnormal muscle tone, which could actually decrease your range of motion.

Proprioceptive Neuromuscular Facilitation (PNF)

PNF is a training method used in the physical therapy setting to promote the response of neuromuscular processes related to voluntary and involuntary movement by stimulating the appropriate proprioceptors. It is beyond the scope of this flexibility chapter to fully discuss the principles and procedures of PNF, but an introduction to the so-called PNF or super-stretch techniques used in athletic conditioning can add to your understanding of exercising for flexibility.

PNF uses specific relaxation techniques to help enhance functional flexibility. Two of these techniques, contract-relax and hold-relax, comprise only a small aspect of PNF flexibility training, but they are popular because they help increase the functional range of motion by promoting relaxation of the working muscle so it can be stretched to increase range of motion. Both techniques are performed with an assisting partner who places the extremity with the tight target muscle in a stretched (lengthened) position.

Contract-Relax. This technique involves an isotonic active contraction of the target muscle against maximal resistance by the partner. The contraction is often carried out for a count of 5 to 10 sec, followed by a relaxation phase. The partner then passively moves the relaxed extremity to stretch the target muscle to its new range of motion limit. The technique is then repeated, each time from a new point of greater elongation. The number of repetitions depends upon the functional goal of the stretch. This technique is often better than hold-relax (described next) for muscles that act over two joints (e.g., hamstrings) instead of a single joint (e.g., pectoralis major).

Hold-Relax. This technique is similar to contract-relax except that it uses an isometric rather than an isotonic contraction against maximal resistance before the relaxation phase and passive movement to the new limit. This technique is helpful when there is some pain in the extremity, possibly with muscle spasms, because the athlete does not have to actively move.

Both the contract-relax and hold-relax techniques are helpful when someone has spasticity in the extremity or is not able to move through the full range of motion. It is often beneficial, however, for the person to perform the full motion actively without any resistance other than gravity or the weight of the extremity after using the techniques.

Flexibility Exercises

The following stretching exercises start with the neck and work through the whole body down to the ankles. Whole-body stretching of all major muscle groups is beneficial for everyone as a warm-up; it is especially important to perform whole-body stretching when you have spasticity or abnormal muscle tone. Again, hold each stretch for 10 to 30 sec and perform the stretch three to five times, depending upon the tightness of the muscle group and the motions or muscle groups that are to be used or have been used in the workout or athletic event.

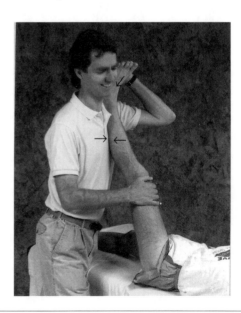

The hamstring stretch with arrows indicating the partner's resistance as the stretcher increases the force of his contraction.

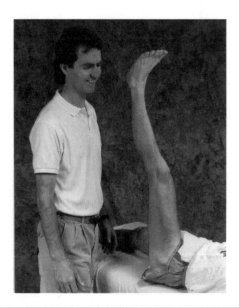

The stretcher actively moves into a deeper stretch with no help from his partner.

Stretching Posterior Neck and Anterior Shoulder

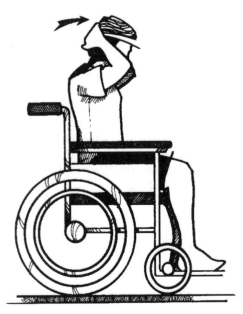

Clasp your hands behind your head at about ear level. Slowly pull your head forward until you feel a slight stretch in the back of the neck.

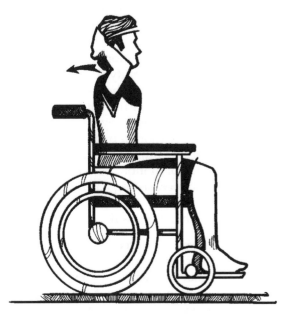

Clasp your hands behind your head and pull your elbows and head back until you feel a stretch in the anterior shoulder and posterior neck area.

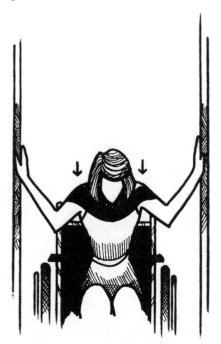

Hold on to both sides of a doorway with your hands behind you at about shoulder level. Lean forward and down to stretch the anterior and top of shoulder.

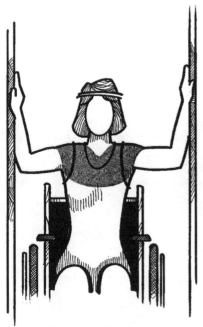

Hold on to both sides of a doorway with your hands behind you at ear level. Lean into the doorway to stretch the chest and anterior shoulder.

Stretching Anterior Shoulder and Inner Forearm

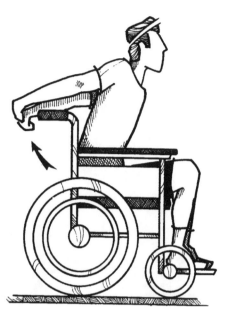

Clasp your hands behind your back, then lift your arms up until you feel a stretch in the anterior shoulder and chest. Keep your chest out and chin tucked.

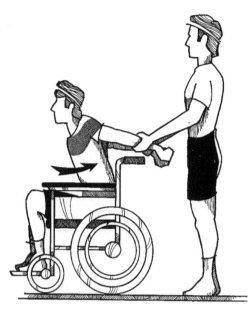

Place your arms behind your back with someone assisting by holding on to both arms above the wrists. Assistant pulls your arms back and up to stretch the anterior shoulder and chest. Keep your chest out and chin tucked.

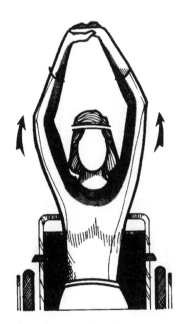

Grasp one hand over the other above your head with palms facing upward. Push your arms up to stretch the anterior and inner arm.

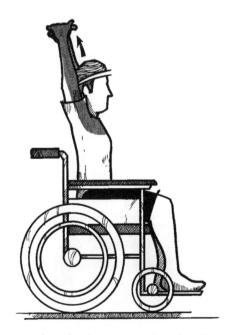

Clasp your hands above your head with palms facing upward. Push your arms up and slightly back to stretch the anterior shoulder and inner forearm.

Stretching Inner Forearm and Posterior Shoulder

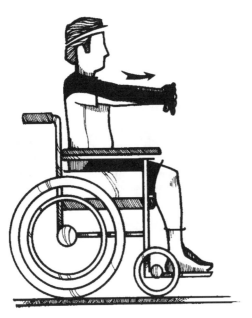

Clasp your hands out in front of you at shoulder height. With palms facing away, extend your arms forward and slightly up to stretch the inner forearm and top of the shoulder.

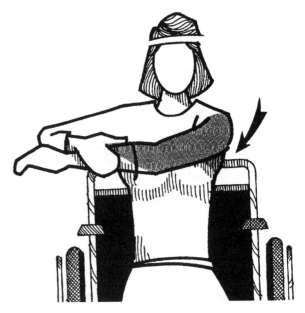

Grasp one arm below the elbow and pull the arm (at shoulder level) across your chest to stretch the posterior shoulder.

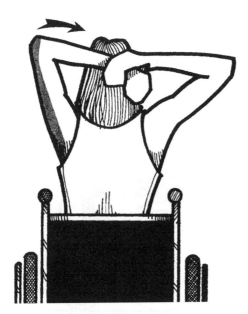

Grasp one arm above the wrist and behind your head. Pull toward the opposite shoulder to stretch the posterior shoulder and side (latissimus muscle).

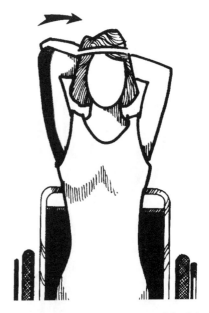

Grasp one arm at the elbow and behind your head. Pull toward the opposite shoulder to stretch the posterior shoulder and triceps.

Stretching Forearm, Trunk, and Buttocks

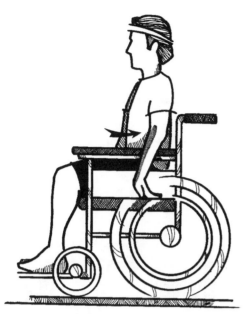

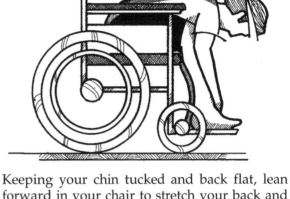

Keeping your chin tucked and back flat, lean forward in your chair to stretch your back and buttocks.

Place your hand on your wheelchair or a supporting surface at hip level. Flex the elbow while keeping your hand flat to stretch the inner forearm. *Caution:* not to be done with quadriplegia.

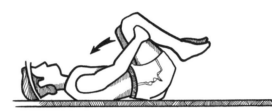

Lying supine (on your back), slowly raise both knees toward your chest, using both arms to stretch the buttocks and lower back.

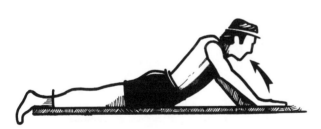

Lying prone (on your stomach) and keeping your hips on the supporting surface, place your hands just above the shoulder level and slowly push up to stretch the abdominals.

Stretching Buttocks, Quadriceps, and Calves

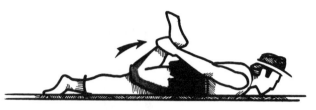

Lying prone (on your stomach), grasp one leg above the ankle with flexed knee to stretch the quadriceps.

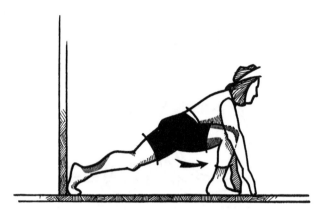

Move into lunge position, with forward knee over the foot and the back leg extended. With arms at your sides, lean forward with a straight back to stretch buttocks, quadriceps, and calf.

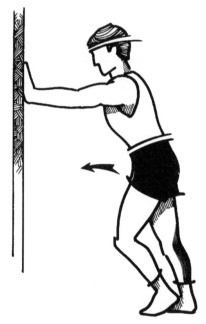

Stand with hands placed on the wall, back leg extended, with foot pointed straight ahead and front leg forward with knee flexed. Keeping the heel on the floor, lean hips toward the wall to stretch the calf of the back leg.

Stretching Hamstrings and Calves

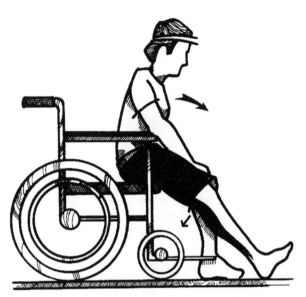

Sitting at the edge of a chair, place one leg straight out with the heel resting on the floor. Apply gentle pressure to the knee to keep it extended and lean the trunk forward, maintaining an erect back, to stretch hamstrings.

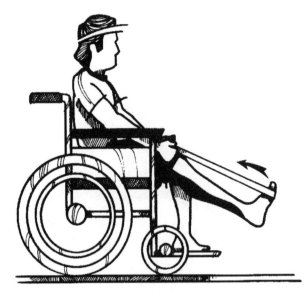

Sitting in a chair or on a mat with legs extended, place a strap around the forefoot, extend your knee, and pull the strap toward your chest to stretch calf.

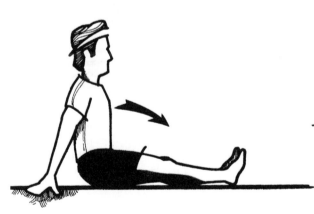

Sit with legs extended and together. Keeping your back straight and arms at your side, slowly lean forward to stretch the hamstrings.

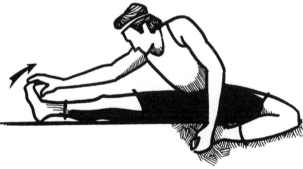

Sit with one leg extended to the side and the other with knee flexed. Keeping your back straight, lean over the extended leg and reach for the foot to stretch the hamstrings and calf of the extended leg.

Stretching Inner Thigh and Posterior Leg

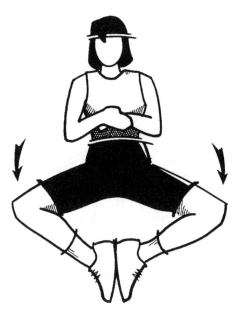

Lying supine (on your back), flex knees up with feet together. Let the knees slowly move apart and down toward mat to stretch inner thighs.

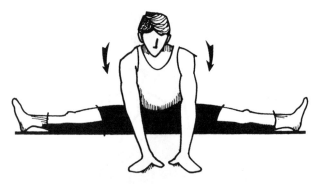

Sit with both knees extended to the side as far as possible. Keeping your back flat, place hands on the mat and lean forward to stretch the inner thighs.

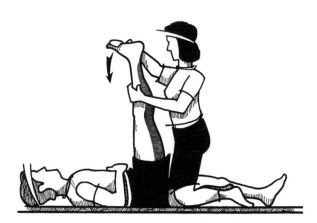

Lying supine (on your back), lift one leg perpendicular to the mat while keeping the other leg flat on the mat. Your assistant applies pressure at the calf to keep the knee extended and at the ankle to keep it dorsiflexed to stretch the hamstrings and calf.

Stretching Posterior Hip and Buttocks

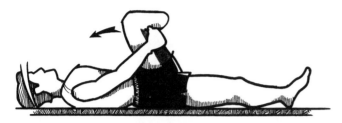

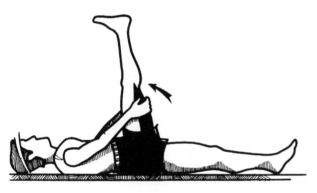

Lying supine (on your back), keep one leg flat on the mat and bring the opposite knee toward your chest, assisting with both arms to stretch the buttocks.

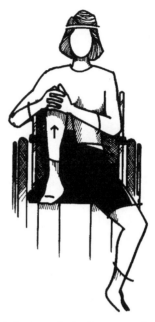

Lying supine (on your back), keep one leg flat on the mat and lift the opposite leg up with the knee extended until perpendicular to the mat to stretch the hamstrings.

Sitting upright in a chair, keep one leg flat as you raise the opposite knee to your chest. Assisting with both arms under the thigh, pull the knee toward the body to stretch the buttocks.

PART II

Disability Profiles and Conditioning Programs

This part of the manual focuses specifically on you. The disabilities covered in this manual are grouped into the United States Disability Sports Organizations (DSOs)—each organization represents a group of disabilities with similar medical and physical characteristics. Every chapter in Part II represents a different DSO. The DSOs and their corresponding disabilities are as follows:

- Chapter 5, "Cerebral Palsy Athletics" (cerebral palsy, stroke, head injury)
- Chapter 6, "Spinal Cord Injury Athletics" (spinal cord injury, spina bifida, polio)
- Chapter 7, "Amputee Athletics"
- Chapter 8, "Other Disabilities" (multiple sclerosis, osteogenesis imperfecta, arthrogryposis, dwarfism, neuromuscular diseases, postpolio disability)

In these chapters, we will deal directly with your disability. In the first portion, we will discuss the medical and physical concerns that may affect your ability to perform exercise. You may already have an in-depth knowledge of your disability, so some of this information may be a review. However, we highly recommend that you review the medical and physical characteristics because the remainder of these chapters (exercise readiness assessment, exercise precautions, exercise modifications, and response to exercise) are all based on this initial knowledge. If you are a family member, friend, coach, or instructor, you may also find this introductory material very useful in your understanding of the disabilities.

Once you have reviewed all the background information to give you a fresh insight into your disability, you will then need to find your own classification and identify the training program that corresponds to it. After making the necessary modifications to your specific exercise program, you can turn to Part III of this manual to learn about the specific exercises you will perform during your workout. Explanations and photographs of these exercises are also provided in Part III.

We also encourage you to consult Appendix B on pages 231-233 for information on the numerous fitness and sport associations for people with disabilities.

CHAPTER 5

Conditioning With Cerebral Palsy, Stroke, and Head Injury

In this chapter we address conditioning for people who have cerebral palsy or have experienced a stroke or head injury. For sports participation, these three conditions fall under the auspices of the United States Cerebral Palsy Athletic Association; they are categorized together because they all result from damage to the brain. This damage results in similar physical characteristics and limitations that affect the body in various patterns. We will address each disability profile separately, but the exercise classifications and routines will be grouped together.

So you can quickly find the information that pertains to you, note the following order:

Cerebral Palsy

The term *cerebral palsy* (CP) applies to a group of medical and physical conditions characterized by an impairment of voluntary movement or motor control. Cerebral palsy is a noninherited, nonprogressive disorder that results from lesions to the upper motor neurons in the brain that control muscle tone and spinal reflexes. Cerebral palsy is primarily a motor deficit, with associated conditions; in other words, it is the ability to move and the quality of movement that characterizes CP.

The motor, or movement, involvement or difficulty with movement varies greatly. A severely impaired individual may not have enough motor control to feed himself or herself, whereas a minimally impaired individual may show no observable movement problems. The motor nature of CP separates it from **autism**, organic brain defects, mental retardation, and psychological disorders. Causes of CP range from disorders during development of the fetus, such as maternal illness, blood incompatibilities, and premature birth, to problems at birth, such as anoxia, trauma, and postbirth disorders (anoxia, malnutrition, trauma, infections, seizures, and poisoning). These causes occur during the period of development and growth of the brain.

Movement and Coordination

Cerebral palsy is classified by motor involvement and its distribution, or pattern. The motor pattern

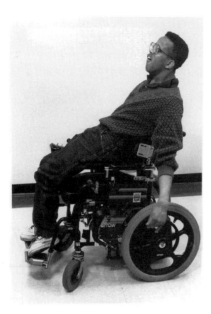

This person goes into an extensor thrust in an attempt to scoot back in his chair.

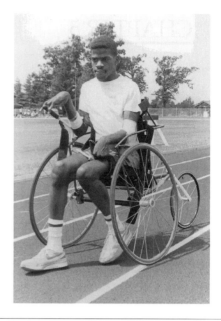

This person uses the dominant extensor pattern in his legs to propel his track wheelchair backward for increased speed and control.

types take several forms, including spastic, athetoid, ataxic, and mixed.

Spastic CP. Spastic CP indicates a fixed lesion in the motor portion of the cerebral cortex. This common form of CP exists in about 70% of all cases. The extent of **spasticity** can vary greatly, from mild to severe. The primary symptom is a state of increased muscle tone, or hypertonicity. For example, in an attempt to scoot back into a wheelchair, someone may set off the body's spasticity, causing the legs and back to extend and the body to slide out of the chair. Spasticity typically involves the flexor muscle groups of the upper extremities and the extensor muscle groups of the lower extremities (see Table 5.1). When spasticity is present, there may be patterns of grouped

Table 5.1
Typical Spasticity Patterns

Upper extremity (flexor pattern)	Lower extremity (extensor pattern)
Humeral adduction	Hip flexion
Internal rotation	Internal rotation
Elbow flexion	Adduction
Wrist and finger flexion	Knee extension
	Plantar flexion
	Inversion

muscle movements (synergies) and an absence of isolated joint control. For example, you may not be able to flex your knee joint with your hip extended but can flex it while flexing both the hip and ankle.

As a result of spasticity, the affected extremities are usually underdeveloped and weak in specific muscle groups, those being the opposing muscle groups to the hypertonic muscles, such as the wrist extensors, hip abductors, and anterior tibialis.

Severe and unmanaged spasticity may lead to a **contracture** (a shortening of muscle and connective tissue). A scissors gait and toe walking are characteristic spastic patterns. In someone just mildly affected, symptoms may be seen only during particular activities, such as running. Spasticity is a dynamic, fluctuating condition; it may fluctuate with stretching, external temperature, positioning, and emotional stress. Slow, maintained stretches of the spastic muscle typically can decrease the muscle tone, whereas quick movements, cold weather, fatigue, and emotional stress often increase it, making it more difficult to move.

Athetoid CP. **Athetosis** indicates involvement of the basal ganglia (an area of the brain); it is the second most common motor disturbance, involving 20% to 30% of all cases of CP. Athetosis is characterized by writhing, involuntary, purposeless movement that occurs primarily in the extremities but can also be seen in the trunk. Involuntary, abrupt, jerky movement (choreiform) may also be seen. These extraneous movements may increase with effort or with emotional stress. Athetosis is most obvious in slow movement, and dysarthria (difficulty with speech) is often associated with it.

Ataxic CP. **Ataxia** involves a lesion in the **cerebellum**, the cerebro-cerebellar pathways, or both. Pure ataxia syndromes are uncommon, involving approximately 5% to 10% of all cases. Ataxia is characterized by unsteadiness and involuntary movements of the trunk and extremities resulting in decreased balance, decreased trunk control, and difficulties with fine or rapid movements. It is most obvious in fast movements, and people with ataxia typically walk with a wide-based gait to compensate for poor balance and trunk control.

Mixed Motor Involvement. Mixed forms of cerebral palsy are most common. The combination of spasticity and athetosis is most often seen, whereas ataxia with athetosis occurs less frequently.

Cerebral palsy can be further categorized by affected body area. Refer to Table 5.2 for the distribution of cerebral palsy types.

Associated Conditions

The specific type and location of motor control impairment generally define cerebral palsy. How-

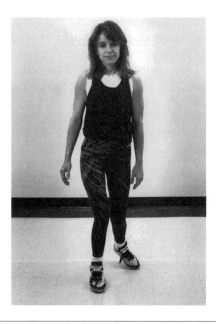

An example of a "scissors gait" caused by spasticity of the hip adductors (inner thigh muscles).

Table 5.2 Topographical Description of Cerebral Palsy Types	
Location	**Description**
Monoplegia	One extremity affected, usually one of the upper extremities.
Quadriplegia	All four extremities and trunk affected. Upper extremities are usually more involved than lower extremities.
Diplegia	Quadriplegia with mild upper extremity involvement.
Triplegia	Primary involvement in three extremities.
Hemiplegia	One-sided involvement, arm usually involved more than leg.

ever, depending on the cause and site of the brain involvement, associated conditions such as convulsive disorders, cognition disorders, perceptual and motor disorders, visual difficulties, speech and language difficulties, or orthopedic problems may occur.

Convulsive Disorders. Convulsive seizures occur in about 25% of the cerebral palsy population and are most often seen in those with **hemiplegia**. Two types of seizures may occur in CP: focal (complex and simple) and generalized (grand mal, tonic/clonic seizures). Focal seizures may further be divided into complex, which involve loss of awareness, staring, and lip-smacking, and simple, which involve involuntary jerking or shaking of one part of the body without loss of consciousness and may become generalized. Grand mal (tonic/clonic) seizures usually involve involuntary jerking or shaking of some or all four extremities, unresponsiveness, and loss of bladder control.

Instructor's Note: If seizures occur, remove potentially hazardous objects from the space around the person. Do not intervene during the seizure, except to lower the person safely to the ground if the seizure began in a standing position. Do not place any objects into the mouth of a convulsing individual.

Seizures are best controlled with standard anticonvulsant medication. In most circumstances, if you are competing in sports, you will have addressed this problem with your physician. Seizures are less likely to occur during sporting activities than at rest.

Cognition. Just 10% to 15% of cerebral palsy athletes have mental retardation. The United States Cerebral Palsy Athletic Association (USCPAA) recognizes this difference by specifying that cerebral palsy sports are intended for those individuals not eligible for the Special Olympics, which is an organization for the mentally handicapped. Children with spastic hemiplegia or diplegia frequently have normal intelligence and a good prognosis for social independence. If you are instructing individuals with learning disabilities or lower IQs in this population, you'll find repetition and demonstration to be useful techniques.

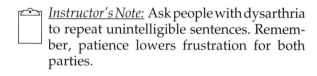 *Instructor's Note:* Do not assume someone is mentally retarded based on appearance or other physical signs. Many individuals with cerebral palsy who were once considered mentally retarded because of communication and other disorders are now known to have IQs within or above the average range.

Perceptual-Motor Disorders. Approximately 60% of cerebral palsy athletes and 25% to 50% of the pediatric cerebral palsy population show perceptual-motor disorders. One such disorder, spatial relations impairment, affects the ability to perceive an object's position in relation to oneself and other objects. Decreased directionality and judgment of distances affect performance in fitness and sport activities in many ways, such as difficulty maintaining a lane on the track or with precision or target sports. Slow demonstrations and repetition may allow you to compensate for your lack of perceptual-motor skills and to increase them. For example, as you increase your accuracy in throwing a ball at a target, move the target to allow you to play the entire field. This technique is useful in training for boccie and other precision sports.

Visual Difficulties. Many individuals with cerebral palsy show associated visual defects. Strabismus (crossed eyes), the most common visual defect associated with cerebral palsy, affects about half of those with cerebral palsy.

Speech and Language. **Dysarthria**, which is difficulty in speech due to impairment in the muscles that produce speech, is the most common speech and language problem. Usually as-

sociated with athetosis, it causes slurred and distorted speech.

Instructor's Note: Ask people with dysarthria to repeat unintelligible sentences. Remember, patience lowers frustration for both parties.

Orthopedic Problems. Decreased flexibility occurs frequently with abnormally increased muscle tone (spasticity) and may result in possible deformities or **contractures**. Stretching the spastic muscles and strengthening the muscle groups opposing the spastic muscles are helpful in maintaining flexibility.

Persistence of Primitive Reflexes. In normal motor development some reflexes appear, mature, and disappear, whereas others become controlled or mediated at a higher level. In children with cerebral palsy or other individuals with motor abnormalities, earlier primitive reflexes can persist and higher level reflex activity can be delayed or absent. Severely involved individuals may primarily move in reflex patterns, whereas those with mild to moderate involvement may be only temporarily hindered by reflexes during extreme effort or emotional stress. The influence of reflex activity is most apparent in class 1, 2, 3, 6, and 7 athletes.

An example of primitive reflex activity is the symmetric tonic neck reflex (STNR). The primitive STNR flexes the upper extremities when the head is moved toward the chest and extends the upper extremities when the head is moved to the back. With normal development this reflex is integrated, but in cerebral palsy it may still be evident, as is seen in the influence of different head positions on power in the bench press. The normal STNR responses in the bench press are characterized by increased muscle tone of the elbow extensors during head extension (toward the back) and decreased muscle tone in the elbow extensors during head flexion (chin to chest). If the primitive tonic reflex persists, performing a free-weight bench press could be potentially dangerous. Extreme muscle effort during a heavy lift may cause lifting the head (head flexion), setting off the STNR of complete elbow flexion.

An inexperienced instructor may mistake this reflex for weakness. If you have the primitive tonic neck reflex, you should choose a safer mode of exercise to work the same muscle groups. The five most prominent primitive reflexes are featured in Table 5.3.

Table 5.3
Primitive Reflexes

Abnormal	Reflexes
Asymmetric tonic neck reflex (ATNR) 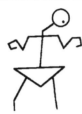	When the head is turned to one side, extensor tone is present in the upper extremity that the face is turned toward. Flexor tone is present in the upper extremity that the back of the head is turned toward. This posture is similar to an archer's or fencer's pose.
Symmetric tonic neck reflex (STNR) 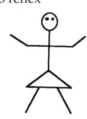 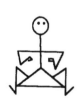	When the chin is brought to the chest, it causes flexion of the upper extremities and extension of the lower extremities. When the head is extended or brought toward the back it causes extension of the upper extremities and flexion of the lower extremities.
Positive support reaction 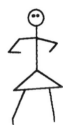	Stimulus to feet will result in a full extension pattern of the lower extremities—hip extension, knee extension, and plantar flexion (posture of standing on pointed toes).
Moro reflex 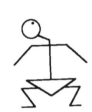	A loud noise, surprise, or a quick dropping of the head causes the extremities to extend out and quickly draw in to a closed position.
Tonic labyrinthine reflex  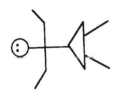 (prone) (supine)	Muscle tone of body is determined by head position. When on stomach (prone), flexion tone dominates. When on back (supine), extension tone dominates.

Note. Adapted from United States Cerebral Palsy Athletic Association (1990).

Exercise Readiness Assessment

Before setting up your exercise program, assess the following areas:

- Coordination
- Presence of primitive reflexes
- Balance and trunk stability
- Muscle tone
- Range of motion

The amount of coordination and control you have in your trunk and extremities will dictate the movements and muscle groups appropriate for exercise, the choice of exercise, and the overall program design. For example, class 1, 2, 3, and 6 individuals will show some coordination difficulties with arm movements. If you fall in these categories, you need to identify the movements over which you have control. If you are unable to touch your knee and then your nose, strengthening the arm is not appropriate. No matter how strong you get it, it does not do you any good if you cannot use it functionally. On the other hand, if you can perform the knee-to-nose movement without too much difficulty, then it may be appropriate to strengthen that arm or muscle group, and you'll have to decide whether you have enough control to safely exercise with free weights. If you can perform the desired movement, but it remains jerky and fast, you will probably be better off using exercise machines that control the path of the exercise movement.

As mentioned earlier, some people with cerebral palsy and head injuries in classes 1, 2, 3, 6, and 7 may show primitive reflexes. It is important to check for primitive reflexes, especially before attempting any free-weight exercise, the bench press in particular. Flex your head forward and then extend your head back to see if your arms and legs move involuntarily with the position changes of your head. If these reflexes are present, then you should not do a free-weight bench press. Maintaining the position of your head in a neutral position can prevent these reflexes from being set off during other exercises.

Your balance and trunk stability determine the mode of strengthening (free weights versus machines) that will be most appropriate as well as whether you'll need external support to stabilize the upper and lower trunk during exercise. With decreased motor control and balance in the upper trunk, you may require some form of support or assistance to stabilize the upper trunk during

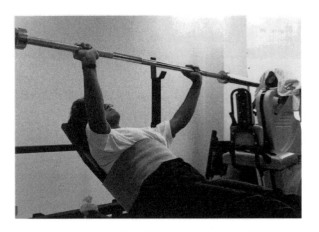

With the use of an elastic binder for trunk stability, you can perform free-weight exercises with mild athetosis in the arms.

overhead activities such as the shoulder press. One simple way to stabilize the trunk is to wrap an elastic binder or strap around you and your chair. If you have decreased standing balance, you should perform upper extremity exercises in a seated position and lower extremity exercises on a mat.

An abnormal increase in muscle tone (spasticity) in specific muscle groups must be observed initially to see the influence of the exercise program. If spasticity increases and interferes with movement or function with specific activities, stop the exercises and reassess them for appropriateness.

Spasticity can also result in decreased range of motion. A quick range of motion assessment helps identify which muscles need to be stretched and strengthened. Tight, spastic muscles require stretching, and the muscles opposing the spastic muscles should be strengthened.

Exercise Modifications and Training Considerations

Most exercise modifications and training considerations depend on your coordination and the nature of any coordination impairments (athetosis, ataxia, spasticity). Your initial program focus should always be on control or coordination rather than muscle strength. If you show mild to moderate athetosis or ataxia, you should be able to touch your knee and then your nose, but your movement will not be in a smooth, direct path. In this situation, assess whether you have enough control to perform exercises with free weights or if you should use machines.

If you are unable to safely perform and control your movements with free weights, you should use exercise machines that control the exercise throughout the range of motion. If you have mild coordination deficits, dumbbells may be appropriate, but you need to be positioned securely to allow for trunk balance during exercise. Strapping yourself in your chair with an elastic binder or belt allows some freedom of movement while providing good trunk stability. Refer to chapter 2, pages 26 to 29, for specifics on positioning and strapping.

If you show moderate to severe coordination difficulties in the form of athetosis or ataxia, a strength program may not be appropriate for you. In this situation, it may seem as though your arms have a mind of their own and will not go where you want them to go. Once again, emphasize controlling your desired movements over strength gains. As previously mentioned, you must take an aligned, secured, and stable position to perform exercises with your extremities. With moderate to severe coordination difficulty, you will not be able to perform exercises with conventional exercise equipment, including exercise machines and dumbbells. You need to assess the movements over which you have control, whether punching motions or biceps curls, and concentrate on them.

If you do not have a functional hand grasp, wraparound weights can help develop both strength and control with some motions, especially elbow flexion. Manual resistance may be a useful mode of exercise for people with moderate coordination difficulties. A partner manually guides the extremity through the exercise range of motion at the start of an exercise program, with the ultimate goal of complete, active control of the movement. Once active control of the exercise movement has been achieved, resistance may be added. This particular routine has been effective in training Class 1 and 2 boccie players.

Strength training usually is not appropriate for moderately to severely spastic muscles. If mild to moderate spasticity is present, the exercise program should focus on the muscles opposing the spastic muscle groups. When you exert extreme effort, your extremity may move on its own in a pattern. If this occurs, focus on exercise movements that move out of the pattern. Try to work on only one joint at a time, and remember that function and control are always the main goals. Spasticity in the involved extremity may temporarily increase with increased muscle effort on the noninvolved side, but it should subside shortly after exercise. Avoid quick movements because fast, ballistic movements can trigger spasms. If spasms do occur, they are seldom detrimental to your function or activities of daily living. Any exercise or activity that sets off or increases abnormal muscle tone or limits function should be stopped immediately and your exercise program

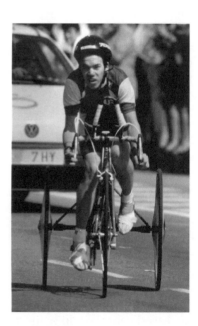

Athletes with limitations in balance can use a three-wheel bicycle or a stationary bike to perform aerobic exercise.

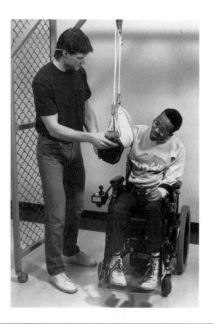

With manually guided resistance from a partner, you can work on strength and coordination for movements you have the most control of.

should be reevaluated. When in doubt, consult your doctor or physical therapist.

Response to Exercise

Cerebral palsy typically limits physical performances because it leads to decreased motor control, abnormal muscle tone (commonly seen as hypertonia or spasticity), nonfunctional activation of primitive reflexes, and difficulty with maintaining an upright posture. These characteristics, coupled with lack of physical activity, predispose people with CP to a lower fitness level.

Research in several areas substantiates observations of lower fitness levels. Studies show subnormal oxidative capacity and low locomotor efficiency in persons with CP and head injury. Lundberg showed that athetoid and ataxia subgroups had low mechanical efficiency during standard submaximal exercise (16% and 12% mechanical efficiency, respectively) compared to a normal control group (mechanical efficiency of 22%). Wasted energy from extraneous movements stemming from decreased motor control results in a high ratio of oxygen consumption to work performed. A study of peak power output and maximum oxygen uptake in CP has shown results up to 30% below those of individuals of the same age and gender without CP. These factors can commonly lead to extreme fatigue, which further lowers physical activity levels and may compromise fitness level.

Recent studies suggest a positive response to progressive resistance exercise for those with CP and head injury; however, some authors emphasize caution because resistance training can increase abnormal muscle tone and reflexes. If spasticity is present, resistance training may inhibit function by increasing spasticity. But resistance training for the muscle groups that oppose spastic muscle groups can improve the strength of those muscles and decrease abnormal muscle tone in the spastic muscle groups through **reciprocal inhibition**. In this case, muscle balance and range of motion should be stressed.

If abnormal tone and reflexes continue despite exercise, an individualized task performance appraisal should determine whether they can be used to accomplish functional skills of daily living. Adult movement patterns are typically well established, making such an assessment easier. Children with CP who are progressing through motor growth and development

should be closely monitored by a physical therapist or physiatrist (a physician trained in rehabilitation techniques). Inhibiting or facilitating muscle techniques performed by a physical therapist may be helpful to prevent or decrease overriding reflexes and abnormal muscle tone, even in early childhood. When in doubt, consult with rehabilitation medicine professionals.

The impact of CP on motor control varies greatly, as indicated by the eight different classes used in the United States Cerebral Palsy Athletic Association. Depending on the severity of presenting signs and medical complications, strength training and community fitness programs may not be appropriate for everyone—some people with CP may require close early monitoring by a physical therapist or other health professional.

Cerebral Palsy and Head Injury Exercise Precautions

- Perform slow, prolonged stretching routines before starting the exercise program and after warming up to help normalize muscle tone and prepare the body for exercise.

- If abnormal, involuntary, or nonfunctional muscle patterns persist with exercise, stop the activity and reassess its role in your exercise program. When in doubt, consult your physical therapist or other medical professional.

- Be sure to determine whether primitive reflexes are present before starting an exercise program. Maintain good body alignment for all exercises. (Refer to Table 5.3, p. 69 for information about primitive reflexes.)

- If tonic neck reflexes (TNR) are easily licited, a bench press with free weights is contraindicated. A machine bench press with a lighter load may be appropriate.

- When strapping for positioning or to control spasticity, use straps at least 2 in. wide. Be sure to check your skin for any reddened areas and identify areas prone to skin breakdown. Be aware of skin color changes, swelling, or decreased sensation in a strapped extremity, which could indicate that the strap is placed over a blood vessel or nerve.

Your Next Move

Now that you have all of the background information, you can turn to pages 81-83 to find your appropriate classification so you can identify your training program.

Stroke

A stroke is compromised blood flow to the brain or bleeding into the brain (hemorrhagic stroke) causing brain damage. Without a continuous supply of oxygen-rich blood, brain cells function poorly and eventually die, resulting in various neurological impairments and associated conditions.

The brain is a highly organized structure with left and right halves or hemispheres that control the opposite side of the body. Specific sections of the brain are responsible for specific functions. In 90% of right-handed persons and 60% of left-handed persons, the left hemisphere is dominant for language reception and expression. As the nondominant hemisphere, the right hemisphere specializes in visual-perceptual, spatial, and constructive tasks. Refer to Table 5.4 for specific differences that result from damage to the right brain and the left brain.

Most strokes (approximately 75%) result from a cerebral thrombosis of the carotid and cerebral arteries. A **thrombosis** is a blockage of a blood vessel by a clot that has formed inside it, usually under **atherosclerotic** conditions in which the artery is narrowed by plaque deposits. Cerebral embolisms and hemorrhages account for most of the remaining strokes. A cerebral **embolism** is a circulating clot in the bloodstream that lodges in an artery of the brain and obstructs blood flow. A cerebral hemorrhage occurs when a diseased artery in the brain bursts as a result of a combination of atherosclerosis and high blood pressure.

Nearly 3 million people alive today have had a stroke, and 500,000 new strokes occur per year in the United States. Of these, 150,000 people will die from stroke each year, making it the third largest cause of death in America, after heart disease and cancer. Stroke is primarily a disease of the elderly, but it ranks third as a cause of death among middle-aged people. The stroke death rate has declined significantly since 1972, with much credit given to prevention efforts aimed at controlling risk factors, especially high blood pressure.

Age, sex, race, diabetes mellitus, and prior strokes are uncontrollable or static risk factors for stroke. The risk of stroke increases with age, men are more likely to have a stroke than women, and blacks have a greater risk than whites. Heart disease and high blood pressure are the primary risk factors for stroke, although heart disease can usually be controlled through medical intervention and lifestyle modification.

The severity of brain damage from a stroke can vary greatly. Not everyone is left with disabilities

---

Table 5.4
Differences Between Right Brain and Left Brain Stroke Damage

Right brain damage ⟍   ⟋ **Left brain damage**
Right Hemiparesis   *Left Hemiparesis*

Right brain damage	Left brain damage
Speech and language deficits Decreased auditory comprehension Decreased reading comprehension Decreased word retrieval skills	**Intellectual deficits** Rigidity of thought Decreased abstract thinking Decreased orientation Decreased short- and long-term memory
Intellectual deficits Difficulty with initiating activities Decreased arithmetic processing Slow processing information Disorganization of thought	**Visual-perceptual deficits** Decreased hand-eye coordination Decreased spatial arrangements and relationships
Behavioral style Slow and cautious Anxious-hesitant	**Behavioral style** Quick and impulsive Short attention span Irritability and confusion Poor judgment and unrealistic behavior

Note. Adapted from American Heart Association (1989).

following a stroke; some can show almost complete recovery with mild residual deficits.

Movement and Coordination

Hemiparesis, partial weakness on the opposite side of the body from the stroke's brain damage, is the most obvious result from a stroke (complete **paralysis** on one side of the body is called hemiplegia). Often the hemiparetic side presents with **flaccidity**, lack of muscle tone. Hemiparesis is followed by a relatively predictable pattern of increasing tone (spasticity) in the muscles, which ranges from involuntary control of the movement patterns to voluntary control of movement in, and ultimately out of, patterns. These patterns of movement are called *synergy patterns* (see Table 5.5).

The last stages of recovery show isolated movement out of these synergy patterns, for example, reaching for an object by flexing the shoulder and extending the elbow. Bobath and Brunnstrom have described these synergistic patterns of movement in detail. The amount of recovery of muscle tone and control varies greatly according to the location and amount of brain damage, as does the amount of time motor recovery takes. Formerly, motor recovery was thought to be complete after 3 to 6 months from stroke onset, but some researchers have shown that functional recovery from a stroke can continue for months and years. For practical purposes, use 6 to 12 months from stroke onset as a general guide, and when in doubt, consult your physician. After medical rehabilitation, you should have at least started poststroke motor recovery before starting a community exercise

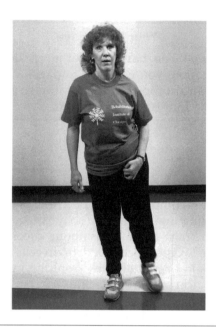

An example of left hemiparesis showing the beginning synergy pattern of the arm.

program. If you are recovering from an acute or recent stroke that has caused movement problems on the involved side, you may not be able to start an exercise program at all. You should be closely monitored by medical professionals until your initial motor recovery is complete.

Associated Conditions

Motor dysfunction is the most obvious result of a stroke; it is not always the most significant or limiting deficit, however. Depending on the location of the brain damage, poststroke conditions can include perceptual problems; visual field, speech, and language problems; shoulder problems; respiratory dysfunction; cardiovascular disease; and anticoagulation needs.

Perceptual Areas and Visual Field

With nondominant hemisphere (usually right hemisphere) poststroke involvement, the ability to perform spatial-perceptual tasks may be distorted. That is, you may have difficulty judging distances from objects, sizes of objects, and positions of objects and body parts. For example, you might reach back for a wall to lean on and misjudge hand contact, or unexpectedly hit the curb during parallel parking.

Neglect, a decreased awareness of the hemiparetic side, can also occur after a stroke. In

Table 5.5 Stroke—Synergistic Patterns of Movement	
Upper extremity	**Lower extremity**
Humeral adduction/ internal rotation	Retracted pelvis
Elbow flexion	Hip flexion/internal rotation
Forearm pronation	Hip adduction
Wrist and finger flexion	Knee extension
	Ankle plantar flexion (tiptoe)
	Foot inversion

Table 5.6 Stroke—Communication Difficulties		
Aphasia	**Apraxia**	**Dysarthria**
Absence or impairment of the ability to communicate through speech, writing, or demonstration due to damage in the brain. Trouble processing all language input and output. **Types** *Expressive (nonfluent)*—knows what to say but cannot say it. Unable to coordinate muscles for speech production to convey thoughts. *Receptive (fluent)*—impaired ability to understand spoken or written words. *Global*—expressive and receptive functions are both impaired.	An inability to plan and execute speech movements on command, even when muscle strength and coordination are preserved. May substitute with inappropriate words.	Weakness of the muscles for speech or decreased control of speech muscles. Speech may be distorted or difficult to understand.

severe cases, you may not attend to activities on the involved (affected) side or even be aware of this side. In mild cases, you may occasionally bump into objects on the involved side.

Following a stroke, you can experience visual field deficits. In minor cases, only the view of the far lateral visual field on the involved side may be limited.

Speech and Language

Commonly, with dominant hemisphere (usually left hemisphere) involvement, you may have difficulty with language, both with speaking and understanding, called **aphasia** (see Table 5.6).

Instructor's Note: Do not underestimate the abilities of people with aphasia. Some of them have full comprehension but cannot verbally express their thoughts (expressive, or nonfluent, aphasia). Others may have intelligible speech but cannot fully comprehend and respond with sensible appropriate sentences (receptive, or fluent, aphasia).

If you're working with someone who has had a stroke and find reciprocal verbal communication to be difficult, body language, gestures, and demonstration can be effective. Do not underestimate an individual's ability to comprehend and communicate, but do not overestimate these abilities either. An individual may use the same gestures for all responses, for example, nodding the head in response to both yes and no questions.

Family members or caregivers are often helpful in suggesting appropriate communication techniques (see Table 5.7). Family members are often a good resource for assisting with information about medical history, precautions, and common communication patterns.

Shoulder Problems

Shoulder pain is the most common and most limiting secondary complication from a stroke.

Table 5.7 Communication Tips and Techniques

- Face the person you are speaking to. Touch him or her on the shoulder and wait until you get attention before speaking.
- Make eye contact when speaking. Be sure to stay within the individual's intact visual field.
- Use demonstrations and gestures to communicate. Nonverbal communication can be very effective.
- Pictures and illustrations can be used to help explain exercises.
- Allow for adequate response time. Some individuals may require more time to process information before responding.
- Speak slowly and pause between important parts of each sentence. Repeat the sentences, if necessary. Patience can decrease or eliminate frustration for both parties.

Shoulder problems include frozen shoulders, subluxation, tendonitis, and reflex sympathetic dystrophy. Positioning of the hemiparetic shoulder during activity or exercise is particularly important—try to prevent gross subluxation at the glenohumeral joint and prevent trauma to the upper extremity by proper static positioning at weight machines or other equipment. Active exercise and passive range of motion can prevent contractures and possibly decrease pain; however, overaggressive range of motion can do shoulder damage. Consult a medical professional for an active shoulder problem or pain, and be alert for reflex sympathetic dystrophy (RSD), which can present as hand and shoulder pain. These problems frequently require rehabilitative medical services.

Respiratory Dysfunction

Spasticity (involuntary increase in muscle tone) can also affect the muscles of respiration on the involved side. Investigations have shown decreased **vital capacity**, inspiratory capacity, maximum breathing capacity, and flow rates in hemiplegic individuals. Exercise programs should emphasize endurance activities and deep rhythmical breathing to increase strength and endurance of respiratory muscles.

Cardiovascular Disease

Cardiovascular disease is commonly found in individuals who have had strokes, and it is also a major risk factor for strokes. A study by Framingham (Roth, 1988) showed that more than 75% of stroke victims have some form of heart disease. It is typical to be on anticoagulation medication such as Coumadin following a stroke, which increases your risk of bleeding with exercise, another important point to monitor. Yet, an investigation by Monga et al. (1988) of the cardiovascular responses to exercise in individuals with strokes and cardiac histories suggests that exercise is not contraindicated or dangerous if progression is slow and monitored. A physician's clearance should be obtained before starting an exercise program, and you should watch closely for abnormal signs and symptoms such as irregular pulse, fluctuating or extremely high or low blood pressure, chest pain, shortness of breath, dizziness, and change in general physical appearance. Cardiac reha-

bilitation may be more appropriate for you than community fitness.

Stroke Exercise Readiness Assessment

Before setting up your exercise program, address the following areas:

- Date of stroke onset
- Strength
- Coordination

Before starting an exercise program in the community, you should have almost complete motor recovery on your involved side, which typically occurs 6 to 12 months after the initial incident. You should allow this time for your natural recovery under the supervision and guidance of medical professionals. Following your rehabilitation, you can begin strength training if you have enough control, strength, and coordination in your affected extremities.

A general survey of your strength and available range of motion will help you identify the muscles that are appropriate to work as well as the most appropriate exercise mode to use. You may typically show residual weakness on the involved side of the body, and you will require gravity-reduced exercises for muscles that you cannot move actively through the full range of motion against gravity. For example, you may have to perform side leg raises on your back to reduce the weight of your leg and gravity.

The amount of coordination and control you have in the involved extremities will also dictate the movements and muscle groups appropriate for exercises, the choice of exercises, and your overall exercise program. Determine which muscles or movements you can actually control by trying to isolate or move one joint at a time. If you are not able to isolate movements and you can only move in a mass pattern, then strength training for that extremity is not appropriate.

Exercise Modifications and Training Considerations

Many factors must be considered before beginning an exercise program after a stroke, including your preexercise or fitness baseline, cardiac precautions, medications, and age. Strokes are more prevalent in the elderly, and elderly, deconditioned individuals may be too weak to perform continuous aerobic exercise and show increases in cardiovascular fitness. On the other hand, a severely deconditioned person may show a significant increase in cardiovascular fitness due to a low initial baseline. Younger people who have had strokes may not exhibit secondary cardiac complications and may be able to perform both anaerobic (weight training) and aerobic exercise without precautions. A strength program emphasizing muscle endurance is often a good starting point for these people before they progress to aerobic activities. A preliminary strength program allows muscle strength and endurance to increase gradually and prepares the person to exercise longer. This program is often less intimidating than aerobic exercise, especially for those starting an exercise program after a period of being inactive.

Heavy or rigorous weightlifting is not recommended. Instead, use moderate to low resistance and a high number of repetitions (10 to 20). This approach decreases the rise in blood pressure during exercise whereas lifting heavy weights can cause your blood pressure to rise excessively and is unsafe, especially if you have a history of cardiac complications. Start slowly and progress gradually. If you have been inactive and are weak, it will not take much resistance to increase your strength. Performing general, active range-of-motion exercises is a good starting point prior to advancing to resistance such as bands and dumbbells.

Do not hold your breath when performing strengthening exercises because it can place excessive stress on your cardiovascular system. It is important to exhale, or breathe out, during exertion. For example, exhale during the up phase of a shoulder press, and inhale on the down phase.

Once you have enough strength to endure longer exercise bouts, you can start aerobic activities or longer duration endurance activities such as walking or riding an exercise bike. If you have a history of cardiac complications or other chronic disorders, initiate your exercise training under medical supervision. Generally, activities that use the larger muscle groups in the legs such as walking and riding a stationary bike, cause less rise in blood pressure than activities that use smaller muscles of the upper body such as arm ergometry (arm crank) or wheelchair rolling.

Appropriate modes for aerobic exercise can vary greatly depending on your needs and interests. Walking is one of the most appropriate exercises and it requires no equipment with the exception of an assistive device such as a cane, if necessary. Walking also has a very low level of stress to the musculoskeletal system. Jogging may be appropriate for some individuals; however, be aware of increased stress on both the musculoskeletal system and the cardiovascular system. If you have other physical impairments such as spasticity, jogging may not be appropriate or even possible. If you have the ability to jog, we highly recommend that you start out with a walking program and gradually progress to fast walking and then to jogging.

Riding a stationary bike is another exercise option. This mode of exercise may be especially useful if balance and coordination difficulties prevent you from walking safely for long distances. Be sure you have adequate balance on the bike before beginning the exercise. Some exercise bikes have foot straps that can help you keep your feet on the pedals. If you have decreased sensation on the involved side of your body, it is important to perform a pressure relief, or a weight shift in your sitting position, every 10 to 15 min to promote circulation and avoid skin breakdown on your buttocks.

Remember that whether you use strength training or aerobic exercise, it is important to work within your limits. The idea that it takes high-intensity exercise to show gains in fitness is a misconception. Submaximal exercise can be very beneficial to your overall health, and high-intensity exercise can actually be very dangerous for anyone with chronic diseases such as diabetes, heart disease, and hypertension. If you are prone to hemorrhagic strokes, high-intensity exercise is definitely contraindicated.

Medications can also greatly influence exercise response. Beta blockers are commonly prescribed following a stroke due to cardiovascular disease, and they can limit the maximum exercise heart rate. If you take beta blockers you should use the rating of perceived exertion (RPE) instead of the heart rate to monitor exercise intensity. (Refer to chapter 3, pp. 45-46 for specifics on RPE.) Your medications should be listed on the medical form you complete before beginning an exercise program.

More studies on the effects of exercise with stroke are needed before specific conclusions or recommendations can be made. However, we believe that exercise is a necessary tool for helping you avoid further medical complications by decreasing risk factors of associated diseases such as heart disease and in maintaining or improving functional daily skills.

Response to Exercise

The exercise response following a stroke has not been studied well. Most exercise stroke literature has focused on various muscle facilitation and inhibition techniques used in rehabilitation to control muscle tone. However, studies show that walking can require significantly more energy for someone with hemiplegia compared to unaffected individuals. Two investigations have shown that individuals with hemiplegia have low physical endurance even long past the acute stroke. The increase in energy demands for walking and other functional activities can compromise an individual's fitness baseline. One investigation by Inaba (1973) involving 77 hemiplegics compared the effectiveness of progressive resistive exercise, simple active exercise, and training in activities of daily living. More patients receiving progressive resistive exercise made significant improvement in activities of daily living following 1 month of treatment than did those who received training in activities of daily living alone or who participated in active exercise in combination with training for the activities of daily living.

> ### Stroke Exercise Precautions
>
> 1. Get a medical evaluation and approval for participation in an exercise program, especially if you have a history of cardiac problems. You should also have checkups at regular intervals.
> 2. Your exercise program should be initially supervised, or at least followed, by your physician.
> 3. Avoid any exercise or activity that causes an irregular rise in your blood pressure.
> 4. Be aware of the medications you are taking and how they alter your body's response to exercise.
> 5. Be sure to develop rhythmic breathing when you are performing your exercises. Do not hold your breath during strengthening exercises because it can cause a steep rise in your blood pressure.

> ### Your Next Move
>
> Now that you have all of the background information, you can turn to pages 81-83 to find your appropriate classification. With the classification information, you can identify your training routine.

Head Injury

The incidence of traumatic brain injuries has been rising. A 1989 estimate from the National Institutes of Health states that 2 million individuals sustain a traumatic brain injury yearly. The mortality rate is relatively low (5%), leaving 95% or 1,900,000 survivors, many of whom may have residual physical (movement), behavioral/emotional, or cognitive impairments, or combinations of those problems. The incidence of head injuries is significantly higher for males than for females, at a ratio greater than 2 to 1. The majority of traumatic brain injuries occurs between the ages of 15 and 24; however, an increasing number of children are being treated for traumatic brain injuries.

Motor vehicle accidents are the primary cause of traumatic brain injuries. Other common causes of head injury include industrial and sporting accidents, attempted suicides, and accidents at home. Some less common causes of brain injury that show similar results include subarachnoid and intracranial hemorrhage, some forms of encephalitis, diffuse hypoxia, and ischemia. Although conditions associated with head injuries can vary greatly in the extent of involvement and areas affected, they can be categorized as physical (both motor and **sensory**), cognitive, behavioral, and other medical involvement.

Movement and Coordination

Most movement disturbances caused by a head injury are complex. Motor function or movement can be limited by decreased strength, impaired coordination, and the presence of involuntary movement. These deficits can range from mild to severe involvement, resulting in different degrees of limitation in functional mobility or movement. Strength may be reduced or absent. **Spasticity** (abnormal involuntary increase in muscle tone) may be present in various degrees. (Refer to p. 66 for further information on the effects of spasticity on movement.) Coordination of movement may also be disrupted by **ataxia** (cerebellar involvement), which is the inability to smoothly coordinate muscle movements. Ataxia produces shaky, irregular, extraneous muscle movements that can interfere with the ability to walk, talk, eat, and perform other activities in daily living.

Primitive Reflexes

Primitive reflexes that were once integrated can reappear and dominate movements following a head injury. Refer to pages 68-69 for a chart on primitive reflexes and guidelines for exercise when they are present.

Sensory Impairments

Head injuries frequently limit by producing double vision (diplopia) and decreasing visual field. Other areas that may be affected include hearing, general sensation (light touch), and kinesthetic sense (balance and the sense of movement).

Cognitive Impairments

The physical impairments following a head injury are generally the most obvious; however, cognitive impairments may be more persistent and limiting. A head injury may result in difficulty in perceiving, interpreting, and processing information. Cognitive impairments may include decreases in attention, memory, perception, thinking, communication, and language.

Attention. Even a minimal head injury can have some deleterious effects on the attention mechanisms in the brain. Many traumatic brain injuries decrease the ability to maintain attention, to focus on a task without being distracted, and to shift from stimulus to stimulus. The amount of impact on attention is directly related to the extent of the brain injury. To appropriately participate in a fitness program, you may require assistance. Participating may be even more difficult if you show a low tolerance to fatigue. Exercising in a calm environment with few stimulations may decrease distractions.

Memory. Memory disturbances are common following a traumatic brain injury.

Instructor's Note: Individuals with traumatic brain injuries may demonstrate difficulties receiving, organizing, and retrieving information. They can usually recall information or remember life events that happened before the injury; however, they may have difficulty remembering events immediately before the injury.

The inability to remember new information is one of the most limiting memory deficits. This decrease in short-term memory makes it difficult to learn new skills. Some improvement can be achieved through rehabilitation; however, many learn to compensate using memory aids such as lists and memory books for dates and activities.

Perception. Many perception disorders resulting from traumatic brain injury can have significant and confusing impacts on everyday performance.

Instructor's Note: Many brain-injured individuals have difficulties in the way they perceive the environment and themselves. Some may be very aware of their physical deficits, but may have poor insight into or be unaware of their cognitive deficits. Misinterpretation of actions or intentions of other people may also be seen as a result of not adequately perceiving and interpreting information.

Communication and Language. Brain-injured individuals may experience more generalized expressive and receptive language and other communication disorders than people with more localized brain injuries, such as those who have had a stroke. (Refer to Table 5.8 for descriptions of communication disorders.) These disorders can result in decreased language comprehension and expression secondary to difficulties processing all language input and output (**aphasia**), word retrieval difficulties, and difficulty forming intelligible, appropriate phrases or sentences when strength and coordination of the muscle of speech are intact (**apraxia**).

Instructor's Note: Some individuals have no problem understanding or formulating language, but may show speech difficulties secondary to weak, uncoordinated muscles of speech (dysarthria). Other communication deficits include an individual's inability to reciprocate in conversation. An individual may talk too much, interfering with communication and irritating others. Difficulty maintaining a topic of conversation, possibly related to an attention deficit, can also hinder communication. Individuals may jump from one topic to another for no apparent reason.

Table 5.8
Communication Guidelines
for People With Brain Injuries

Aphasia
- Get the individual's attention before starting the conversation.
- Do not speak too quickly. Allow the individual ample time to comprehend and respond.
- Do not overpraise someone for efforts at communication.
- When possible, questions should be simple, direct, and answerable by "yes" or "no." For example, "Did you stretch prior to working out?"

Apraxia
- Allow the individual sufficient time when speaking. It may be necessary to politely remind the individual to speak more slowly.
- If you are not sure of words ask for clarification. For example, you may hear "scurching" for "stretching."

Dysarthria
- Ask the individual to repeat the sentence if you are unable to understand what was said.
- An individual with speech difficulties probably has normal hearing. Do not speak louder in an attempt to improve communication.
- When speech is unintelligible, use nonverbal forms of communication such as writing or demonstrations.

Behavior

Behavior disturbances may include confusion, irritability, outbursts of rage, anxiety, aggression, depression, egocentricity, impulsiveness, dementia, and hyperactivity.

Instructor's Note: Aggression is one of the most troublesome behavior disorders following a head injury. It typically manifests itself as a result of initial confusion, which gradually changes to irritability. Irritability, impatience, restlessness, and agitation can result from increased difficulty in performing tasks that were once quite simple, such as balancing a checkbook.

Depression is also common after a traumatic brain injury. It may result as individuals gain more insight into their deficits.

TIPS AND STRATEGIES
FOR COGNITIVE AND
BEHAVIORAL DIFFICULTIES

1. Use visual cues such as exercise charts to facilitate remembering exercises and exercise technique.
2. Use exercise checklists or written programs to help you remember the exercises and sequences. Enhance your ability to recall exercises by performing the same exercise sequence—each exercise will then be a cue to perform the next one.
3. Use verbal instructions with written, illustrated exercise sheets.
4. Demonstrations can help you learn exercise skills and techniques more efficiently.
5. Carry a small notebook to record important information and list your emergency contacts and physician's number.

Seizures

Seizures are common conditions with head injuries. Seizures are categorized into many types. The symptoms can vary greatly from a focal seizure, involving only a lapse in attention, to a grand mal (tonic/clonic) seizure, involving the total body. Most individuals competing in sports or participating in fitness will address the issue of seizures with their physicians. Seizures are less likely to occur during sporting activities than at rest. Refer to page 67 for further information on convulsive disorders.

Due to the similarities in the effects of cerebral palsy and head injuries, the exercise readiness assessment, exercise modifications, and response to exercise apply to both. Review this information on pages 70-72 prior to proceeding to the classification section of this chapter.

Classification and Exercise Guidelines

Now you can identify your classification and locate the corresponding exercise program. Because of the great variability in cerebral palsy, head injury, and stroke, the classification system uses eight functional profiles (see Table 5.9). To use the following exercise programs and exercise index, you need to identify the class appropriate for you. The following charts will help you select the profile that best fits you. Once you have found the appropriate class, photocopied the training log on page 84, identified your training program, and made the necessary modifications to it, you can learn about the specific exercises you will perform during your workout. Part III provides explanations and photographs of these exercises.

Table 5.9 Classification Chart for CP Athletics				
Class	Upper extremities	Trunk control	Lower extremities	General
1	Severe limitation in active range of motion is the major limiting factor in all sports. Poor follow-through and shortened throwing motion. Often, only opposition of thumb and one other finger is possible, allowing athletes to hold a beanbag, boccie ball, etc.	Very poor to nonexistent static and dynamic trunk control. Difficulty regaining balance back to a midline upright position. Cannot sit unsupported.	Severely limited in strength, range of motion, and control. Legs considered nonfunctional for sports movements. Little to no purposeful, functional movement.	Severe spasticity and/or athetosis with poor strength and range of motion in trunk and four extremities. Unable to propel manual wheelchair due to poor motor control. Dependent on an electric wheelchair for all mobility.
2	Demonstrates sufficient dexterity to manipulate and throw a ball. Throwing motions must be tested for effects on release of grasp or hand function. Wheelchair propulsion with upper extremities is present but with moderate to severe limitations of control and range of motion for the push stroke.	Static trunk control is fair, but dynamic trunk control is poor, seen by extraneous movements of the arms and legs to regain balance back to midline.	Can walk with help for short distances but walking is not functional for sport. Can propel wheelchair with lower extremities.	Severe to moderate spastic and/or athetoid movements with involvement in trunk and all four extremities. Individuals are able to propel a manual wheelchair independently. Severe hemiplegics with fair function on the involved side are included in this class.

(continued)

Table 5.9 (continued)				
Class	Upper extremities	Trunk control	Lower extremities	General
3	Moderate involvement in dominant arm exemplified by limitation in extension and in follow-through with throwing activities. Rapid grasp-and-release hand movements are usually slow and labored. Dominant hand shows normal grasp of cylindrical and spherical objects, but the release in throwing motion is more involved than Class 4.	Fair trunk control during wheelchair propulsion. Extension tone in trunk limits forceful forward wheelchair stroke. Most throwing motions are from the arm with little or no trunk rotation.	Short distance walker with an assistive device. Can usually perform all transfers from standing.	Moderate quadriplegic, triplegic, or severe hemiplegic with fair to normal functional strength and movement in one arm. Propels a wheelchair independently with one or two arms but is slow.
4	Good functional strength and minimal control problems in both arms. Some minimal limitations in range of motion may be seen but a normal follow-through is observed with wheel-chair propulsion and throwing.	Trunk movements in both wheelchair propulsion and with throwing. Good dynamic trunk control with all activities. May demonstrate poor balance when standing with crutches.	Legs have moderate to severe involve-ment. Usually not a functional ambulator for long distances.	Basically a diplegic, uses a wheelchair for most daily activities and sport. Presents as a paraplegic.
5	Upper extremities are generally within normal limits. These individuals show a normal cylindrical, spherical, and prehen-sile grasp.	When throwing a ball or field implement, the athlete shows fair to poor balance without an assistive device.	Moderate to severe involvement in one or both legs. May show decreased balance with high-level balance activities.	Moderate to severe diplegic or hemiplegic. Ambulates and does not use wheelchair for daily activities. Athlete may or may not require an assistive device for ambulation.
6	Grasp and throwing release may be significantly affected by moderate to severe athetosis. With sports involvement, the throwing follow-through is further limited.	Trunk control may be functionally better than Class 5. Athetosis of trunk and proximal muscles limit balance during dynamic sport movement.	Lower extremity function varies, gait coordination difficulty is common. May show less coordination and balance problems when running.	Moderate to severe ambulatory quadriplegia, spasticity, and athetosis are common. All four extremities show involvement in all sport activities. Tone usually fluctuates.

Class	Upper extremities	Trunk control	Lower extremities	General
7	Nonaffected extremity typically shows no limitations. Affected arm may show spasticity, which is exacerbated with effort.	Involvement primarily on one side of trunk. May show spasticity with inability to shift weight on hip and elongate trunk on the affected side.	Spasticity usually present on affected extremity. Nonaffected leg shows normal strength and development. Runs with an asymmetric gait (marked difference between the legs). Spasticity in affected leg usually increases with running.	Moderate to minimal hemiplegia with good functional ability on nonaffected side. Hemiplegia may be congenital (as in cerebral palsy) or acquired (as in stroke). Usually walks with an asymmetric gait without an assistive device.
8	May show only minimal involvement in one arm. Normal grasp and release present in both extremities. Normal follow-through with throwing.	Minimal to no involvement, good strength and coordination for all dynamic sport activities.	Minimal to no involvement. Runs with a symmetric gait and without a limp. May show slight loss of coordination in one leg or minimal shortening of the Achilles tendon.	Ambulatory without an assistive device. Minimal physical limitations. Displays good balance with both running and jumping.

Note. Adapted from United States Cerebral Palsy Athletic Association (1990).

Conditioning With Cerebral Palsy, Stroke, and Head Injury

Date	Weight						Sets/reps	Exercises	Notes

CP CLASSES 1 AND 2 EXERCISE GUIDELINES

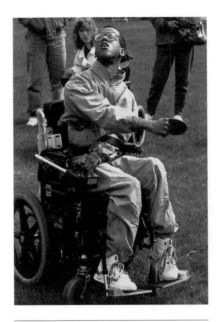

Cerebral Palsy Class 1.

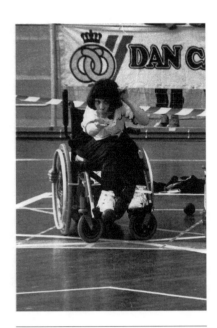

Cerebral Palsy Class 2.

Due to differences in coordination and associated conditions within this class, outlining a strict routine for everyone is not possible. Everyone in classes 1 and 2 must have a customized program. Refer to these guidelines when designing your program.

POSITION All exercises will be performed from your wheelchair, the optimal position to allow adequate balance and support for exercise. Strapping may be useful to maintain your balance (refer to pp. 26-29).

EXERCISE OPTIONS Suggesting specific exercises for this class is not appropriate because each of you will be able to control different muscle groups or movements and your exercise options will be limited to these movements. Emphasize movements that are, or can be, functional for you. Most of your exercises will focus on your arms, but if you have some purposeful movements in the legs you can also focus on them. Typically, lack of coordination or the hand-grasp function will keep you from using conventional exercise equipment. Your exercise options include manually guided resistance from a workout partner and your use of wraparound weights for movements that you can safely perform independently with adequate control. Although exercise choices are limited in these two classes, exercise training can enhance sports performance (i.e., boccie, slalom) and can have a positive psychological effect.

EXERCISE VARIABLES With decreased coordination, exercise intensity, or resistance, is less important. Emphasis should be on reinforcing smooth, isolated movements. Your workout partner can guide your arm through the exercise range of motion instead of directly resisting the movement with wraparound weights.

You can apply resistance in planes perpendicular to the desired movement, which is sometimes helpful to decrease extraneous movements out of the desired exercise pattern. If you achieve better control of the exercise movement, then the perpendicular resistance can be decreased or eliminated.

CP CLASS 3 EXERCISE GUIDELINES

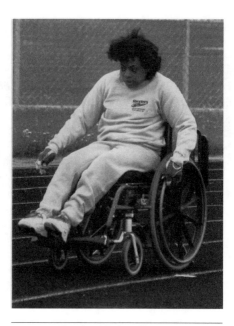

Cerebral Palsy Class 3.

POSITION You can perform exercises in your wheelchair, on a bench or mat, or possibly on your stomach. Strapping may be beneficial for many of you, especially if you are performing heavy lifts such as on the bench press. Some of you in this class may have a history of hip dislocations or other hip disorders. If this is the case, strapping should be at or above the waist level versus directly on the hips. Refer to pages 26-29.

EXERCISE OPTIONS You should be able to perform all upper extremity exercises with free weights or conventional exercise machines. If you have decreased coordination in your arms, you will have to determine whether you can safely control free weights with proper technique. Otherwise, exercise machines will be the preferred mode for the movements you have difficulty controlling, typically over-the-head exercises such as the shoulder press. Lower extremity exercises will be limited by spasticity and should be individualized to your abilities. Your lower extremity emphasis typically will be stretching. If you do have active, controllable movements in your legs, you should work these muscle groups, emphasizing the muscles that oppose the spastic ones. The following are suggested exercises for your class.

Upper Extremity
Bench press   p. 176
Straight-arm back raise   p. 187
Shoulder overhead press   p. 164
Lat pull-downs   p. 178

Lower Extremity
Leg side raises   p. 214
Leg back raises   p. 216
Knee extensions   p. 218

EXERCISE VARIABLES Your exercise intensity should start out low. Make sure you have selected the appropriate exercise mode (free weights or machines) and that you perform the exercises with proper technique prior to adding more resistance.

CP CLASSES 4 AND 5 EXERCISE GUIDELINES

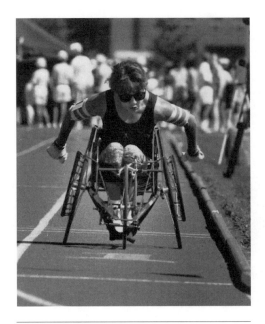

Cerebral Palsy Class 4.

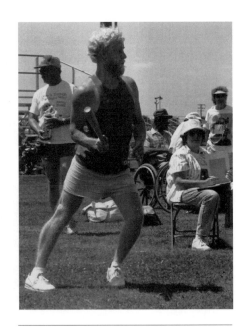

Cerebral Palsy Class 5.

POSITION You can perform exercises sitting in your wheelchair, on your stomach, on your back, and possibly standing, if your balance allows. Position and secure yourself in the desired position. Lower extremity muscle tone and range of motion usually do not limit the performance of upper extremity exercise.

EXERCISE OPTIONS You should be able to perform all upper extremity exercises with free weights. The type of equipment available to you will be the only limiting factor in selecting the mode of your upper extremity exercises. Spasticity can limit lower extremity exercises, which should be individualized to your abilities. Your lower extremity emphasis should include stretching for your spastic muscles and working to strengthen the muscles that oppose the spastic ones. The following are suggested exercises for your class.

Upper Extremity
Bench press   p. 176
Straight-arm back raise   p. 187
Shoulder overhead press   p. 164
Lat pull-downs   p. 178
Dips   p. 173
Triceps extensions   p. 188
Biceps curl   p. 191

Lower Extremity
Leg side raises   p. 214
Leg back raises   p. 216
Knee extensions   p. 218

CP CLASS 6 EXERCISE GUIDELINES

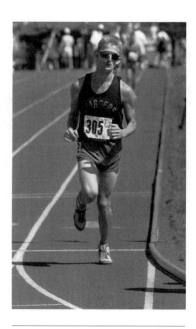

Cerebral Palsy Class 6.

POSITION   You can perform sitting in your wheelchair, on your stomach, or on your back. Position and secure yourself in the desired position. You may require strapping to stabilize your trunk while exercising with your arms and legs. Refer to pages 26 to 29 for information about strapping.

EXERCISE OPTIONS   You should be able to perform exercises for both your arms and legs. The amount of coordination you have will dictate your selection of exercises—if you cannot safely perform the exercise through its complete range of motion, you should not include it in your program. Exercise machines and equipment that evenly apply resistance and limit extraneous movement throughout the exercise range of motion are the preferred modes of exercise because of your decreased coordination. Some of you may have enough control to use free weights for specific exercises; however, you must consider the use of weights separately with every exercise. The following are suggested exercises for your class, but keep in mind that your exercise program needs to be customized to your abilities.

Upper Extremity
Machine bench press   p. 177
Machine biceps curls   p. 191
Machine triceps extensions   p. 189
Shoulder overhead presses   p. 164
Lat pull-downs   p. 178

Lower Extremity
Machine leg curls   p. 212
Machine knee extensions   p. 218

CP CLASS 7 EXERCISE GUIDELINES

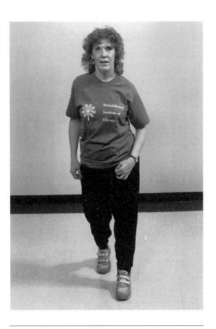

Cerebral Palsy Class 7.

POSITION You can perform exercises sitting in your wheelchair, on your stomach, on your back, and possibly standing, if your balance allows. Strapping may be required—refer to pages 26 to 29 for more information.

EXERCISE OPTIONS You should have no limitations on your nonaffected side and should be able to use free weights and machines as your balance allows. Typically, people in this class perform free-weight unilateral exercise because of the strength and coordination differences between the two sides of the body. Your coordination and muscle tone will dictate the choice of exercise for your involved extremity. The exercises you choose should involve movement patterns you can use functionally. If they elicit involuntary movement in nonfunctional patterns, stop immediately and reassess whether they are appropriate for you. When in doubt, consult your physician or physical therapist. The following are suggested exercises for your class, but keep in mind that your exercise program needs to be customized to your abilities.

Upper Extremity	*Lower Extremity*
Front shoulder raise p. 179	Leg side raises p. 214
Lateral shoulder raise p. 180	Leg back raises p. 216
Back shoulder raise p. 181	Straight leg raise p. 213
Triceps extensions p. 188	Knee extensions p. 218
Biceps curl p. 191	Leg curls p. 212
	Ankle curls p. 219

EXERCISE VARIABLES Your exercise intensity should start out low. Make sure you have selected the appropriate exercise mode (free weights or machines) and perform the exercises with proper technique prior to adding more resistance.

CP CLASS 8 EXERCISE GUIDELINES

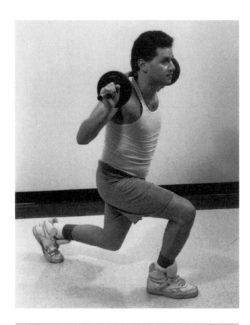

Cerebral Palsy Class 8.

POSITION You show no limitations and can assume all positions; strapping for balance is rarely required.

EXERCISE OPTIONS No limitations. You can use free weights with all exercises. Initial supervision may be required. Your exercise routine should reflect muscular balance. The following are suggested exercises for your class.

Upper Extremity
Bench press   p. 176
Bent-over rows   p. 174
Straight-arm back raise   p. 187
Shoulder overhead press   p. 164
Lat pull-downs   p. 178
Dips   p. 173
Triceps extensions   p. 188
Biceps curl   p. 191

Lower Extremity
Squats   p. 210
Lunges   p. 211
Leg curls   p. 212
Knee extensions   p. 218
Heel raises   p. 220
Ankle curls   p. 219

CHAPTER 6

Conditioning With Spinal Cord Injuries, Spina Bifida, and Poliomyelitis

In this chapter, we will cover the conditions of spinal cord injury, spina bifida, and poliomyelitis. The National Wheelchair Athletic Association (NWAA) supervises sports participation for people in these categories. These three conditions are grouped together because they all result from damage to the spinal cord, which produces similar physical characteristics and limitations of muscle function. We will address each disability profile separately but group the exercise classifications and routines together because they apply to all three conditions.

So you can quickly find the disability information that pertains to you, note the following order:

Spinal Cord Injury

Spinal cord injury (SCI) is one of the most life-altering traumas anyone can sustain. The most obvious effect of damage to the delicate spinal cord tissue is loss of voluntary muscle use—paralysis. However, as you know, other systems can also be affected, including sensory, bowel and bladder, circulation, temperature regulation, and sexuality. The resultant loss of function from spinal cord damage can range from an all-encompassing complete injury to a less-involved incomplete injury. A complete spinal cord injury means there is no muscle or sensory function more than three segments below the neurological level of cord damage. Incomplete injuries occur when parts of ascending and descending tracts in the spinal cord are able to send their messages through the damaged area and muscle, or sensory function exists below the level of injury, or both.

Classification of the level of spinal cord injury should be based on the level of lowest functioning musculature (neurological level) rather than the level of vertebral bone damage (vertebral level), because where the spine is broken may not be a true indication of what remaining muscle function you have. This is because the nerves from the spinal cord that supply the muscles exit from the bony spine below their numbered segment. So the real concern is the level of spinal cord damage, not the vertebral bone fracture.

Most damage from a spinal cord injury is secondary to swelling in the spinal cord area that results in nonfunctional spinal cord tissue. The nerves that exit below this level of spinal cord damage no longer stimulate the associated muscles. Subsequently, a spinal cord injury is classified according to the lowest region of the spinal cord that is actually intact or functional (cervical, thoracic, lumbar, or sacral) and the number of the nerve segment that exits from the spinal cord (C1-8, T1-12, L1-5, and S1-5). For example, a fracture to the sixth cervical vertebra (C6) can cause incomplete or complete spinal cord damage at that segment. Incomplete damage to the spinal cord could leave an individual with muscle and sensory function to the C7 level in the right arm and to the C8 level in the left arm. The person with this injury would be classified with C7 quadriplegia on the right and C8 quadriplegia on the left even though the original fracture was at the C6 level.

A neck injury (to the cervical part of the spinal cord) or an injury to the upper thorax is referred to as **quadriplegia**, which means complete or incomplete spinal cord damage that causes neurological impairment of all four extremities and the trunk. Although all four extremities are affected in quadriplegia, this does not mean that the affected person has no use of the arms. The amount of working musculature depends on the level and extent of the spinal cord damage. The levels for quadriplegia are referenced to their neurological level in the cervical area, C1 to C8, and thoracic involvement at T1. An injury to the lower part of the neck at C8 results in the loss of most hand muscles but spares the function of the shoulder, forearm, and wrist musculature. In contrast, injury to the spinal cord at level C4 is the highest lesion that a person can sustain and remain alive without artificial breathing support. Those with an injury at C4 have use only of neck muscles, two shoulder girdle muscles, and the diaphragm for breathing. The diaphragm is supplied by the phrenic nerve at C3, 4, and 5 so even breathing may be impaired. In wheelchair athletics these individuals are in classes 1A, 1B, and 1C.

An injury below the neck, to the thorax or lower spine, is referred to as **paraplegia**, which means that the person has full use of the upper extremities including the hands, with neurological impairment to their lower extremities, often involving part of the trunk. Paraplegia also can be complete or incomplete depending on the extent of damage to the spinal cord. The levels for paraplegia are referenced to their neurological level in the thoracic (T2-T12), lumbar (L1-L5), or sacral spine (S1-S5). In wheelchair athletics they are in classes 2 to 5.

Associated Conditions

Paraplegia and quadriplegia after spinal cord injury can lead to a degenerative cycle that results in decreased lean body mass, low **aerobic capacity**, increased risk of cardiovascular disease, osteoporosis, renal dysfunction, and possible contractures or skin pressure sores. This degenerative process is similar to the problems those having a very sedentary lifestyle encounter. This section introduces the following associated conditions: body composition, aerobic capacity, thermoregulation, orthostatic and exercise hypotension, cardiovascular disease, spasticity, osteoporosis, bowel and bladder function, contractures and decreased range of motion, **heterotopic ossification**, pressure sores, autonomic hyperreflexia, thrombophlebitis, and tenodesis.

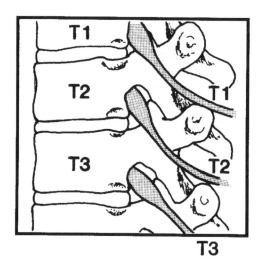

Spinal cord vertebrae and exiting nerve roots from the spinal cord.

Body Composition. Decreased lean body mass is a long-term change in overall body composition that may follow a spinal cord injury. Muscle wasting (atrophy) from motor loss or paralysis is the primary reason for decreased lean body mass. Atrophied muscle is eventually replaced with connective tissue and filled with fat and water, resulting in an increased percent of body fat and weight gain. This decrease in available working muscle slows down the body's metabolism and can limit potential for cardiovascular fitness with aerobic exercise.

Aerobic Capacity. Many studies associate a decrease in cardiovascular fitness (VO_2max) with spinal cord injuries due to the decreased large active muscle mass of the lower extremities and, in some cases, loss of sympathetic neural regulation of the heart and vasomotor tone. In addition, many people with spinal cord injuries emphasize short-duration tasks in rehabilitation and lifestyle, such as developing muscles required for transfers, activities of daily living, and self-care. Often, not much attention is paid to longer duration activities using the muscle groups of the upper extremities, which constitutes aerobic exercise.

Any spinal cord damage above T6 is capable of disrupting the sympathetic nervous system's control of the heart. The **sympathetic nervous system** is one branch of the **autonomic nervous system**, a regulatory control system that maintains the internal environment of the body at an optimal level (homeostasis) and governs involuntary visceral or internal function. As a branch of the autonomic nervous system, the sympathetic nervous system is partially responsible for increasing the heart rate and shunting blood to the working muscles during exercise; it plays a major role in preparing the body for stressful events. Stimulation of the sympathetic system prepares the body for movement and emergency situations by alerting the body's organs as needed.

Stimulation of the **parasympathetic nervous system**, the other branch of the autonomic nervous system, promotes relaxing and vegetative (resting) functions of the body. This system plays a major role in returning the body's internal environment to a normal level after a stressful event has occurred. These two systems normally act reciprocally.

If injury occurs above the T6 level, the spinal cord is unable to maintain control of the sympathetic pathways, and the other half of the autonomic nervous system, the parasympathetic, with its opposite functions from the sympathetic system, takes unopposed control. The parasympathetic system exerts effects outside of the brain and spinal cord through cranial nerve number 10 (the vagus nerve). Control by the parasympathetic system limits maximum exercise heart rate to approximately 110 to 130 beats per minute. People with paraplegia due to an injury at level T6 or below may be able to reach a higher maximum heart rate, but they may still have difficulty achieving an aerobic training effect because of the inability to use the large muscle groups of the lower extremities. An aerobic training effect can also be hindered by the pooling of blood in the inactive legs due to a loss of vasomotor tone and the loss of the pumping action of the muscles. The small musculature of the upper extremities is not enough to challenge the heart. In addition, untrained upper extremity musculature often fatigues before an aerobic training effect can be achieved. People with spinal cord injuries can still enhance cardiovascular fitness because training allows improved peripheral extraction of oxygen from the blood. Oxidative enzymes increase with training, so more oxygen-rich blood can supply exercising muscles and metabolic by-products can be cleared to permit longer exercise.

Thermoregulation. The autonomic nervous system is also responsible for temperature regulation (**thermoregulation**) of the body. The higher and more complete the spinal cord damage above T6, the greater the strain to the cardiovascular system and temperature regulation when the body is exposed to environmental extremes of heat or cold. This is because there is no sympathetic vasomotor control of heat transport from warm internal structures to the skin (which is needed in extreme cold weather) or of the rate of heat loss from the body surface via sweating (which is needed to cool the body in extreme heat). Experts also speculate that damage to the spinal cord with subsequent absent voluntary muscle use may prevent shivering, which increases the body temperature in individuals with no sympathetic nervous system damage. Depending on exercise intensity, you may need to be monitored in extremely hot and cold weather for increased or decreased body temperatures that could lead to overheating (hyperthermia) or excessive cooling (hypothermia). Keep cool, damp cloths available during exercise in warmer temperatures or for long-duration aerobic activities to help your body cool down in the absence of the sweating mechanism.

Orthostatic and Exercise Hypotension. The sympathetic nervous system also maintains and controls the muscle tone of the blood vessels (**vasomotor tone**). The degree of loss of sympathetic vasomotor tone again depends on your level of injury. Spinal cord injuries above L1 show a complete separation of lower extremity vasculature from central nervous system control (brain and spinal cord). Spinal cord injuries at L1 to L2 result in partial separation, and injuries below L2 have no effect on the normal vasomotor tone in the lower extremities. Pooling of blood in the inactive lower extremities because of the loss of vasomotor tone and muscle pump reduces the blood return to the heart. The term *muscle pump* refers to pumping blood back to the heart by actively contracting the muscles of the legs, a process that is absent in the majority of spinal cord injuries. During exercise, this results in a lower **stroke volume** (blood pumped out) from the heart, because the amount of blood returned to the heart is reduced.

Exercise hypotension, or low blood pressure, can result from blood pooling in the legs in conjunction with the shunting of blood to the working muscles of the upper extremities during aerobic activities. Exercise hypotension is exhibited by a drop in blood pressure, which may cause you to feel faint or even pass out because of the decrease in oxygen from decreased blood circulation reaching the brain. Get assistance to recline in your chair or lie on your back to relieve symptoms by elevating your blood pressure.

You can prevent exercise hypotension by starting exercise slowly, with a warm-up period that gives the body's blood pressure time to adjust. Slowly increasing the intensity and duration of the exercise session can help build up a tolerance to aerobic exercise and enable proper blood pressure adjustments.

This problem of exercise hypotension can be exacerbated when exercising in a seated upright position if you already have **orthostatic hypotension**—an intolerance to an upright position because of insufficient blood reaching the brain—at rest. You may need to exercise from a reclining position or gradually build up consistent tolerance to regular exercise in an upright position. Elastic, pressure-gradient stockings and abdominal binders can decrease venous pooling and help you adapt to the upright position. However, some people with orthostatic hypotension

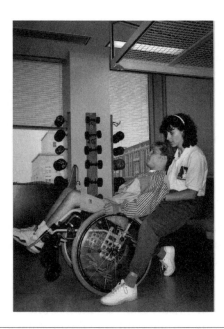

Have someone help you recline in your chair to relieve symptoms of exercise hypotension by elevating blood pressure.

at rest may never tolerate long periods of aerobic activity.

Cardiovascular Disease. One investigation found that acute spinal cord injury is a possible direct risk for cardiovascular disease. This investigation suggested that spinal shock, excessive release of myocardial norepinephrine, emotional stress, and the vascular effects of **autonomic hyperreflexia** contribute to the development of cardiovascular disease. Individuals with paraplegia are at greater risk than their non-disabled counterparts for atherosclerosis or "hardening of the arteries," which a 1986 report called one of the greatest risk factors in their decreased life expectancy. **Hypertension** has been well documented as the predominant type of cardiovascular disease found in individuals with paraplegia. Studies have shown significantly lower concentrations of HDL-C ("good" cholesterol) in sedentary people with spinal cord injuries than in nondisabled groups and athletes with spinal cord injuries, and higher levels of HDL-C have been shown to contribute to a decreased risk of cardiovascular disease. These studies suggest that physical inactivity in sedentary people with spinal cord injury can in part explain their lower HDL-C values; this supports the need for and benefit of exercise for individuals with spinal cord injury.

Spasticity. Spasticity tends to increase for the first 2 years following a spinal cord injury and then appears to plateau. Spasticity is an abnormal increase in muscle tone and is velocity dependent—the faster you try to move a spastic extremity through a range of motion, the more resistance you may encounter. Spasticity may originate in loss of control from the injured brain or spinal cord, hypersensitivity of nerve receptors that no longer are being supplied with control after the injury, or growth of new nerve pathways. Spasticity can be mild, moderate, or severe, and it may interfere with range of motion (ROM), transfers, and proper positioning.

Spasticity may be controlled through proper use of medication and daily range-of-motion exercise to maintain optimum flexibility. Stretching twice a day remains the cornerstone of spasticity control. During exercise, spasticity may be controlled through proper positioning and assistive strapping. In some cases, extensor tone can be used to help with transfers and weight-bearing activities.

Osteoporosis. Bone demineralization or decrease in skeletal mass is another result of an inactive lifestyle. Growth and resorption of bone, particularly in the lower extremities, are balanced by activity and weight bearing through the long axis of the bones, so immobilization from recumbency, paralysis, or periods without weight bearing leads to decreased bone mass. Initially following paralysis the entire skeleton suffers mineral loss, and eventually localized **osteoporosis** can be found in the immobilized extremities. Researchers suggest that the combination of voluntary muscle contraction with

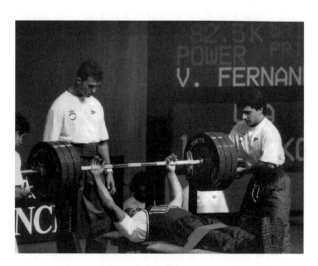

A strap below the hips or knees assists a lifter to stabilize the spastic lower extremities when lifting heavy loads with the upper extremities.

weight bearing through the long axis of bones can effectively prevent and possibly reverse osteoporosis. Further, volitional contractions contribute to a positive balance in bone maintenance, whereas spasticity has no such effect. Weight bearing alone is not sufficient to prevent or retard osteoporosis in paralysis, but active weight-bearing activities or exercise, such as walking with braces, can possibly contribute to the prevention of osteoporosis.

Bowel and Bladder Function. Because the sacral level of the spinal cord controls the bladder and bowels, most people with spinal cord injuries do not have control of these organs. Instead, they may use indwelling **catheters**, intermittent catheterization, or external catheters to empty the bladder. A fluid schedule can provide a consistent, regulated delivery of fluid to the kidneys and prevent excessive buildup. A consistent pattern of emptying is also important in bowel care, often promoted with stool softeners, a high-fiber diet, and suppositories.

Persons with spinal cord injuries are at higher risk for urinary tract and kidney infections. If signs of infection, such as a flushed face or elevated temperature, are noticed, stop exercise and arrange for a medical evaluation. It is always a good habit to empty a leg bag before exercise as a precaution against overdistending the bladder with a full leg bag that can reverse the flow of the urine.

Good skin care is important. This includes keeping the skin dry and relieving pressure frequently. If urine spills, the area involved needs to be changed or dried. If incontinence is a problem, keep a change of clothes available.

Contractures and Decreased Range of Motion. As with other persons with disabilities who require a wheelchair, you must be aware of the possibility of developing **contractures** (shortening of muscles and other connective tissue). Extended time spent sitting combined with significant spasticity can cause the hip, knee, and ankle flexors to become too tight, leading to difficulty with transfers, dressing, and basic hygiene. The anterior shoulder is another area prone to muscle tightness because of poor posture while sitting or excessive wheelchair pushing. Contractures can be prevented with regular, sustained stretching or range of motion exercise and proper positioning of the trunk, arms, and legs. Lying on the stomach can stretch out the trunk, hip, and knee flexors, and appropriate back support in the wheelchair can facilitate proper posture. Adjust or replace stretched-out wheelchair upholstery.

Depending on the severity of the contracture and how long it has existed, surgical intervention may be needed; joint capsules may need to be released or tendons may need to be lengthened. Be aware that muscle contractures left unmanaged can eventually lead to changes around the involved joint including joint fusion or **ankylosis** at their most severe.

Heterotopic Ossification (HO). HO, the excessive laying down of bone in soft tissues around joints, has also been referred to as *ectopic* or *hypertrophic bone.* HO can cause a problem when it limits available range of motion (ROM). The cause is unknown, but it usually occurs in people who have had neurological injury or trauma, including complete spinal cord injuries, myelo-**meningocele**, poliomyelitis, multiple sclerosis, stroke, and head injury. Current theories of its cause include decreased oxygen to the tissue from poor circulation, the presence of abnormal calcium metabolism, the presence of **pressure sores**, and trauma from excessive, aggressive passive range of motion exercises or repeated force generated by muscle spasticity. In spinal cord injuries HO appears most frequently near the hip joints of males, unilaterally or bilaterally; however, it can also be found commonly below the shoulder or near the elbow and knee joints. With spinal cord injury, HO is always found below the level of the spinal cord injury. The suggested treatment is proper medication and consistent gentle stretching exercises to maintain ROM.

Ectopic bone formation, if not managed properly, can progress to involve joint fusion, again, most often in the hip joint. In this case, pressure sores often develop as a secondary complication due to the excess bone formation that makes proper positioning difficult or to a new bony protrusion in a weight-bearing area, for example in the buttocks behind the hip. If HO is present, aggressive ROM exercise is contraindicated due to the possibility of muscular tears. Consult a physician regarding precautions. Surgery may be indicated if an ankylosed joint causes severe limitations in activities of daily living and transfers. Surgery could remove the mature bone formation to restore functional ROM at the joint.

Pressure Sores. Breakdown of skin and other connective tissues from continuous sitting or lying are a potentially fatal complication that can be avoided. Pressure sores are most often seen in conditions such as quadriplegia because of decreased sensation and limited movement. This is why care must be taken to avoid skin trauma when transferring in and out of the wheelchair and it is essential to perform pressure reliefs to reduce pressure on the sitting surface. One of the following pressure reliefs can be used according to mobility level: wheelchair push-ups, shifting weight in the wheelchair by leaning forward or sideways, having someone assist by tipping the wheelchair back, or using a motorized recliner wheelchair. One of these techniques should be performed every 15 to 20 min to allow for blood circulation needed to nourish the skin and other tissues. Participation in wheelchair sports and fitness programs can also decrease the incidence of pressure sores. Pressure sores can be life threatening and often may require surgical repair. An admission to the hospital for a pressure sore can cost up to $30,000.

Autonomic Hyperreflexia. **Autonomic hyperreflexia** or **dysreflexia** is an exaggerated autonomic response to irritating stimuli to the skin and viscera below the level of the spinal cord damage that occurs with a complete or incomplete spinal cord lesion above T6. It is most often caused by a distended bladder (possibly from kinked catheter tubing) or a distended rectum. The symptoms are a pounding headache, high blood pressure, flushed skin, and sweating above the level of the spinal cord injury due to parasympathetic vasodilation. In addition, sympathetic vasoconstriction causes paleness, clamminess, and coolness below the level of the injury. Nasal obstruction and a slow pulse are common features due to overriding parasympathetic response. All symptoms are aggravated by lying flat, which tends to increase blood pressure. These symptoms signal a medical emergency. Failure to respond immediately can result in elevated blood pressure high enough to potentially produce a stroke.

You should respond in the following manner:

1. Immediately sit straight up and elevate your head to create postural hypotension, which is a decrease in blood pressure.
2. Identify and remove the irritating stimulus:
   - Check the catheter and tubing for plugging or kinking.
   - Empty the leg bag if it is full—a leg bag should never be left completely full.

- Check for bladder and lower bowel distension.
- Check for tight clothing or an abdominal binder, leg bag strap, brace, or shoe that is too tight.

3. If symptoms persist, get immediate medical attention.

Thrombophlebitis. Thrombophlebitis or **deep vein thrombosis (DVT)** is a swollen area of a vein due to a clot that has formed inside it; this clot frequently obstructs blood flow. This may often occur in the calves and thighs following a spinal cord injury and resulting inactivity in the presence of one of the following conditions: absence of pumping action in the leg musculature, trauma, or increased age with decreased activity level over time. The symptoms may be a painful, swollen, warm calf or thigh. People who have no sensation will not feel pain, and the clinical exam is often inaccurate, so people at risk must check closely for symptoms on a regular basis.

Treatment of thrombophlebitis consists of blood anticoagulant therapy and no range of motion in the affected area for about a week to prevent the blood clot from dislodging and causing further complications, such as a **pulmonary embolism**. During this time care should also be taken not to put pressure or place straps over the involved area. Exercise can be performed with the uninvolved extremities, but the affected extremity must remain immobilized until cleared by the doctor.

Anticoagulant medication is generally used for up to 3 to 6 months after a spinal cord injury along with pressure-gradient elastic stockings, passive range-of-motion exercise, and early mobilization, to prevent a DVT.

Tenodesis. **Tenodesis** allows people who don't have use of the hand muscles for a functional grasp (as in Class 1A, B, and C) to passively pull the fingers into flexion by extending the wrist. These individuals must *never* stretch the finger flexor muscles in this position or they will take away the grasp that they have. To range the fingers properly, work on moving them into flexion with the wrist extended or work on moving them into extension with the wrist flexed.

Exercise Readiness Assessment

Before setting up your exercise program, assess the following areas:

- Functional range of motion
- Strength
- Balance and trunk stability
- Muscle tone
- Tolerance to aerobic activity

Look at functional range of motion to identify which muscles or muscle groups need stretching. Tight muscles influence your posture, and proper posture is a must for correct exercise technique. Go through the functional range of motion tests in chapter 1 to see what limitations you have. Then look at chapter 4 to see which stretches can help you with your "tight spots." You might need assistance for some stretches, so find an exercise partner and make stretching part of your warm-up and cool-down.

Knowing the level of your spinal cord injury and whether it is complete or incomplete will help determine which muscles need strengthening and the type of exercises and adaptive equipment you should use. For example, if

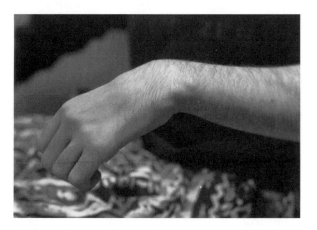 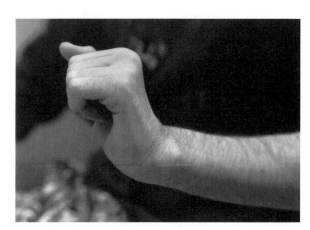

Tenodesis grip: The tight finger flexors are passively pulled into flexion by extending the wrist.

muscles cannot actively move through their full range of motion against gravity you may require gravity-reduced exercise, a supporting table, or an exercise partner. If you have quadriplegia, you should assess your triceps strength—weak or absent triceps may require elbow bracing to work on shoulder musculature. With strong triceps, you should be able to perform all shoulder and arm exercises with the use of exercise machines, pulleys with wrist cuffs, wraparound weights, and the like. Remember that periodically reevaluating your strength can help you evaluate your exercise performance and program effectiveness.

The amount of trunk balance that you have determines which exercise options will be most appropriate for strengthening and aerobic activity (free weights vs. machines, and so on). Evaluating your trunk balance will also help you determine if you need external support, such as binders and straps, to stabilize the trunk with exercise. If you do not have working abdominal musculature, you usually will require support or assistance to stabilize the upper trunk during overhead activity such as the shoulder press. Spasticity, or an increase in muscle tone, can occur with exertion or exercise, most often in the lower extremities, and may require strapping. If extensor tone causes the legs to kick out, strapping below the knees while sitting can help you maintain the proper position for exercise. On the bench, strapping below the hips, knees, or both can assist with controlling the lower extremities.

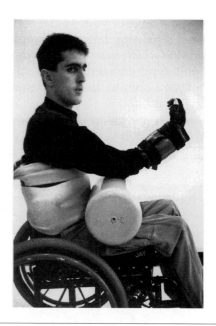

Nonelastic and elastic straps and binders can help maintain trunk balance with exercise.

Before initiating long-duration continuous aerobic activity such as the arm crank, check for a history of orthostatic hypotension, which is a decreased tolerance to the upright position. Everyone with quadriplegia should perform a 1- to 2-min exercise trial on the wheelchair rollers or arm crank before beginning aerobic activity. If you become light-headed or dizzy, stop the activity immediately. If dizziness does not soon resolve, recline or get assistance to recline in your chair. Some people may have to build up a tolerance to continuous activity by starting with short periods of exercise, then increasing the time as tolerated. You also may need to start exercise in the reclined position. If you have a history of orthostatic hypotension at rest, long-duration continuous activities may not be appropriate for you. Individuals with paraplegia generally do not experience exercise hypotension.

Exercise Modifications and Training Considerations

Depending on the level of spinal cord injury and the trunk musculature that remains, varying degrees of assistance are needed for sitting balance with exercise. The most common assistive device is a binder, with or without elasticity, that you can wrap around you and your chair. If you do not have adequate trunk balance in your wheelchair, you may need a rigid, nonelastic binder with no "give" so you can perform resisted arm exercise without the risk of falling forward or to the side. If you have limited trunk musculature and you want to challenge the strength of these muscles, you can use an elastic abdominal binder that is tight enough so there is some "give" but no risk of falling forward or to the side. The elastic binder is preferred because when you use it at the abdomen just above the hips it can support in the same way as the abdominal muscles, which helps those with absent or weak abdominal musculature. Binders or strapping can also be used below the waist during the bench press to aid in trunk stability and balance or to help control lower extremity spasticity.

You can maintain your balance by hooking one arm around your wheelchair push handle to stabilize your trunk so you can perform an exercise with your free arm. This technique is commonly used when performing biceps curls or triceps overhead extensions with free weights or sand bags. You may also brace one arm locked in extension against the wheelchair tire to help sta-

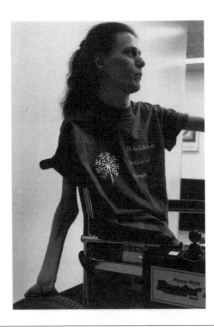

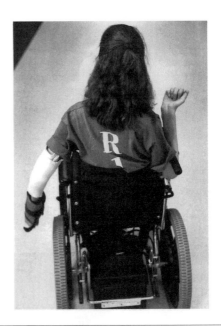

You can stabilize your balance by using the tire unit or push handle of your wheelchair.

bilize your trunk for exercise with the opposite arm.

Exercises on your stomach can be modified to be performed in the wheelchair by placing a pillow in the abdominal area for support and then leaning forward into the pillow. If you are in Class 1A (with an injury at C4-6), 1B (C7), and occasionally Class 1C (C8), you may prefer to stay in your wheelchair for exercises on the stomach if transferring out is difficult or time consuming. Don't use the forward position in the chair, however, if you have difficulty breathing in this position or if you have stabilization rods in your spine from spinal surgery; the rods are placed to stabilize the spine and you have to

be careful when bending or rotating it. You should not force movements.

When a muscle or muscle group attempts to compensate for a lack of movement in a weak or paralyzed muscle, it produces a substitution movement. Substitutions for paralyzed muscles are helpful because they can assist with functional activity that would be impossible otherwise. Tenodesis and elbow locking are two examples. In **tenodesis**, an active hand grasp with the fingers is absent, and the action of the wrist extensors is used to produce passive finger flexion through the tension placed on the tight finger flexors. Tenodesis does not allow for a complete grasp, but it does give more control to the wrist and hand so eating and writing are possible with adaptive equipment. Elbow locking is used when triceps are absent; it uses the external rotators of the shoulder (supraspinatus, infraspinatus, teres minor) to place the arm in a position where gravity will straighten the elbow. Locking the bones of the elbow joint then keeps the elbow extended. In a weight-bearing position you can use elbow locking to assist with sitting balance or transfers. A similar movement is to use the anterior deltoid of the shoulder in the weight-bearing or closed-chain position to move the upper arm forward by using shoulder flexion when the triceps is absent.

During exercise, substitutions must be eliminated if they are compensating for lack of movement in a weak muscle. If you permit substitutions, the weak muscle will not improve in strength and muscle imbalances will remain unresolved.

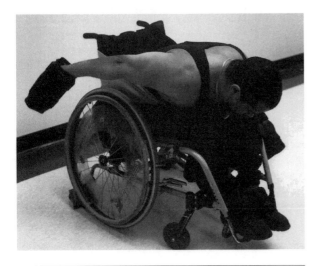

Exercises on the stomach can be modified and performed in your wheelchair.

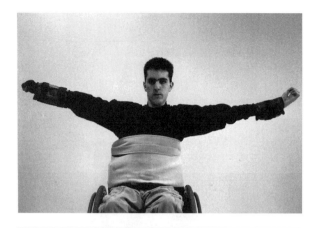

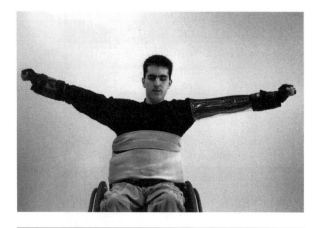

The left arm is externally rotated substituting the biceps, clavicular pectoralis, and anterior deltoid for the middle deltoid during a lateral raise.

The left arm is in a neutral position with an air splint to maintain elbow extension and correctly perform a lateral raise.

A common example involves weakness of the triceps when performing a lateral shoulder raise aimed at strengthening the middle deltoid. The external rotators of the shoulder rotate the arm so that the palm is facing up, passively locking the elbow in extension. In this position, weak triceps have caused the biceps, clavicular portion of the pectoralis, and anterior deltoid to substitute for the middle deltoid in laterally raising the arm out to the side. To prevent substitution, you must use proper technique (see p. 180). Exercising in front of a mirror can provide helpful feedback, but you may need an elbow splint to perform the exercise correctly.

With a spinal cord injury, you must maximize the strength of the existing functional musculature without causing overwork injuries. Using a variety of exercises, which prevents overuse injuries and promotes muscular balance, is beneficial. For example, to prevent overuse injuries

such as a painful shoulder from biceps tendonitis, which is common with weak or absent triceps, you should concentrate on strengthening the shoulder girdle and scapular muscle instead of overworking the biceps. Make sure the scapular muscles are strong before you perform overhead activity or you will run into shoulder impingement and rotator cuff injuries.

Splinting with upper extremity exercise can help you perform a wider variety of isolated shoulder movements. For example, if you have weak or absent triceps and are not able to keep the elbow extended, the elbow can be splinted with an air cast or solid Velcro splint to allow for correct technique and to reduce the possibility of substitution when trying to focus on shoulder, chest, and back exercises. If you have weak or absent wrist flexion and extension, the wrist can be supported during the exercise with a custom-made hand splint or a strap-on weight.

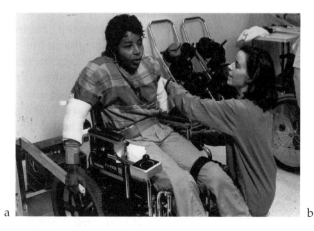

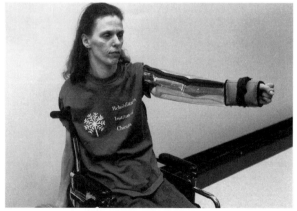

a b

(a) Elbow splints and (b) air casts maintain the elbow in extension, allowing access to more shoulder, chest, and back exercises.

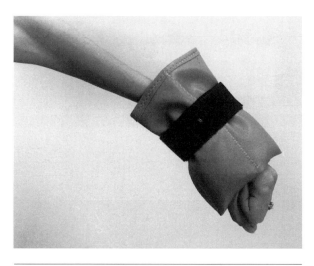

The wraparound weight over the wrist joint supports and protects the joint during arm exercise.

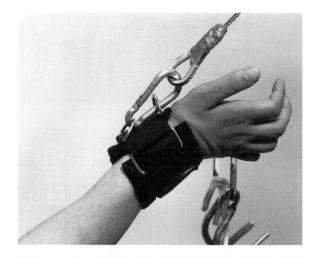

The use of wrist cuffs allows people with quadriplegia to access pulley exercise systems.

To make exercise machines and upper body ergometers accessible if you do not have full hand function, some adaptations are necessary. The exercise machine's lat pull-down bar and pulley system must have accessible hooks for a wrist cuff, which is placed around the wrist to substitute for absent hand function. Be very careful to put wrist cuffs on properly so the line of pull of the exercise does not cause wrist hyperextension. For the upper body ergometer, you can use adaptive gloves with Velcro fasteners or adaptive handles. Due to varying hand size and function, however, we have found that an ace wrap is often the best way to keep the hand secure on a handle.

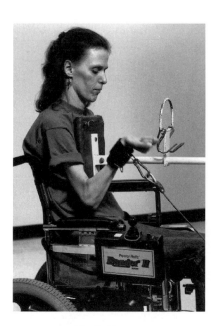

Exercising with the wrist cuff.

Response to Exercise

As previously mentioned, physiological responses to exercise and exercise testing with spinal cord injury depend on the amount of active muscle mass engaged in exercise and the degree of sympathetic nervous system dysfunction. Researchers have recently studied cardiovascular responses to exercise with spinal cord injury extensively, specifically

- voluntary arm cranking ergometry (ACE),
- wheelchair ergometry (WERG),
- functional electrical stimulation leg cycle ergometry (FES-LCE), and
- combined arm crank with E-stim leg cycle ergometry (hybrid).

It is beyond the scope of this manual to outline the results of these studies because they most often relate to research and the exercise testing lab setting. Although it is important to be aware of the forms of exercise being studied, our focus is on what you are actually able to perform in your exercise facility.

In quadriplegia (C5 to T1) and paraplegia, you can exercise on both the ACE and WERG. In the clinic or gym, that means using an upper body ergometer and a stationary wheelchair roller. Remember from chapter 3 that arm cranking ergometry is more mechanically efficient than stationary wheelchair rolling—it will often allow you to achieve a higher training heart rate before muscle fatigue sets in.

Functional electrical stimulation leg cycle ergometry is used in some hospital or rehabilitation

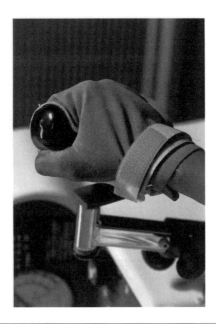 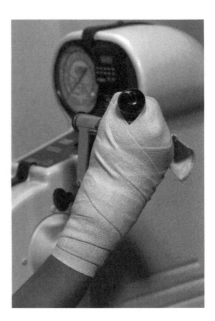

Commercial Velcro gloves or an ace wrap allows people with quadriplegia to access aerobic exercise equipment.

settings as well as in exercise testing labs. Electrodes are placed on the large paralyzed muscle groups of the legs (quadriceps, hamstrings, gluteal muscle groups) to stimulate them to propel an exercise bike. FES-LCE has been found to be more effective than ACE and WERG in increasing the volume load for the heart in quadriplegia and paraplegia, probably because larger muscle groups are used and the muscle pump of the legs is partially reactivated. The benefit of FES-LCE over arm cranking ergometry for central cardiovascular training is this cardiac loading and a longer duration than arm cranking, where fatigue sets in sooner. Some studies have found that this type of aerobic training may produce central cardiovascular fitness in conditions of quadriplegia and paraplegia.

Some studies have shown that only individuals with paraplegia who have an injury at T6 and below are able to efficiently train aerobically and achieve central training effects. Central cardiovascular training produces an increased capacity to circulate blood and to obtain a lower resting heart rate; in other words, the heart becomes a more efficient pump. These benefits cannot be achieved without exercising for a prolonged period in your target heart rate range. This central effect is most likely produced by exercise on the hybrid system, which involves using the large muscle mass of the legs plus the arms to create an adequate volume load for the heart. The hybrid system is a combined arm crank ergometer and electrical stimulation to the large muscle groups of the legs so the latter are also active in a recipro-

cal, aerobic exercise. This is an expensive and time-consuming set-up that has been used mostly in the laboratory setting for aerobic testing. This method allows the individual with paraplegia to achieve target heart rates at an aerobic level that produces central training effects.

With a complete spinal cord injury above T6, you may not be able to achieve central cardiovascular training because sympathetic nervous system dysfunction and limited active muscle mass prevent you from reaching target heart rates and from stressing the central circulation. In people with quadriplegia, hybrid exercise may cause difficulty or may not be tolerated because ACE and FES-LCE may interfere with each other at the higher output levels needed to raise your already restricted heart rate. However, training at an elevated heart rate during continuous aerobic exercise such as upper arm ergometry or long-distance wheelchair racing may increase aerobic capacity ($\dot{V}O_2$max). Besides increasing aerobic capacity with endurance exercise, you may also benefit from the peripheral effects, including increased exercise tolerance, improved muscle endurance, increased "good cholesterol" (HDL-C), decreased risk of cardiovascular disease, increased lean body mass, and decreased fat.

Spinal Cord Exercise Precautions

• With an injury to the spine, be aware of restrictions because of surgically placed rods or spinal fusions. In these cases, forced flexion and rotation of the spine with exercise are contraindicated.

- To preserve tenodesis in the hand, do not stretch out finger flexors.
- In conditions of quadriplegia with limited hand function, be careful not to hyperextend the wrist with strap-on weights or adaptive wrist cuffs.
- If you have heterotopic ossification, a contracture, or osteoporosis in an extremity, understand your medical restrictions for stretching and strengthening exercises.
- If you have thrombophlebitis or deep vein thrombosis in an extremity, exercise with the uninvolved extremities, but keep the affected extremity immobilized until cleared by your doctor. Take care not to put pressure on or place straps over the involved area.
- When strapping for positioning or to control lower extremity spasticity, use padded straps at least 2 in. wide. Be sure to observe your skin for any reddened areas and identify areas prone to skin breakdown. Be aware of skin color changes, swelling, or decreased sensation in a strapped extremity; this could indicate that the strap is placed over a blood vessel or nerve.
- Exercise hypotension is exhibited by a drop in blood pressure, which may cause you to feel faint or even pass out. Get assistance to recline in your chair or lie on your back to relieve symptoms by elevating your blood pressure.
- Empty your leg bag before exercise to avoid overdistending the bladder as you drink water with exercise.

Your Next Move

Now that you have all of the background information, turn to page 106 of this chapter to find your appropriate classification. With this classification, you can identify your training program.

Spina Bifida

Spina bifida is a congenital spinal cord injury that occurs while the embryo is developing in the uterus during the first trimester of pregnancy and is present at birth. Spina bifida is a defect in the spinal column caused by the failure of one or more of the posterior vertebral arches or more simply, the back part of the vertebrae, to close appropriately before birth. The cause of spina bifida is unknown, but there is some evidence that environmental factors, combined with genetic predisposition, may trigger the development of spina bifida; however, this evidence is not conclusive.

The more common and severe form of the defect is called **myelomeningocele** (*myelo* denoting relationship to the spinal cord, *meningo* referring to the membranous covering of the brain and spinal cord or meninges, and *cele* denoting a tumor or swelling). When the parts of the word are put together they describe what occurs: The spinal cord and its membranes protrude through a defect in the vertebrae in the form of a tumor that is called a sac. Within the sac, abnormal growth of the spinal cord makes normal connections of nerve pathways impossible. The result is sensory and muscular impairment at the level of the sac and below similar to a spinal cord injury.

Myelomeningoceles are most common in the lower thoracic, lumbar, or sacral areas of the spine. Individuals with myelomeningocele are the ones that most often require rehabilitation. Thus the terms *spina bifida* and *myelomeningocele* (MM) are often used interchangeably.

Many children with MM have other complications, and it is important to keep in mind the total effect of spina bifida on the growing child. After adolescence, the rehabilitation of an individual with spina bifida can be handled similarly to the rehabilitation of an adult with a spinal cord injury.

Associated Conditions

Orthopedic Deformities of the Spine. Besides the malformation of the vertebrae at the site of the spinal cord damage, deformities of other vertebral bodies or the ribs attached to the thoracic vertebral bodies may also be present. These deformities of the vertebrae and associated ribs can lead to three different types of abnormal spine curvatures.

Most commonly, a thoracic kyphosis may be present as a result of the original deformity and subsequent absent trunk musculature to hold the spine properly. A *kyphosis* is an abnormally increased convexity in the curvature of the spine as viewed from the side (i.e., hunchback). Similar to a spinal cord injury with absent trunk musculature, a kyphosis can become worse in someone with spina bifida because of the increased weight of the trunk when sitting.

With a large spinal defect and hip flexor tightness a lordosis or lordosoliosis is often seen in the adolescent. A **lordosis** refers to an abnormally increased curvature of the lumbar spine as viewed from the side (i.e., swayback). A scoliosis may be present at birth because of vertebral abnormalities, or it may become evident as the child grows older if he or she does not have the proper trunk musculature to hold the spine in correct alignment. **Scoliosis** is a large lateral deviation in the normally straight vertical line of the spine as it is viewed from the back. This lateral deviation is accompanied by rib cage rotation because the ribs attach to the vertebrae.

These abnormal curvatures of the spine often exist at birth and progress with the effects of gravity as a child grows; however, the subsequent trunk and postural deformities can sometimes be prevented or minimized. Proper positioning in and out of the wheelchair, with assistive supports as needed, is often helpful. Attention to good body alignment, especially with the spine, can also help minimize postural deformities. Often bracing or an **orthosis** is needed to help with proper spinal support. Proper stretching of tight musculature and strengthening of weak musculature can help minimize muscular imbalances.

Orthopedic Deformities of the Hips and Feet. The type and extent of a deformity in the lower extremities will depend upon what musculature is available. With total flaccid paralysis, deformities may be present at birth from the result of passive positioning in the uterus. Common deformities are hip flexion with hip adduction and internal rotation, which leads to subluxed or dislocated hips. With lower level damage to the spinal cord (L2, L3, L4), a hip abductor brace may be worn for a few months after birth to prevent hip dislocation. But with higher level damage to the spinal cord (T1 to T12), dislocated hips are not treated because they often have no effect on later rehabilitation efforts.

Foot deformities also occur, and casting or taping can correct the position of the foot as the child grows. Short leg braces or splints may be used to maintain and prevent foot deformities once the individual has grown.

Hydrocephalus. **Hydrocephalus** develops in 80% to 90% of children who have myelo-

meningocele. Again the word itself describes what hydrocephalus is: *hydro* refers to the accumulation of fluid in a body part, and *cephalus* refers to the head. Hence hydrocephalus is an increased amount of cerebrospinal fluid in the **ventricles** of the brain. It results from some type of blockage in the flow of **cerebrospinal fluid (CSF)** between the ventricles of the brain and the spinal canal that surrounds the spinal cord. Cerebrospinal fluid is a clear fluid that surrounds the brain and spinal cord and acts as a protective shock absorber. The most obvious effect of the increased CSF in the brain's ventricles is increased head size. Unless this buildup of CSF is reduced, brain damage and death may result because the skull can tolerate only minimal increases in brain mass before irreversible compression of the tissues results in permanent damage.

After an individual has been diagnosed as having hydrocephalus, a surgically placed ventricular **shunt** is indicated. This procedure involves diverting (shunting) the excess CSF away from the ventricles of the brain to some other site for reabsorption, most often the abdominal cavity. Hydrocephalus can usually be reduced or it improves on its own. Some individuals have shunt complications that occur frequently and require revisions for obstructions, infections, or both.

Hydrocephalus may cause some brain damage, and those with hydrocephalus, particularly those requiring shunts, are likely to have below-average intelligence or learning disabilities. Although some individuals may show normal intelligence, their learning process may be impaired by lack of physical mobility, lack of proprioception (a sense of where the body or the extremities are positioned), attention disorders, visual-motor perceptual deficits (inability to coordinate eye and hand movements), and auditory-language problems.

Due to the similarities in the nature of spina bifida and spinal cord injury, the associated conditions, exercise readiness assessment, exercise modifications, response to exercise, and precautions apply to both . Refer to pages 92 to 103 for this information prior to proceeding to the classification section of this chapter.

Poliomyelitis

Poliomyelitis (polio) is caused by a virus that enters into the stomach and intestines and is then absorbed into the bloodstream. This virus travels in the bloodstream and can affect parts of the brain or the motor neurons (anterior horn cells) that are located in the front part of the spinal cord. Polio may produce permanent paralysis, and until the late 1950s polio was the leading cause of disability for children in the United States. In the late 1950s and early 1960s the Salk and Sabin vaccines were developed and polio became an almost completely preventable disease.

In the United States, new cases of polio are no longer common, but there are people with polio paralysis and postpolio syndrome. Postpolio syndrome or progressive polio develops on average 30 to 40 years after the initial onset of polio. Postpolio may or may not be related to the original disease. It has a different physical presentation than acute polio and is covered under the Les Autres sports classification. (See chapter 8 for complete information on postpolio syndrome.) Polio is classified under the National Wheelchair Athletic Association (NWAA) system because the resultant muscle paralysis is similar to the effects of spinal cord injury and spina bifida.

Poliomyelitis may have no symptoms, be nonparalytic (causing no paralysis) but with symptoms, or be paralytic (causing paralysis) with symptoms. The symptoms at onset usually include headache, malaise, generalized muscular aches, and nonspecific systemic symptoms common to many viral infections. The virus attacks motor neurons in the anterior part of the spinal cord and may destroy them, which causes a permanent muscle weakness and paralysis of the muscles that the neurons supply. The infection can also produce a temporary inflammatory swelling in the anterior horn cell (where the motor neurons are), which may cause reversible neuron damage and temporary paralysis. Unlike spinal cord injury and spina bifida, sensation is not affected because the virus attacks only motor neurons.

During the acute phase of paralytic poliomyelitis, flaccid paralysis develops in those muscles supplied by the damaged motor neurons. The extent of the paralysis can range from weakness of one muscle, to weakness in one muscle group, to complete paralysis of the muscles for all four extremities and the trunk. If the polio virus affects the **brain stem**, the muscles that supply breathing become paralyzed and mechanical respiration is necessary. However, the virus tends to affect the lower extremities more often than the upper extremities or the trunk.

Gradual recovery of any temporary paralysis takes place during the recovery phase, which can last up to 2 or 3 years. Usually most of the recovery occurs within the first 6 months, and approximately half of the affected individuals will make a complete recovery during this phase. The last phase, residual paralysis, continues for life and no further recovery of motor function is expected. Approximately half of individuals with remaining paralysis have moderate involvement, but the remainder have extensive paralysis. No form of treatment is able to affect the extent of the paralysis or the degree to which an individual recovers.

Associated Conditions

Polio is very similar to spinal cord injury and spina bifida in that the same associated conditions that apply to trunk and extremity muscle paralysis and resultant atrophy exist, at least in people with paralytic polio who have sedentary lifestyles. However, polio differs in that paralysis is typically patchy and **asymmetrical**. Please refer to the spinal cord section of this chapter for detailed information on body composition, heterotopic ossification, osteoporosis, contractures and decreased ROM, and thrombophlebitis.

Unlike spinal cord injury and spina bifida, polio does not damage the entire spinal cord at a certain neurological level. The polio virus attacks motor neurons that are located outside the spinal column and leaves sensation and the sympathetic nervous system intact. So whereas the muscle paralysis may be similar in spinal cord injury, spina bifida, and polio, with polio the associated conditions relating to the absence of sympathetic or central (brain and spinal cord) nervous system control do not exist. Polio does not cause problems with thermoregulation, autonomic hyperreflexia, spasticity, or exercise hypotension.

Polio, however, has a variety of associated conditions depending on how much paralysis exists. The causes of these associated conditions include muscle atrophy, muscle imbalance, and muscle contracture. With the severe paralytic form of polio, 2.5% of children and 15% to 30% of adults die. So those in rehabilitation often have a less extensive paralytic form of polio. If polio has developed during childhood, it can slow bone growth in the involved extremity.

Leg Length Discrepancy. When polio affects just one of the lower extremities it often causes a leg length discrepancy—the affected leg is shorter. External shoe lifts are commonly used on the involved polio leg. In extreme cases leg length equalization surgery can be performed.

Orthopedic Deformities. Depending on the extent and distribution of the paralysis, several orthopedic conditions can exist. Similar to spina bifida, if polio develops at an early age during childhood, the lack of active movement and muscular support fosters abnormal growth of bones and possible deformities. For example, extensive paralysis of one upper extremity and part of the thoracic trunk can lead to a thoracic kyphosis (i.e., hunchback). Paralysis of the trunk can lead to scoliosis, or an abnormal curvature of the spine. If one lower extremity is involved, paralytic subluxation of the involved hip or deformities at the knee or ankle may exist.

These conditions should be treated on a preventive basis, using active exercises to strengthen recovering muscles, stretching exercises to maintain available range of motion in affected joints, and proper bracing to stabilize a weak trunk or extremity. For some, the remaining paralysis in the lower extremity is so extensive that permanent bracing is required to provide stability for standing or walking.

Role of Exercise

Before setting up your exercise program, you need to assess your functional range of motion, strength, balance, and trunk stability. This part of the exercise readiness assessment as well as exercise modifications and training considerations are similar to those for spinal cord injury. Please refer to pages 92 to 103 for this background information.

Poliomyelitis produces selective damage to the anterior horn cells of the spinal cord, leaving the sympathetic nervous system unaffected. Individuals with polio consequently are able to achieve higher exercise heart rates than the spinal cord–injured population. Spinal cord injury above the T6 level involves dysfunction of the sympathetic nervous system, which is partly responsible for elevating heart rate during exercise. That is not the case for people with polio. Therefore, someone with polio is limited only by the extent of paralysis when it comes to aerobic exercise.

Poliomyelitis Exercise Precautions

- Properly protect the joints during all exercise. Know if you should wear your braces or orthoses during strengthening exercises.
- Pace your activity because your body is still recovering 2 to 3 years after your diagnosis. Intersperse activity and exercise with rest. Intermittent strength training and aerobic training are best to avoid overfatigue.
- To preserve hand function in a weak arm, be careful not to hyperextend your wrist with strap-on weights or adaptive wrist cuffs.
- If you have a contracture or osteoporosis in an extremity, know your medical restrictions for stretching and strengthening exercises.

Your Next Move

Now that you have all of the background information, find your appropriate classification so you can identify your training program.

Classification and Exercise Guidelines

It is time to identify your classification and locate the corresponding exercise program. The National Wheelchair Athletic Association (NWAA) uses the classification system to help determine your level of muscle function and allow for equality in competition. In this manual, we will use the national classification system to clearly present your physical capabilities for field event competition, which is most similar to the strength training you will be doing in your exercise program.

The NWAA classification system groups people with spinal cord injuries into seven different classes based on the level of injury. This neurological level influences the strength of remaining extremity and trunk muscles, which in turn influence sitting balance. The classes are labeled 1A, 1B, 1C, 2, 3, 4, and 5 (see Table 6.1). The lower the class number, the higher the spinal cord damage. The progression of functional strength and trunk stability is from the least functional, class 1A, to the most functional, class 5. Because the system is anatomically based, classes 1A, 1B, and 1C represent the quadriplegic classes in which damage occurs in the cervical or high thoracic area of the spinal cord. Classes 2, 3, and 4 include paraplegic classes in which damage occurs in the thoracic area (class 2 and class 3) or the lumbar area of the spinal cord (class 4). Class 5 includes the paraplegic class with damage to the low lumbar or sacral area of the spinal cord, including those who have enough power to ambulate with assistive devices (the majority of whom are disabled by polio).

To use the following exercise programs and the exercise index, you need to determine the class that is appropriate for you. Tables 6.2 and 6.3 will help you select the profile that best fits you. Once you have found the appropriate class, photocopied the following training log, identified your training program, and made the necessary modifications to it, you will learn about the specific exercises you will perform during your workout. Part III provides explanations and photographs of these exercises.

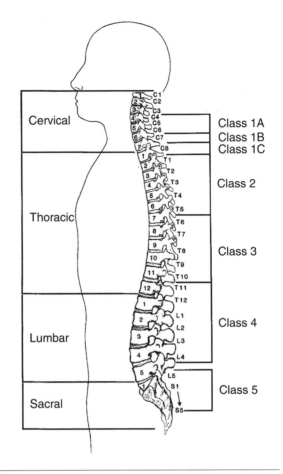

The NWAA classification system is based on the level of your injury.

Table 6.1		
NWAA Classifications and Muscle Movements		
Class	**Neurological level**	**Key available muscles/movements**
1A	C4-6 (cervical spine)	Diaphragm; Trapezius, levator scapulae; Rhomboids, serratus anterior; Rotator cuff; Deltoid, biceps; Pectoralis major; Latissimus dorsi; Supinator, pronator; Wrist extension (partial to complete)
1B	C7	Triceps (partial to complete); Wrist flexion (partial); Finger and thumb extension
1C	C8	Triceps (complete); Finger and thumb flexion; Finger abduction/adduction
2	T1-5 (thoracic spine)	Intrinsic hand function; Upper back extensors
3	T6-10	Upper abdominals; Middle back extensors; Trunk rotation (partial)
4	T11-L4 (low thoracic and upper lumbar spine)	Abdominals (complete); Trunk rotation (complete); Quadratus lumborum (hip hiker); Iliopsoas (hip flexion); Hip adduction; Quadriceps (knee extension); Ankle dorsiflexion (may be partial)
5	L5-S5 (low lumbar and sacral spine)	Gluteus maximus (hip extension); Gluteus medius (hip abduction); Hamstrings (knee flexion); Ankle dorsiflexion (heel walking); Ankle plantarflexion (toe walking); Bowel and bladder control

Table 6.2
Description of Neurological Level and Differences Between Classes

Neurological level	Description/class	Primary mode of mobility	Transfers out of wheelchair
C4-C6	• May have shoulder weakness • May have functional elbow flexion and wrist extension • May have weak elbow extension by using mechanical positioning of arm, but do not have wrist flexion • Require upper extremity support to maintain sitting balance *Class 1A complete injury*	• SCI level C4 will use an electric wheelchair with sip and puff, head, or chin control • SCI level C5 will use an electric wheelchair with an assistive wrist splint for hand control • Have the potential to propel a manual wheelchair with oblique projections on level indoor surfaces • SCI level C6 can propel a manual wheelchair on level surfaces, with vertical projections or with rubber coated hand rims and wheelchair gloves to assist with grip control for pushing	• SCI level C4 will be a dependent transfer, the type of dependent transfer determined by the size of the individual and the assistance available: one-man pivot, two-man lift, lateral sliding board with one person, or a hoyer lift • SCI level C5 most often is a dependent one-man pivot or lateral sliding board with one person to assist • SCI level C6 will use a lateral sliding board with assist or may be able to transfer independently with a prone push-off transfer using a sliding board
C7	• Has good shoulder muscle function • Has functional elbow and wrist flexion/extension • May have some finger flexion/extension movement, but it is not functional *Class 1B complete injury* • Impaired sitting balance *Class 1A incomplete injury* • Ability to lift back off of wheelchair and perform backward and forward movements of the trunk • May be able to rotate trunk	• SCI level C7 will propel a manual wheelchair with some assistance needed for environmental obstacles	• SCI level C7 can perform an independent lateral transfer to all level surfaces, with or without a sliding board
C8	• Has full function at elbow and wrist joints • Has full or almost full function of finger flexion/extension • Has functional, but not normal, intrinsic muscles of the hand	• SCI level C8 will propel a manual wheelchair with some assistance needed for environmental obstacles	• SCI level C8 can perform an independent lateral transfer to all level surfaces, with or without a sliding board

Note. Adapted from National Wheelchair Athletic Association (1990).

	Table 6.3		
	Description of Neurological Level and Differences Between Classes		
Neurological level	**Description/class**	**Primary mode of mobility**	**Transfers out of wheelchair**
T1-5	• Have intrinsic muscles of the hand for complete function of the upper extremities • Have partial function of back extensor muscles *Class 2 complete injury* • Has normal upper extremities but no functional trunk movements *Class 1C incomplete injury* • Has trunk movements and hand function where they are able to make a good fist but spreading and closing the fingers is not with normal function	• Will propel a manual wheelchair on level and uneven surfaces (e.g., wheelies to go up and down curbs) • May begin to stand with long leg braces and upper extremity support	• Will perform an independent lateral transfer without a sliding board
T6-10	• Have normal upper extremity function • Have partial abdominal muscles, trunk rotators and spinal extensors *Class 3*	• Will propel a manual wheelchair on level surfaces • With supervision, can work on ambulation (swing to gait pattern) with long leg braces and forearm crutches on level surfaces	• Will perform an independent lateral pivot transfer
T11-L4	• Have very good balance and movement in the backward and forward plane • Have good trunk rotation • Can lift the thighs (hip flexion) and press the knees together (hip adduction) • May have the ability to straighten the knees (knee extension) and some ability to bend the knees (knee flexion) *Class 4*	• SCI levels T11-L4 will propel a manual wheelchair on level and uneven surfaces for long distances • SCI levels L1-3 can ambulate for short distances, on level surfaces and elevations, using forearm crutches and long leg braces • SCI level L4 can ambulate for short distances, on level surfaces and elevations, using forearm crutches and short leg braces	• Will perform an independent lateral pivot transfer
L5-S5	• Have very good balance and trunk movement forward, backward, and rotational • Usually have very good balance and side-to-side trunk movement secondary to the presence of hip abduction to stabilize the hip backward (hip extension) • Usually can bend one ankle downward (ankle plantarflexion)	• SCI level L5 will ambulate in short leg braces or ankle foot orthotics without an assistive device • SCI levels S1-5 will ambulate without any braces or assistive devices • Lower extremity is intact at level S2, and beyond this level bowel and bladder function may be the only problem	• Often no wheelchair is needed for this class as they are ambulatory • Some individuals may use a wheelchair for long distances; use an independent stand-pivot transfer

Note. Adapted from National Wheelchair Athletic Association (1990).

Conditioning With Spinal Cord Injury, Spina Bifida, and Polio

Notes	Exercises	Sets/reps	Date	Weight

SCI CLASS 1A EXERCISE GUIDELINES
C4-C6 (Cervical Spine)

| POSITION | Most, if not all exercise, will be performed in your wheelchair. If your SCI is at level C6, you may transfer out to do shoulder exercises lying on your back using air casts or elbow splints to keep your elbow locked and help isolate the shoulder muscles. Strap your trunk as needed for each exercise (refer to pp. 26-29). If your SCI is at level C4, you will most often need a stiff trunk support, while those of you at levels C5 and C6 will hook one arm around your wheelchair push handle or use an elastic abdominal support or binder. It is important to keep your shoulders back with exercise so gravity helps place the scapula more appropriately on the chest wall.

| EXERCISE OPTIONS | If your SCI is at level C4, you may use gravity-reduced exercises that allow you to exercise weak muscles on a supporting surface such as a table or with an exercise partner. If your SCI is at level C4, you must be extremely cautious about overtraining and overusing your limited musculature. Your main concern will be respiratory training and therefore you will benefit most when working with medically trained personnel.

If your SCI is at levels C5 or C6, you may use gravity-reduced exercises, strap-on weights, the rickshaw, exercise machines with wrist cuffs to access pulley systems, the machine shoulder press, and the upper body ergometer.

Your choice of exercise will depend on how much ability is left in your triceps; the triceps may be very weak or you may have to mechanically position the arm to lock the elbow straight. Focus on multijoint *pull* exercises to develop back muscles; use single-joint exercise to counter them with elbow splints substituting for the absent triceps. However, triceps limitation may mean that you have to focus on single-joint exercise. Be cautious not to overwork the biceps and cause elbow flexion contractures or a painful shoulder from biceps tendonitis. Exercise available back musculature (latissimus dorsi) to build shoulder (rotator cuff) and scapular stability and prevent forward posture and shoulder impingement syndromes. To assist in your functional mobility and transfers, focus on antigravity musculature (shoulder depressors on the rickshaw, serratus anterior by performing bench press punches on your back. Work on muscle balance of trunk and shoulders to maximize strength before exercising the arms above shoulder level.

The following are some suggested exercises for your class:

Shoulder depressors p. 182	Lateral shoulder raise p. 180
Lat pull-downs p. 178	Straight-arm back raise p. 187
Upright rows p. 166	Shoulder external rotation p. 184
Biceps curl p. 191	

SCI CLASSES 1B AND 1C EXERCISE GUIDELINES
C7 and C8 (Cervical Spine)

POSITION   Most of your exercises will be performed in your wheelchair, using an elastic abdominal binder as needed. You can transfer out of the wheelchair to perform exercises lying on your stomach or modify the exercises to perform them in the wheelchair by leaning forward over your knees. You may transfer out of your wheelchair to perform the bench press. If you do not have adequate hand function to grip the bar, use the machine bench press. When you use the bench for free weight bench press exercise, secure your legs with proper strapping for balance (refer to pp. 26-29).

EXERCISE OPTIONS   If your SCI is at level C7, you may use gravity-reduced exercise on a supporting surface, such as a table, to strengthen the triceps. Other exercise options include strap-on weights, the rickshaw, machine exercises with wrist cuffs to access a pulley system, the machine shoulder press, and the upper body ergometer.

If your SCI is at level C8, you may use strap-on weights, the rickshaw, machine exercises with wrist cuffs to access pulleys if your hand function is not complete, the shoulder press, barbells or dumbbells with spotting, and the upper body ergometer. If trunk balance is a problem, even with strapping, the exercise machine will be the preferred mode of exercise, rather than strap-on weights or barbell exercise.

Focus on back musculature and scapular stabilizers like the serratus anterior and lower trapezius to prevent forward posture and shoulder protraction. Focus on shoulder depressors (latissimus dorsi) to assist with transfers out of the wheelchair. Focus on muscle balance to strengthen weaker trunk and upper extremity shoulder musculature before you exercise your arms above the shoulder level. This will help prevent rotator cuff injuries and shoulder impingement syndromes. If your triceps (which extends the elbow) does not have full function, it will need concentrated strengthening. If you have full triceps, use multijoint exercises for most core exercises.

The following are some suggested exercises for your class:

Class IB—Partial Triceps

Shoulder depressors   p. 182
Lat pull-downs   p. 178
Upright rows   p. 166
Bent-over rows   p. 174
Straight-arm back raise   p. 187
Shoulder overhead press   p. 164
Triceps extensions   p. 188
Shoulder external rotation   p. 184

Class IC—Complete Triceps

Shoulder depressors   p. 182
Lat pull-downs   p. 178
Upright rows   p. 166
Bent-over rows   p. 174
Straight-arm back raise   p. 187
Shoulder overhead press   p. 164
Bench press   p. 176
Wrist flexion/extension   pp. 192-193

SCI CLASS 2 EXERCISE GUIDELINES
T1-5 (Thoracic Spine)

POSITION   Most of your exercises will be performed in your wheelchair with an abdominal binder or with spotting for overhead exercises with heavier weights. You may transfer out to do free-weight bench press using strapping to stabilize your legs. You may also transfer onto the mat to perform exercises on your stomach for back musculature.

EXERCISE OPTIONS   With complete hand grip, you may use dumbbells, barbells, exercise machines, and the free-weight bench press. When your trunk balance allows, use free-weight exercises to challenge your upper back extensors and the smaller stabilizing muscles of your shoulder girdle.

Focus on back musculature for improved posture and shoulder girdle musculature to maximize strength and wheelchair mobility.

The following are some suggested exercises for your class:

Lat pull-downs p. 178	Bench press p. 176
Dips p. 173	Bent-over rows p. 174
Shoulder overhead press p. 164	Straight-arm back raise p. 187
Upright rows p. 166	Wrist flexion/extension pp. 192-193

SCI CLASS 3 EXERCISE GUIDELINES
T6-10 (Thoracic Spine)

| POSITION | Most of your exercises will be performed in your wheelchair without an abdominal binder. You may transfer out to do free-weight bench press using strapping to stabilize your legs. You may also transfer onto the mat to exercise your back musculature on your stomach.

| EXERCISE OPTIONS | You may use dumbbells, barbells, exercise machines, and the free-weight bench press. When your trunk balance allows, use free-weight exercises to challenge the smaller stabilizing muscles of the shoulder girdle, abdominal muscles, trunk rotators, and back extensors.

Focus on antigravity muscles that you need to walk with long leg braces and forearm crutches, including the triceps, shoulder girdle depressors, and abdominal and back musculature.

The following are some suggested exercises for your class:

Lat pull-downs   p. 178
Dips   p. 173
Shoulder overhead press   p. 164
Upright rows   p. 166

Bench press   p. 176
Bent-over rows   p. 174
Straight-arm back raise   p. 187

SCI CLASS 4 EXERCISE GUIDELINES
T11-L4 (Lower Thoracic and Upper Lumbar Spine)

| POSITION | Your exercises will be performed in your wheelchair, in a regular chair, or, if your trunk balance is adequate, sitting at the edge of a mat with single arm support. Stabilize your legs with strapping for the free-weight bench press. Perform exercises on your stomach to focus on back musculature.

| EXERCISE OPTIONS | You may use dumbbells, barbells, exercise machines, and the free-weight bench press. Focus on free weights and exercise machines to provide resistance for your available lower extremity musculature. Gravity-reduced exercises on a supporting surface, such as an exercise mat, may be used to strengthen lower extremity muscles that are not able to move against gravity.

Focus on antigravity muscles that you need to walk with long or short leg braces and forearm crutches, including the triceps, shoulder depressors, abdominal and back musculature, and available lower extremity musculature.

The following are some suggested exercises for your class:

Upper Extremity

Lat pull-downs   p. 178
Dips   p. 173
Shoulder overhead press   p. 164
Upright rows   p. 166
Bench press   p. 176
Bent-over rows   p. 174
Straight-arm back raise   p. 187

Lower Extremity/Trunk

Straight leg raise   p. 213
Knee extensions   p. 218
Posterior pelvic tilt   p. 197
Upper abdominals #1   p. 202
Lateral abdominal crunch   p. 204
Upper back extension #1   p. 205
Upper trunk rotation   p. 207

SCI CLASS 5 EXERCISE GUIDELINES
L5-S5 (Lower Lumbar and Sacral Spine)

POSITION Your exercises may be performed in all positions, although you may require strapping to stabilize the legs for the free-weight bench press.

EXERCISE OPTIONS You may use dumbbells, barbells, exercise machines and the free-weight bench press. Use strap-on weights and exercise machines to provide resistance for your available lower extremity musculature and supported exercises to strengthen lower extremity muscles that are not able to move against gravity.

Focus on back musculature and muscular balance for the upper extremity. Strengthen the weak lower extremity muscles that you need for a stable walking pattern. Choose single-joint exercises on the mat or exercise machines for lower extremities if you do not have the strength and balance needed to perform multijoint exercises such as squats and lunges. Focus on strengthening abdominal and lower back musculature, which will assist with your balance during walking.

The following are some suggested exercises for your class:

Upper Extremity	Lower Extremity/Trunk
Lat pull-downs p. 178	Knee to chest p. 213
Dips p. 173	Leg back raise p. 216
Upright rows p. 166	Leg side raise p. 214
Shoulder overhead press p. 164	Leg curls p. 212
Bent-over rows p. 174	Knee extensions p. 218
Bench press p. 176	Heel raises p. 220
Straight-arm back raise p. 187	Ankle curls p. 219
	Posterior pelvic tilt p. 197
	Upper abdominals #1 p. 202
	Lateral abdominal crunch p. 204
	Upper back extension #1 p. 205
	Upper trunk rotation p. 207

CHAPTER 7

Conditioning With Amputations

In this chapter, we will cover upper and lower extremity amputations, both congenital (present at birth) and acquired. Sports participation with an amputation is under the jurisdiction of the National Handicapped Sports Association, which assigns a classification according to the number of amputations, the location of the amputation, and whether the amputation is unilateral or bilateral.

The following abbreviations are commonly used when referring to the location of an amputation:

AK Above or through the knee joint

BK Below the knee, but through or above the ankle (talocrural) joint

AE Above or through the elbow joint

BE Below the elbow, but through or above the wrist joint

This chapter is arranged in the following order:

About Amputations

Amputation refers to a condition in which part or all of one or more extremities is missing. A *major amputation* is defined as an amputation in the lower extremity through or above the ankle joint or in the upper extremity through or above the wrist joint. Amputations may be **congenital**, or they may result from trauma or disease. An estimated 1 of every 250 people in the United States has had a major amputation; of these about 700,000 are in the lower extremities. Additional amputations occur at the rate of 35,000 to 40,000 annually with a ratio of 5 in the upper extremities for every 20 in the lower extremities.

Congenital amputations can result from surgical revision of a malformed extremity or from absence of part of the extremity. If you have a congenital anomaly, you may have an extremity that is fully or partially present but with malformations. Prophylactic amputation in infancy depends on the nature and extent of the malformation and how it will influence the functioning of the extremity. Prophylactic amputation can also be indicated for congenital absence of an extremity when an undeveloped part of the extremity exists at the end portion of the stump. If the undeveloped portion serves no useful purpose or interferes with fitting a **prosthesis**, the portion is then removed and the stump reshaped.

Acquired amputations may be caused by trauma or disease. The traumatic amputation, like the congenital amputation, usually occurs in an otherwise healthy individual. This contrasts with a vascular amputation, which may be associated with cardiovascular disease. Traumatic amputations may occur as a result of accidents, burn or cold injuries, or specific nerve injuries that leave the extremity without sensation and susceptible to ulceration and infection. Amputations in the upper extremity predominantly result from traumatic accidents (industrial, thermal) and occur in a much younger average age group than do amputations involving the lower extremity.

Amputations due to disease may be the result of a malignant tumor (cancer), a severe infection of tissues or bone, or vascular insufficiency. Peripheral vascular insufficiency or disease (PVD) accounts for about 80% of all lower extremity amputations in adults. A variety of causes for circulatory failure lead to amputation. The most common causes are related to diabetes, arteriosclerosis, emboli, arterial thrombi, and arteriovenous aneurysm that have failed to respond to medical or less extensive surgical procedures. Individuals with vascular amputations tend to be older and can have significant medical histories, including cardiovascular disease or other heart conditions. If you have a vascular amputation and a history of heart disease, you will have lower tolerances for physical activity and greater likelihood of manifesting abnormal cardiac responses to exercise.

Associated Conditions

Amputations can change your activity level and ability to walk. You need to monitor the affected extremity for range of motion and skin integrity, and you need to be aware of altered balance with activity. Next we introduce associated conditions related to these changes, including contractures and decreased range of motion, orthopedic deformities of the spine, impaired sensation and skin care, and impaired balance or coordination.

Contractures and Decreased Range of Motion.   After an amputation, proper positioning and active range of motion exercises are essential to avoid developing tight musculature that can decrease range of motion (ROM). With a below-

knee amputation, more time spent sitting and less time spent ambulating can cause hip and knee flexion tightness. With an above-knee amputation, it is important to avoid tight hip flexors and hip adductors—lying on your stomach is encouraged to stretch out the trunk, hip, and knee flexors. With an upper extremity amputation, the anterior shoulder is the main area susceptible to muscle tightness, usually due to improper posture or muscle imbalances that develop because of the amputation.

Contractures (shortening of muscles and other connective tissue) can be prevented with regular sustained stretching or range of motion (ROM) exercise, strengthening antagonist muscle groups, and proper positioning of the trunk, arms, and legs. Contractures and decreased ROM can lead to problems with proper prosthetic fit and can cause abnormal walking patterns. Impaired walking mechanics often result in increased energy expenditure during walking and decreased control of dynamic balance. Impaired walking mechanics can cause skin breakdown or sores on the stump that can restrict you from walking until the skin is completely healed.

Orthopedic Deformities of the Spine.   **Scoliosis** and deviations of head position are not uncommon following upper extremity amputations. To compensate for the discrepancy in weight across the shoulder girdles by loss of part or all of the upper extremity, you should do trunk and postural exercises regularly. These exercises focus on midline control and your new center of gravity. For example, with an amputation above the elbow on one side, it is important to strengthen the back extensors and lateral flexors on that side to compensate for the tendency to lean toward the heavier side without the amputation.

Impaired Sensation and Skin Care.   Wearing a prosthesis requires good skin care, including frequent skin checks when you begin new activities or exercise. This is especially true if you have an amputation due to peripheral vascular disease or a nerve injury because decreased sensation and a tendency for skin breakdown can accompany those conditions. You must be responsible for monitoring proper wear and fit of your prosthesis to avoid skin stress due to abnormal shearing forces. Use appropriate stump sock thickness and contact your prosthetist, physical therapist, or physician if you cannot obtain proper fit with stump sock or **edema** management. Most exercises are performed with the prosthesis off, but if

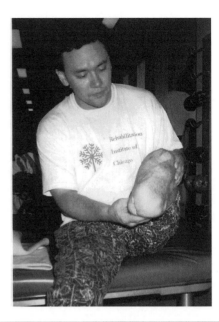

Check the skin of your stump following new exercise activities with your prosthesis.

done properly weight-bearing exercises in the prosthetic extremity (e.g., bench press, shoulder press, rickshaw, squats, lunges) create minimal to no shear force.

Impaired Balance and Coordination. The **proprioceptive** functions of your foot and hand are derived from skin receptors that detect weight bearing and displacement of your center of gravity. An amputation of the upper or lower extremity removes these receptors, making balance the one aspect of motor performance that probably will give you the most trouble. You must be trained with your new prosthetic extremity to adjust to the challenges of new weight-bearing surfaces and frequent adjustments of your center of gravity. Balance activities and coordination exercises are essential to maximize the use of your prosthesis and enhance your adaptation to the environment.

Exercise Readiness Assessment

Before setting up your exercise program, assess the following areas:

- Type of amputation
- Functional range of motion
- Strength
- Balance and trunk stability
- Skin integrity

If your amputation is congenital or due to trauma, you probably will not have specific exer-

cise restrictions. If your amputation is the result of a vascular complication and you have associated conditions such as diabetes, hypertension, or heart disease, medical assessment and clearance are essential before starting an exercise program. Often, individuals with vascular amputations, cardiopulmonary disease, or both will need exercise testing by a medical or exercise professional to predict possible therapeutic risk before engaging in an exercise program. You need to follow their precautions and exercise parameters in your exercise program design.

Look at your functional range of motion so you can identify which muscle or muscle groups need stretching. Tight muscles influence your posture and the positioning of your amputated extremity, and proper posture and extremity positioning is required for correct exercise technique. Go through the functional range of motion tests in chapter 1 to see what limitations you have. Then turn to chapter 4 to see which stretches can help you with your "tight spots." You might need assistance for some stretches so find an exercise partner and make stretching part of your warm-up and cool-down.

Assessing your strength is important for setting exercise intensity and goals. Improving your strength in weak spots can help you control your new center of gravity. The control you have with your center of gravity is referred to as *balance*. The amount of balance you have determines which

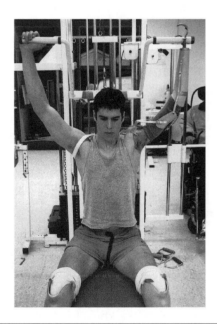

Weight-bearing exercise with your prosthesis can be performed without shearing forces that may compromise skin integrity.

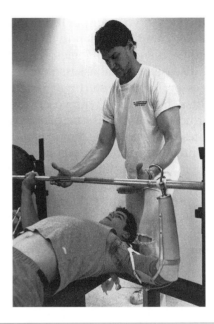

The bench press is a safe exercise if you have a BE amputation and perform it correctly with weight through the long axis of the forearm.

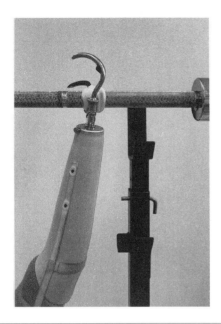

A piece of rubber wrapped around the metal bar prevents the metal prosthetic hook from sliding.

exercise options will be most appropriate for you, both for strengthening and for aerobic activity. Evaluating your trunk balance will also help you determine if you need external support to stabilize your trunk with exercise.

When assessing what exercises are appropriate with the use of a prosthesis, observe the skin of the stump for possible reddened areas before and after exercise. At the beginning of an exercise program, make frequent skin checks to be sure that the skin can tolerate the exercise and that shearing forces are not excessive. This is especially important if you have a new amputation because the skin may still be tender with weight-bearing activities. You'll also need to assess your skin frequently with exercise if you have decreased or compromised circulation or sensation. Progress your exercise program only as skin tolerance permits.

Exercise Modifications and Training Considerations

To improve flexibility and perform an adequate warm-up and cool-down, include stretching exercises in all routines. Pay special attention to stretching the hip and knee flexors if you have an amputation below the knee, to the hip flexors if you have an amputation above the knee, and to the shoulder and scapular range of motion if you have an amputation in the upper extremity.

Use correct technique with your weight displaced evenly through the extremity and prosthesis when performing weight-bearing activity or exercise. Avoid quick twisting motions or perpendicular forces to the prosthesis because they can cause shearing forces on your skin. Hanging weights or using other forms of resistance, such as Theraband or pulleys, on the prosthesis is not recommended. Resultant shearing forces can compromise your skin's integrity.

Restrict prosthetic use during resistance training with equipment to weight-bearing exercises only. These exercises may include performing a bench press with a below-elbow prosthesis or

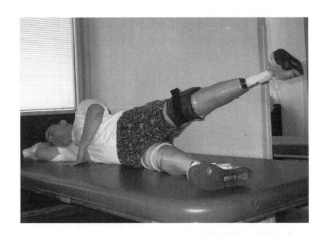

Performing a side leg raise with a wraparound weight *above* the prosthesis, with the prosthesis adding additional resistance.

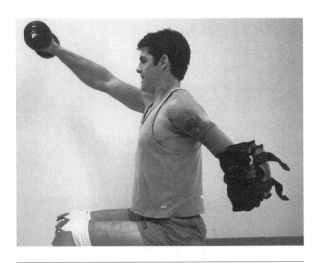

Adding resistance to the amputated extremity.

performing a squat with a below-knee prosthesis. Remember to frequently monitor your skin when engaging in a new exercise that requires use of your prosthesis.

The prosthesis itself may be used as a form of resistance—for example, you can perform leg lifts with a below-knee prosthesis to strengthen the abdominals or side leg raises to strengthen the hip abductors. Again, never place a wraparound weight, cable, or other form of resistance that does not include a weight-bearing force on the prosthesis. This can cause excessive shearing forces on your stump from the prosthesis; these shearing forces result in skin breakdown or sores that can severely limit or restrict the use of your prosthesis. This can be especially difficult if you have a lower extremity amputation and skin breakdown restricts your walking.

Wraparound weights on your residual extremity are a good form of resistance. You may need more resistance on the residual extremity com-

pared to the unaffected extremity because of a shorter lever arm on your amputated extremity. If you have an upper extremity amputation and cannot access conventional exercise equipment, such as lat pull-downs and dumbbell flys, slings with resistive springs or exercise tubing can be used as an alternative set-up. Wraparound cuffs can also allow you to access pulley exercise machines. However, some standard exercise machines will require no modifications.

If you have a unilateral lower extremity amputation, you can perform resistance exercises in a standing position when appropriate. If you have bilateral lower extremity amputations, you may need to perform resistance exercises in a sitting position to maintain your balance and proper exercise technique.

Response to Exercise

Amputations can compromise your fitness status, regardless of the cause. Exercise conditioning and endurance training can increase your fitness level and help you maintain an optimal level. Close monitoring and assessment of your response to exercise is essential if you have a vascular amputation or cardiopulmonary disease. With an appropriate aerobic exercise and conditioning program, however, you can gain significant cardiovascular and total body benefits. These benefits are especially important because mobility tends to decrease after the amputation, and deconditioning, weight gain, and suboptimal lipid status can become significant secondary complications that increase cardiac risk. Exercise progression should be slow because of deconditioning from disuse and possible cardiovascular conditions. Aerobic activities are

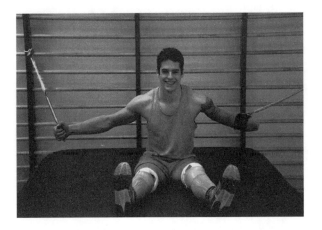
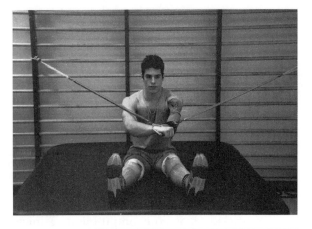

Resistance tubing or springs of varying tension can be used to simulate conventional exercise.

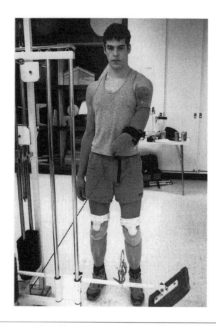
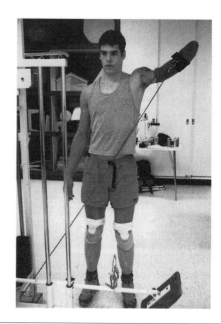

A wraparound cuff can improve the effectiveness of your strength training program.

encouraged to decrease the conditions associated with disuse and to assist in weight management. Weight fluctuations can affect the fit of your prosthesis.

Your fitness level may vary according to the cause of your amputation. Congenital or traumatic amputations often have minimal or no associated conditions, whereas vascular amputations can be the result of vascular disease with many associated cardiac conditions. The latter type of amputation is often called dysvascular because it results from a "disease of the vessels." Peripheral vascular disease (PVD) is the most common cause of lower extremity amputation in the elderly. Elderly individuals with vascular amputations commonly suffer from multiple disorders related to diabetes, cardiovascular disease, and the many complications of a sedentary lifestyle. Most adults with vascular amputations show significant associated cardiovascular disease, and some may show myocardial ischemia or abnormal cardiac responses during exercise. Studies show that the aerobic capacity of elderly individuals with dysvascular amputations is quite low in comparison to those with congenital or traumatic amputations and the general public. People with amputations also have substantially greater energy demands and cardiac workloads for functional activities than the nondisabled population.

Maximum aerobic capacity is influenced not only by your age and present physical state, but also by the level of your amputation. Clinical studies commonly show that the lower the ampu-tation, the more efficient physical performance and walking. Studies also show that maximum aerobic power for individuals with dysvascular amputations is progressively higher in lower levels of amputation. Younger individuals with traumatic amputations show a similar trend, but they have a higher fitness level than their dysvascular counterparts.

Whether vascular or traumatic, people with lower extremity amputations can require up to 50% more oxygen during walking than the general public. The rate of oxygen utilization is influenced by age, existing medical complications, stump length, and mode of mobility. One study suggests that individuals with dysvascular and traumatic BK amputations and traumatic AK amputations who walk with a prosthesis can keep energy costs within normal limits, if they

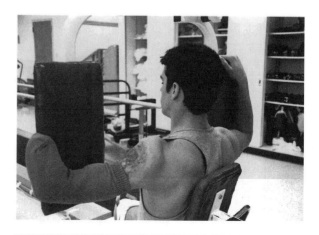

Some exercise machines require no modifications.

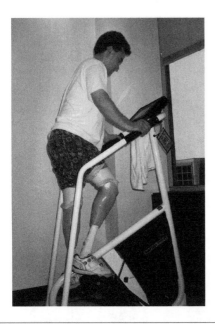

Regular aerobic exercise can decrease risks of cardio-vascular disease and assist in weight management.

modify their walking speed. Individuals with dysvascular AK amputations showed significant increases in walking energy costs in comparison. Other investigations have shown that the physical work capacity of individuals with an amputation is low in comparison to the general public.

Amputee Exercise Precautions

- Medical clearance and assessment are essential before implementing an exercise program if you have a vascular amputation, cardiovascular disease, or both. You must identify precautions, exercise parameters, and restrictions.
- When exercising with your prosthesis on, observe the skin of the residual extremity before and after exercise. Progress your exercise program only as skin tolerance permits.
- Hanging weights or other forms of resistance (Theraband, etc.) on your prosthesis is not recommended because of possible compromise of skin integrity from shearing forces.
- Watch out for muscle exhaustion in weight-lifting exercises that require strenuous reliance on your sound leg or arm. If you don't immediately rest when you feel a burning sensation, the leg or arm may collapse.

Your Next Move

Now that you have the background information you need, you can find your appropriate classification in the section that follows. With the classification, you can identify your training program.

Classification and Exercise Guidelines

Now you can identify your classification and locate the corresponding exercise program. The National Handicapped Sports Association (NHS) uses a classification system that helps you determine your available extremity use and allow for equality in competition. The NHS classification system is based on nine classes according to the number of amputations, the location of the amputation in the upper or lower extremity and above or below a specified joint, and whether the amputation is unilateral, on one side, or bilateral, involving both sides.

To use the following exercise programs and the exercise index, find the class appropriate for you. The following list will help you select your profile. Once you have found the appropriate class, photocopied the following training log, identified your training program, and made the necessary modifications to it, it is time to learn about the specific exercises you will perform during your workout. Part III provides explanations and photographs of these exercises.

Classification Code:

Class A1   Double AK
Class A2   Single AK
Class A3   Double BK or combined BK and AK
Class A4   Single BK
Class A5   Double AE
Class A6   Single AE
Class A7   Double BE or combined BE and AE
Class A8   Single BE
Class A9   Combined lower plus upper extremity amputations

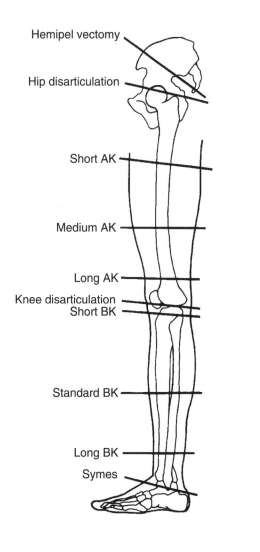

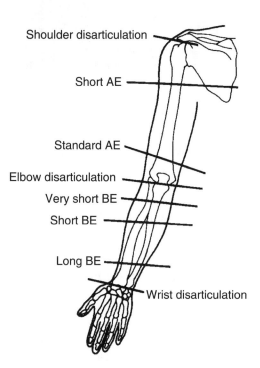

Conditioning With Amputations

Weight					Date	Sets/reps	Exercises	Notes

CLASS A1 EXERCISE GUIDELINES
Double AK (Above or Through the Knee Joint)

POSITION You may exercise in your wheelchair, in a regular chair, or if your trunk balance is adequate, sitting at the edge of a mat table. You should also exercise on your stomach to strengthen back musculature and on your back to strengthen abdominal musculature. You may require strapping to stabilize your lower trunk for the free-weight bench press. No exercises should take place in stance, unless they are balance and coordination activities prescribed by a medical professional for improving walking skills.

EXERCISE OPTIONS You may use free weights (dumbbells, barbells) and conventional exercise equipment for upper extremity exercise. Free weights are preferred to help develop trunk control and proximal shoulder stability. Focus on wrap-around weights, Theraband, or set-ups with springs and cuffs to provide resistance for your available lower extremity musculature.

Focus on antigravity muscles that you need for walking with prostheses and forearm crutches, including the triceps, shoulder depressors, wrist extensors, abdominal and back musculature, and available lower extremity musculature.

The following are some suggested exercises for your class:

Upper Extremity	*Lower Extremity/Trunk*
Dips p. 173	Leg back raises p. 216
Lat pull-downs p. 178	Leg side raises p. 214
Upright rows p. 166	Posterior pelvic tilt p. 197
Shoulder overhead press p. 164	Upper abdominals #1 p. 202
Bent-over rows p. 174	Lateral abdominal crunch p. 204
Bench press p. 176	Upper back extension #1 p. 205
Straight-arm back raise p. 187	Upper trunk rotation p. 207

CLASS A2 EXERCISE GUIDELINES
Single AK (Above or Through the Knee Joint)

POSITION You may exercise in all positions, but you may require strapping to stabilize your lower extremities for the free-weight bench press.

EXERCISE OPTIONS You may use free weights (dumbbells, barbells) and conventional exercise equipment for upper extremity exercise. Free weights are the preferred mode for developing trunk control and proximal shoulder stability. Focus on wraparound weights, Theraband, or set-ups with springs and cuffs to provide resistance for available lower extremity musculature. Your unaffected lower extremity has no limitations and can be strengthened as needed.

Focus on your upper back musculature and muscular balance for the upper extremity. Strengthen your weaker lower extremity musculature for a more stable walking pattern. Use single-joint exercises on the mat for your AK stump and conventional exercise equipment for the unaffected lower extremity. Depending on your AK prosthesis, you may perform small squats and lunges with upper extremity support. Strengthen abdominal and lower back musculature to assist with balance during walking.

The following are some suggested exercises for your class:

Upper Extremity
Dips   p. 173
Lat pull-downs   p. 178
Upright rows   p. 166
Shoulder overhead press   p. 164
Bent-over rows   p. 174
Bench press   p. 176
Straight-arm back raise   p. 187

Lower Extremity/Trunk
Leg back raises   p. 216
Leg side raises   p. 214
Squats   p. 210
Lunges   p. 211
Leg curls   p. 212
Knee extensions   p. 218
Heel raises   p. 220
Ankle curls   p. 219
Posterior pelvic tilt   p. 197
Upper abdominals #1   p. 202
Lateral abdominal crunch   p. 204
Upper back extension #2   p. 206
Upper trunk rotation   p. 207

CLASS A3 EXERCISE GUIDELINES
Double BK (Below Knee
but Through or Above the Ankle [Talocrural] Joint)

| POSITION | You can exercise in your wheelchair, in a regular chair, or if your trunk balance is adequate, sitting at the edge of a mat table. Exercise lying on your stomach to strengthen back musculature and lying on your back to strengthen abdominal musculature. Determine whether exercises in stance are appropriate by your balance control.

| EXERCISE OPTIONS | You may use free weights (dumbbells, barbells) and conventional exercise equipment for upper extremity exercise. Free weights are the preferred mode for developing trunk control and proximal shoulder stability. Focus on wraparound weights, Theraband, or set-ups with springs and cuffs to provide resistance for your available lower extremity musculature.

Focus on strengthening your upper back musculature and promoting muscular balance in the upper extremity. Strengthen your weaker lower extremity muscles with single-joint exercises on the mat. Depending on your balance control and your BK prostheses, you may do modified squats and lunges with or without upper extremity support. Focus on strengthening abdominal and lower back musculature, which will assist with balance during walking.

The following are some suggested exercises for your class:

Upper Extremity	*Lower Extremity/Trunk*
Dips p. 173	Leg back raises p. 216
Lat pull-downs p. 178	Leg side raises p. 214
Upright rows p. 166	Squats p. 210
Shoulder overhead press p. 164	Lunges p. 211
Bent-over rows p. 174	Leg curls p. 212
Bench press p. 176	Knee extensions p. 218
Straight-arm back raise p. 187	Posterior pelvic tilt p. 197
	Upper abdominals #1 p. 202
	Lateral abdominal crunch p. 204
	Upper back extension #2 p. 206
	Upper trunk rotation p. 207

CLASS A4 EXERCISE GUIDELINES
Single BK (Below Knee,
but Through or Above the Ankle [Talocrural] Joint)

POSITION   You can exercise in all positions.

EXERCISE OPTIONS   You may use free weights (dumbbells, barbells) and conventional exercise equipment for upper extremity exercise. Free weights are the preferred mode for developing trunk control. Focus on wraparound weights, Theraband, or set-ups with springs and cuffs to provide resistance for your available lower extremity musculature on your BK stump. Your unaffected lower extremity has no limitations and can be strengthened as needed.

Focus on strengthening your upper back musculature and promoting muscular balance for the upper extremity. Strengthen your weaker lower extremity muscles for a more stable walking pattern. Use single-joint exercise on the mat for your BK stump and conventional exercise equipment for the unaffected lower extremity. Depending on your balance, you may perform squats and lunges with or without upper extremity support.

The following are some suggested exercises for your class:

Upper Extremity

Dips   p. 173
Lat pull-downs   p. 178
Upright rows   p. 166
Shoulder overhead press   p. 164
Bent-over rows   p. 174
Bench press   p. 176
Straight-arm back raise   p. 187

Lower Extremity/Trunk

Leg back raises   p. 216
Leg side raises   p. 214
Squats   p. 210
Lunges   p. 211
Leg curls   p. 212
Knee extensions   p. 218
Heel raises   p. 220
Ankle curls   p. 219
Posterior pelvic tilt   p. 197
Upper abdominals #1   p. 202
Lateral abdominal crunch   p. 204
Upper back extension #2   p. 206
Upper trunk rotation   p. 207

CLASS A5 EXERCISE GUIDELINES
Double AE (Above or Through the Elbow Joint)

POSITION You can exercise in all positions.

EXERCISE OPTIONS Focus on wraparound weights, Theraband, or set-ups with pulleys, springs, and cuffs to provide resistance for your available upper extremity musculature. Use strap-on weights and conventional exercise equipment for your lower extremity exercise.

Focus on strength, coordination, and full active range of motion of the shoulder girdle (scapulothoracic) and shoulder joint (scapulohumeral). Strengthening shoulder flexion, extension, and protraction will help you use your upper extremity prostheses.

The following are some suggested exercises for your class:

Upper Extremity
Front shoulder raise   p. 179
Lateral shoulder raise   p. 180
Back shoulder raise   p. 181
Straight-arm back raise   p. 187
Open to cross   p. 171
Cross to open   p. 172

Lower Extremity/Trunk
Squats   p. 210
Lunges   p. 211
Heel raises   p. 220
Leg back raises   p. 216
Leg side raises   p. 214
Posterior pelvic tilt   p. 196
Upper abdominals #1   p. 202
Lateral abdominal crunch   p. 204
Upper back extension #2   p. 206

CLASS A6 EXERCISE GUIDELINES
Single AE (Above or Through Elbow Joint)

POSITION You can exercise in all positions.

EXERCISE OPTIONS Focus on wraparound weights, Theraband, or set-ups with pulleys or springs, using cuffs to access and to provide resistance for available upper extremity musculature on your AE stump. You may use free weights for the unaffected upper extremity. For your lower extremity, you can use strap-on weights or conventional exercise equipment.

Focus on strength, coordination, and full active range of motion for your shoulder girdle (scapulothoracic) and shoulder joint (scapulohumeral). Strengthening shoulder flexion, extension, and protraction will help you use your upper extremity prosthesis. Focus on strengthening your upper trunk and perform postural exercises to promote muscular balance and to compensate for the discrepancy in weight across your shoulder girdles from your prosthesis.

The following are some suggested exercises for your class:

Upper Extremity	*Lower Extremity/Trunk*
Front shoulder raise p. 179	Squats p. 210
Lateral shoulder raise p. 180	Lunges p. 211
Back shoulder raise p. 181	Heel raises p. 220
Straight-arm back raise p. 187	Leg back raises p. 216
Open to cross p. 171	Leg side raises p. 214
Cross to open p. 172	Posterior pelvic tilt p. 196
	Upper abdominals #1 p. 202
	Lateral abdominal crunch p. 204
	Upper back extension #2 p. 206

CLASS A7 EXERCISE GUIDELINES
Double BE (Below the Elbow, but Through or Above the Wrist Joint)

| POSITION | You can exercise in all positions.

| EXERCISE OPTIONS | Focus on wraparound weights, Theraband, or set-ups with springs and cuffs to provide resistance for the available musculature on your BE stumps. Use strap-on weights and conventional exercise equipment for lower extremity exercise.

Focus on strength, coordination, and full active range of motion for your shoulder girdle (scapulothoracic), shoulder (scapulohumeral), and elbow joints. Strengthening shoulder flexion, extension, and protraction; elbow flexion and extension; and forearm pronation and supination will help you operate your upper extremity prostheses.

The following are some suggested exercises for your class:

Upper Extremity

Front shoulder raise   p. 179
Lateral shoulder raise   p. 180
Back shoulder raise   p. 181
Straight-arm back raise   p. 187
Shoulder external rotation   p. 184
Biceps curl   p. 191
Triceps extensions   p. 188
Open to cross   p. 171
Cross to open   p. 172

Lower Extremity/Trunk

Squats   p. 210
Lunges   p. 211
Heel raises   p. 220
Leg back raises   p. 216
Leg side raises   p. 214
Posterior pelvic tilt   p. 196
Upper abdominals #1   p. 202
Lateral abdominal crunch   p. 204
Upper back extension #2   p. 206

CLASS A8 EXERCISE GUIDELINES
Single BE (Below the Elbow, but Through or Above the Wrist Joint)

POSITION You can exercise in all positions.

EXERCISE OPTIONS Focus on wraparound weights, Theraband, or set-ups with springs or pulleys, using cuffs to access and to provide resistance for the available musculature on your BE stump. Use free weights (dumbbells, barbells) for the unaffected upper extremity. Some conventional bilateral upper extremity equipment can be used with the prosthesis on (shoulder press, free-weight bench press) or with the prosthesis off (chest flys, reverse flys, modified lat pull-downs). Use strap-on weights and conventional exercise equipment for lower extremity exercise.

Focus on strength, coordination, and full active range of motion for the shoulder girdle (scapulothoracic), shoulder (scapulohumeral), and elbow joints. Strengthening shoulder flexion, extension, and protraction; elbow flexion and extension; and forearm pronation and supination will help you operate your upper extremity prosthesis. Focus on strengthening the upper trunk and performing postural exercise to promote muscular balance and compensate for the discrepancy in weight across your shoulder girdles from your prosthesis.

The following are some suggested exercises for your class:

Upper Extremity
Front shoulder raise   p. 179
Lateral shoulder raise   p. 180
Back shoulder raise   p. 181
Straight-arm back raise   p. 187
Shoulder external rotation   p. 184
Biceps curl   p. 191
Triceps extensions   p. 188
Bench press   p. 176
Open to cross   p. 171
Cross to open   p. 172

Lower Extremity/Trunk
Squats   p. 210
Lunges   p. 211
Heel raises   p. 220
Leg back raises   p. 216
Leg side raises   p. 214
Posterior pelvic tilt   p. 196
Upper abdominals #1   p. 202
Lateral abdominal crunch   p. 204
Upper back extension #2   p. 206

CLASS A9 EXERCISE GUIDELINES
Combined Lower Plus Upper Extremity Amputations

| POSITION | Your exercise position depends upon your available trunk balance for sitting and standing with or without support. You will benefit from exercises on your back and stomach to strengthen your back and abdominal musculature.

| EXERCISE OPTIONS | Focus on wraparound weights, Theraband, or set-ups with springs and cuffs to provide resistance for your available musculature on lower and upper extremity stumps. You may use free weights (dumbbells, barbells) for the unaffected upper extremity and strap-on weights or conventional exercise equipment for the unaffected lower extremity.

The following are some suggested exercises for your class:

Trunk

Posterior pelvic tilt   p. 196
Upper abdominals #1   p. 202
Lateral abdominal crunch   p. 204
Upper back extension #2   p. 206

Upper/Lower Extremity

Please see the upper extremity and lower extremity programs of other classes that apply to your specific amputations.

CHAPTER 8

Conditioning With Other Physical Disabilities

In this chapter, we will cover the main disabilities that fall under the jurisdiction of the Les Autres (French for "the others") Athletic Association. Les Autres athletics is the national sports organization for those with disabilities resulting from a condition other than spinal cord injury, cerebral palsy, closed head injury, stroke, amputation, visual impairments, hearing impairments, or mental impairments. Disabilities included in Les Autres competition manifest some level of locomotor dysfunction due to either muscle weakness or constricted joints. Refer to Table 8.1 for a list of eligible disabilities.

Tremendous individual differences characterize the **Les Autres** disabilities. Due to the number of disabilities, many with low incidence, it would be impractical to cover each one. We will cover multiple sclerosis, the neuromuscular diseases, postpolio syndrome, dwarfism, osteogenesis imperfecta, and arthrogryposis because of their prevalence in sports for the disabled (characterized by the higher percentage of athletes attending the national games in the 1991-92 season).

To turn to the disability that directly affects you, please use the following guide:

Visual Impairments

Visual handicap may result from loss of central vision, loss of peripheral vision, or both. Visual handicaps are defined by visual acuity, which measures central vision function and the sharpness or clearness of vision (designated as a numerical ratio). The definition of blindness is vague because most legally blind people are partially sighted with some functional vision.

Table 8.1
Les Autres Disabilities

All arthritis and rheumatic diseases	Ehler's-Danlos syndrome	Neoplasms with motor impairment
Any traumatic neural injury	Fibrous dysplasia	Neurofibromatosis with motor impairment
Ankylosis of any joint	Guillian-barre disease	
Ankylosing spondylitis	Hemophilia with motor involvement	Orthopedic malformations of muscle, ligament, or bone
Amyotonia congenita	Huntington's chorea	Osteochondrosis, including Legg-Perths, Panners, Friebergs, and Schauermanns
Arthrogryposis	Junior rheumatoid arthritis	
Ataxia telangectasia	Lou Gerhig's disease	
Brachial plexus injuries	Lyme disease	Osteogenesis imperfecta
Burn injuries with resulting motor impairment	Marfan's syndrome	Paget's disease/osteitis deformans
Congenital hip dislocations	Multiple combinations of disabilities that do not fit elsewhere	Parkinson's disease
Cushing's syndrome with bone involvement	Multiple extoses	Polyostotic fibrous dysplagia
	Multiple sclerosis	Polymyositis
Dwarfism—all types	Muscular dystrophy—all 40 neuromuscular diseases covered in this category	Postpolio syndrome
Dysmelia/phocomelia		Rheumatic fever with motor/joint involvement
Dysoutoanomias	Myasthenia gravis	
Dystonia	Myelodysplagia	Rickets

Note. This is an incomplete list.

Adapted from Sherrill (1981).

Causes

Blindness and visual impairments are largely problems of the elderly population. Common causes of visual impairments in the elderly (people age 65 and older) include senile macular degeneration, chronic glaucoma, and cataracts. Diabetic retinopathy is a common cause of visual impairment in adults under age 65. Most visual impairments in school-age children are attributed to birth defects. Other less common causes of visual impairments include infectious diseases, tumors, injuries, and neurological disorders (e.g., strokes with possible visual field loss and multiple sclerosis with possible optic neuritis leading to optic atrophy and progressive loss of visual acuity).

Physical and Health Characteristics

Many young blind individuals show low proprioceptive awareness, decreased postural control, and low stamina because of a lack of physical activity. They also may develop "blindisms," general mannerisms resulting from physical and movement deprivation. Common blindisms include rocking back and forth, putting the fist to the eyes, and twitching and shaking the head to release tension.

Studies show that some individuals with visual impairments or blindness have significantly lower physical fitness levels compared to their peers with unaffected vision. These studies indicate that low physical work capacity in the young visually impaired is due to the lack of physical activity, which contributes to age-related obesity, muscular weakness, and low tolerance for exercise. Blind individuals show a normal response to exercise with increases in both cardiovascular and muscular fitness. Other benefits of physical activity (such as cross country running) include improved posture and gait developed from heightened awareness of sensory cues.

Exercise Readiness Assessment

Preexercise assessment should closely parallel the assessment people without visual impairments use, including flexibility, muscular strength

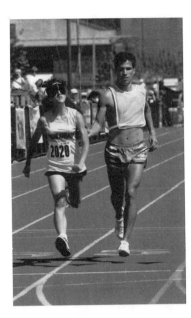

A visually impaired runner maintains her track lane with assistance from a guide runner.

and endurance, cardiorespiratory endurance, and a general survey of body composition. Refer to chapter 1.

Exercise Modifications and Training Considerations

Exercise program design including frequency, duration, and intensity for the visually impaired should follow the guidelines for those without visual impairments; however, some modifications may be needed for exercise:

- Running activities may require the use of a guide wire or rope or a running partner.
- Strength training can be easily performed with a workout partner.
- When teaching new exercises to the visually impaired, kinesthetic teaching will replace visual demonstrations. For example, teach a barbell upright row by assisting the individual with the exercise movement to feel how the skill is performed in slow motion.
- When teaching, think in terms of sound and feel rather than sight.
- Introduce the individual to the size and shape of the workout area or weight room and establish a point of reference for each room or space that the athlete will be using.

Classification for Sports

In sports all legally blind are classified according to visual acuity in one of the groups listed in Table 8.2.

Table 8.2 Vision Classifications	
Legal blindness (20/200)	The ability to see at 20 ft what the normal eye sees at 200 ft.
Travel vision (5/200 to 10/200)	The ability to see at 5 to to 10 ft what the normal eye sees at 200 ft.
Motion perception (3/200 to 5/200)	The ability to see at 3 to 5 ft what the normal eye sees at 200 ft. Vision is limited almost entirely to motion.
Light perception (less than 3/200)	The ability to detect a strong light 3 ft from the eye with the inability to detect movement at that same distance.
Total blindness (lack of visual perception)	The inability to detect a strong light shining directly into the eyes.

CLASSIFICATION AND EXERCISE GUIDELINES

POSITION You can assume all positions; strapping for balance is rarely required.

EXERCISE OPTIONS No limitations. You can use free weights with all exercises. Supervision may be required. Your exercise routine should reflect muscular balance. The following are suggested exercises for your class.

Upper Extremity
Bench press   p. 176
Bent-over rows   p. 174
Straight-arm back raise   p. 187
Shoulder overhead press   p. 164
Lat pull-downs   p. 178
Dips   p. 173
Triceps extensions   p. 188
Biceps curl   p. 191

Lower Extremity
Squats   p. 210
Lunges   p. 211
Leg curls   p. 212
Knee extensions   p. 218
Heel raises   p. 220
Ankle curls   p. 219

Use the following training log to record your progress.

Conditioning With Visual Impairments

Exercises	Sets/reps	Date	Weight

Notes

Multiple Sclerosis

Multiple sclerosis (MS) is one of the most common neurological diseases of young adults, usually appearing first during middle age. MS is a progressive demyelinating disease that affects the central nervous system (CNS) and causes loss of physical function. MS destroys the **myelin** sheath that surrounds nervous tissue to insulate the nerves. The destruction of the myelin disrupts neurotransmission, the signals traveling through the nerves, causing motor impairments including loss of muscle power, ataxia (cerebellar dysfunction), and spasticity. The involvement within the CNS is patchy and not localized, resulting in great variability in physical manifestations. The disease course is unpredictable with varying degrees of severity that take three general patterns:

• The first pattern is characterized by periods of exacerbations (worsening of the condition) and remissions (recovery of the condition). Mild cases may show mild regressions with complete recovery of function, whereas other cases show more regressions with nearly complete recovery, leaving mild residual deficits or restrictions.

• A second pattern is a slow progression of MS without periods of recovery (remission). New symptoms can appear as the disease progresses and old symptoms can become more severe.

• A third pattern is a combination of the first two, resulting in a progressive course of exacerbation and remissions. This pattern of MS, with more debilitating regressions and incomplete recovery, is the most common and results in significant deficits or movement restrictions. Exercise will not reverse or stop the progression of the disease; however, it does help maintain function for longer periods of time.

Associated Conditions

Associated conditions with MS correlate with localized areas of demyelination in the central nervous system (brain and spinal cord). Some common changes that take place include ataxia, spasticity and muscle weakness, impaired sensation, fatigue, and heat intolerance.

Ataxia. MS commonly involves the fibers from the cerebellum as they run through the brainstem causing ataxia, a loss of muscular coordination in the trunk or limbs that can be characterized by

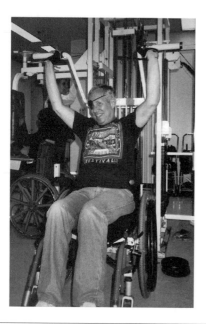

Fitness activities can have both positive psychological and physiological benefits for MS participants.

shakiness and decreased balance during walking. If ataxia affects you, you may find it necessary to walk with your feet farther apart to allow for a greater base of support. You may also have tremors of the head, trunk, and extremities that increase with precise, purposeful efforts. For example, your hand may shake more and more as you attempt to comb your hair. No medications have been found to eliminate these tremors although some medications have been successful in reducing them. Keeping your arms close to your body if tremors occur helps to stabilize your arms. Using a wrist splint sometimes helps wrist tremors.

Spasticity and Muscle Weakness. Loss of strength is a prominent condition of MS and varies greatly with the degree and progression of weakness. This decrease in strength is due to difficulties in transmitting electrical impulses from within the spinal cord and occasionally within the brain. Weakness is typically asymmetrical. Spasticity caused by damage to the brain and central nervous system can also be present, producing an unsteady, stumbling walking pattern. This spasticity may produce foot drag, poor control of one or both legs, or stiffness. When muscles are stiff, more work is required to move them so the energy costs for walking can be significantly higher for those with spasticity in the legs. This can result in early fatigue and increased weakness. Spasticity usually appears in grouped movements called synergy patterns. If spasticity is present, you may not be able to isolate movements to just one joint. For example, you may not be able to flex the knee with the hip extended, but you may be able to flex the knee when simultaneously flexing the hip and dorsiflexing the ankle. This is the flexor synergy pattern. The extensor synergy pattern in the lower extremities is hip flexion, hip adduction, knee extension, and ankle plantarflexion. Spasticity is a dynamic condition and can be increased by anxiety, fear, temperature, fatigue, and other external factors. Stretching routines are helpful to maintain range of motion. Refer to page 25 for specifics on exercise and spasticity.

Impaired Sensation.   Complete loss of sensation is rare, but you may experience numbness, tingling (paresthesias), and blunting of sensation or pain. Disturbances in position sense—knowing where your body parts are in space—and proprioception—knowing where your body parts are with movement—can also occur, contributing to problems with coordination of the extremities. These sensory problems can occur in any part of the body and are most frequent in the legs and trunk.

Fatigue and Heat Intolerance.   MS often limits energy level and endurance. The presence of demyelinating areas decreases the ability of the nerve fibers to conduct repetitive impulses and increases the rate of fatigue. In addition, a small elevation of core temperature blocks an increasing number of conducting fibers. The temperature at which conduction block occurs is proportional to the degree of demyelinization. Exposure to heat or humidity can thus increase MS symptoms and promote rapid fatigue. On the other hand, however, some people with MS are in no way affected by heat. In either case, the tendency for fatigue to increase with MS means that you must pace your activities and conserve energy and strength for those that are productive and meaningful. All activities should be designed to your energy level. Endurance exercises may or may not be appropriate. Swimming may be an excellent activity because it does not lead to increased core temperature if the water temperature is not too warm. The specific heat of the water conducts away body heat.

Exercise Readiness Assessment

Before setting up your exercise program, assess the following areas:

- Coordination
- Balance and trunk stability
- Muscle tone
- Your activity level

The amount of coordination and strength you have in the trunk and extremities will dictate the movements and muscle groups appropriate for exercise, the choice of exercises, and the overall exercise routine. Before starting your exercise program, identify your ability to control your movements. If you cannot perform a shoulder overhead press exercise without your arms going significantly "off course," then exercise machines will be the preferred mode for you.

Balance and trunk stability also help determine what mode of strengthening would be most appropriate and whether external support is needed to stabilize the trunk during exercising. If you have impaired coordination and balance in your upper trunk, you may require some form of support or assistance for stabilizing the upper trunk, especially during overhead exercises such as the shoulder press.

Many people with MS may also show spasticity. If spasticity increases and interferes with movement, function, or both in specific exercises, stop and reassess whether they are appropriate for you. Consult your physician or physical therapist if you are in doubt.

A personal survey of your typical daily activity level can help you determine the appropriateness and timing of exercise. You may have more or less energy at certain times of the day. Your exercise program volume, intensity, and scheduled time should coincide with your normal daily activities to avoid periods of fatigue or times of higher environmental temperature. Remember also that body temperature is normally lowest in the morning and higher in the afternoon.

Exercise Modifications and Training Considerations

Your exercise program will vary greatly depending on your capability. What is appropriate for one person may not be appropriate for another. It is extremely important to customize your exercise program to fit your lifestyle and capabilities. A strengthening program can improve or prolong function in your working muscles, especially when muscles are weak simply from being inactive. However, when weakness is primarily due to poor transmission from your nerves, strength training may not be appropriate due to the potential of fatiguing the nervous system, which can cause further weakness. Rigorous exercise can also increase core body temperature, speeding up the "short-circuiting" of your nervous system caused by demyelinization. To avoid this phenomenon, modify the **overload principle**. Use only moderate intensity or less to prevent overfatigue. The resistance or intensity that you will tolerate is relative to your degree of strength and your fatigability. Be sure to tailor your exercise program specifically to your needs!

Although your choice of exercises should consider your specific needs, some general guidelines apply to almost everyone. Your exercises should focus on your trunk and the muscles of the shoulder and pelvic girdles. These muscles include the scapular, back, and abdominal muscles. Increased strength in these areas may give you more control of your arms and legs when ataxia is present. Antigravity muscles, including the knee extensors, hip extensors, and low back muscles, should also be strengthened. Weakness in these postural muscles can decrease your ability to walk by demanding more effort from your muscles and causing faster onset of fatigue.

Use multijoint exercises, which limit the number of exercises needed for a complete, balanced workout, instead of single-joint exercises. Multijoint exercises can decrease the duration and volume of the exercise session, reducing the possibility of fatigue. Bilateral activities can help build trunk and proximal strength to control or restrict unrelated body movements as seen in ataxia.

Progressive muscle weakening and lack of function can lead to muscle tightness and possibly **contractures**, which are shortening of muscles and other connective tissues. The hip flexors, knee flexors, and plantar flexors are very susceptible to contractures if you are a wheelchair user. In that case, you should include stretches in your exercise routines. Active stretches that you perform yourself may be very physically demanding so use rest periods judiciously. You may also have a family member or workout partner assist (passive range of motion) to conserve energy for the active exercise program or other functional activities. If you have moderate to severe spasticity in conjunction with low endurance, flexibility exercises may be the primary—or only—exercise program focus. Tight spastic muscles require stretching.

In advanced stages of MS it may be impossible for you to obtain an aerobic training effect because the muscles may be too weak to stress the cardiovascular system to obtain a greater fitness level. When appropriate, an exercise bike is a good mode for aerobic training, especially for those of you with impaired balance or minor motor control problems. The exercise bike aids in balance and controls or guides the movement of the exercise. A treadmill or walking program is also appropriate. Discuss endurance activities such as swimming or biking with a physician or physical therapist before beginning them. An interval approach to aerobic exercise is often recommended. The interval approach involves performing a short exercise bout—walking, wheelchair rolling, or similar activities—for 2 to 5 min. Follow this session with a short rest period of 1 to 2 min before the next exercise bout. In interval training as with any aerobic activity, exercise and rest time must be geared to your endurance level.

Visual disturbances and tremors can impair balance. Exercise on a stable surface and give yourself visual feedback exercising in front of a mirror. If you have tremors in the trunk or extremities, stabilize the trunk with a belt or an elastic binder when you exercise the proximal muscles of the arm or legs. If you have decreased standing balance, you may want to perform your upper extremity exercises in a seated position or on a mat.

Your choice of mode of resistance depends on the amount of control or presence of tremors. Exercise machines that control the exercise throughout the full range of motion may be more appropriate than using free weights for people with moderate to severe ataxia (tremors). If you have minimal or no motor control difficulties, you can use free weights such as dumbbells, barbells, or wraparound weights if the effect is within your exercise tolerance.

Do not set off spasticity. Try to strengthen the muscles opposing the tight spastic muscles. If exercise promotes spasticity and prevents purposeful voluntary movements, stop immediately and reevaluate your exercise routine. When in doubt, consult with your physician or physical therapist.

The environment can drastically affect your exercise tolerance. If you are heat sensitive, keep your exercise room cool to avoid overheating and fatigue. Wear light, comfortable clothes, such as cotton T-shirts, and avoid heavy sweatshirts. Reduce your exercise intensity on hot, humid days.

Be sure to investigate the water temperature in community swim programs or classes—the water should be cool, not warm or hot. Your skin temperature is about 91°F; if the water temperature is less than 90 °F, prolonged immersion can decrease your core body temperature. Some researchers suggest that the water temperature should be in the low to mid 80s.

The progression of your exercise program will be influenced by your response to the exercise, the degree of MS severity, and the rate of progression of the disease process. Modify your exercise program as needed. If your symptoms worsen, adjust the exercise program to your capabilities or stop completely in case of severe decline in function. Following an exacerbation, you may be increasingly sensitive to fatigue, in which case exercise may be detrimental. Overfatigue may prevent performance of functional activities such as transfers, wheelchair propulsion, dressing, and so on. Reinitiation of the exercise program may be appropriate after recovery (remission) from the exacerbation; however, you must have medical clearance first.

MS Exercise Precautions

- Wear loose-fitting, light clothes—do not exercise in heavy sweatshirts or jackets.
- Avoid warm temperatures. If swimming or exercising in the water, check the water temperature. It should be cool, not warm or hot.
- Take rest periods as needed.
- Maintain a moderate to less-than-moderate exercise intensity to avoid fatigue.
- If balance is impaired, exercise seated or on a mat rather than in stance.
- Do not exercise through exacerbations (worsening of symptoms). Obtain medical clearance before restarting your exercise program.
- Modify or adjust your exercise program as needed according to your condition and capability. The exercise program must be geared to you, not you to the program. You must customize your own program.

Note: The National Multiple Sclerosis Society offers literature regarding exercise and movement with multiple sclerosis. You can contact the National Multiple Sclerosis Society for more information:

National Multiple Sclerosis Society
733 Third Ave.
New York, NY 10017
(800) 532-7667

Your Next Move

Now that you have all the background information, turn to page 153 to determine your classification. With your classification, you will be able to identify your training program.

Neuromuscular Diseases

Neuromuscular disease (NMD) generally refers to a group of disorders that can be individually classified according to the pathologic course of the disease. Included in this general category are the muscular dystrophies (Duchenne, facioscapulohumeral, myotonic, Becker's, limb-girdle, etc.), amyotrophic lateral sclerosis (ALS), Charcot-Marie-Tooth disease, and others. Refer to Table 8.3 on page 144 for a list and description of some neuromuscular diseases. A common complaint of those with a neuromuscular disease is fatigue during low intensity activities of daily living, including dressing and walking. Many people are forced to alter their lifestyles by avoiding physical activity, which further diminishes their capacity to perform these daily activities. Many of these disorders have similar associated conditions, whether muscular or neurological in etiology. These include muscle weakness and atrophy, extremity contractures, spinal deformity, restrictive lung disease, and cardiovascular complications.

Associated Conditions

The primary conditions associated with neuromuscular diseases are the following.

Muscle Weakness and Atrophy.   Muscle weakness is present in most neuromuscular diseases, but its rate of progression varies—it may be rapidly progressive, as in Duchenne dystrophy and amyotrophic lateral sclerosis (ALS), or slowly progressive in other diseases, such as facioscapulohumeral dystrophy and spinal muscular atrophy. In Duchenne dystrophy, strength loss progresses rapidly in a linear fashion, and

Disease	Onset	Progression	Initial distribution	Cardiac involvement
Duchenne MD	Early childhood	Rapid	Pelvic and femoral	Yes
Becker's MD	Late childhood	Fast, but slower than Duchenne	Pelvic and femoral	Occasional
Facioscapulo-humeral MD	Adolescence or later	Very slow	Facial, periscapular, perihumeral	Rare
Myotonic MD	Late	Intermediate	Facial, ocular, distal limbs	Common
Limb-girdle MD	Early or late	Intermediate to slow	Shoulder or hip girdle	Rare
Friedreich's ataxia	Late	Slow	Trunk, shoulder or hip girdle	Common
Amyotrophic lateral sclerosis (ALS)	Late	Intermediate to rapid	Distal limbs	Rare
Progressive spinal muscular atrophy	Early or late	Slow	Distal to proximal limbs	Rare
Progressive bulbar palsy	Late	Intermediate to rapid	Muscles of mastication and swallowing	Rare
Charcot-Marie-Tooth disease	Middle childhood	Slow	Distal limbs	Rare

Table 8.3
Summary of Features Seen in Neuromuscular Diseases

approximately 50% of normal strength remains at about age 10. The pattern and progression of weakness in both fast- and slow-progressing disorders varies greatly, and you should consider your individual strengths and weaknesses before starting an exercise program.

Extremity Contractures. Extremity contractures are shortening of muscles and other connective tissue. Contractures are common in Duchenne dystrophy and early-onset spinal muscular atrophy, but are rare in the other diseases. Contractures develop because of muscle weakness characterized by muscle imbalances. For example, you may lose significant muscle strength in the knee extensors with less involvement in the knee flexors. Habitual posture with the knees flexed predisposes you to a knee flexion contracture. Any joint that is not moved through its full range of motion can develop a contracture. Limited joint range of motion and contractures can decrease or limit function, including walking. Management of contractures includes early initiation of range-of-motion management programs by medical professionals. Flexibility exercises, passive stretches, or both must be continued throughout life.

Spinal Deformity. Neuromuscular disease also affects the muscles supporting the spinal column. Progressive weakness of the paraspinal muscles, the muscles supporting the spine, can result in abnormal spinal curves varying from mild to severe, depending on the progression and severity. Abnormal spinal curves—scoliosis, kyphoscoliosis, and lordosis, should be managed by medical professionals as soon as the curvature is discovered. In many cases, adequate positioning, bracing, or both can help prevent progression of spinal deformity.

Restrictive Lung Disease. Pulmonary complications are related to the progression of weakness in the muscles of respiration. People with Duchenne dystrophy and amyotrophic lateral sclerosis will have greater difficulties in respiration than people with the slowly progressing disorders.

Cardiovascular Complications. Cardiac complications in neuromuscular diseases may include cardiac arrhythmias, congestive heart failure, and right and left ventricular dilation. Cardiomyopathy has also been reported in some neuromuscular diseases. People with neuromuscular diseases may also be at risk for cardiovascular disease because of obesity and a sedentary lifestyle. Medical clearance before starting an exercise program can identify potential cardiac risks or precautions.

Exercise Readiness Assessment

Before developing an exercise program, assess the following areas:

- The date of onset of the disorder and medical clearance for exercise
- Strength and available active range of motion
- Balance and trunk stability
- Flexibility
- Your activity level

The date of onset of your condition will help identify the rate of progression and the severity of muscle atrophy. Exercise is not appropriate for everyone with a neuromuscular disease. If your condition is a fast-progressing disorder, you probably should not use resistive exercise. Slower

progressing disorders may allow you to participate in exercise programs. Please refer to Table 8.4 for a general profile of appropriate and nonappropriate participation in exercise.

You should initially assess your ability to perform active range-of-motion exercises with the upper extremities. If you have difficulty with simple active movements, an exercise program may not be appropriate. A manual muscle test will assess the strength of the remaining muscles. If you have a significant muscle loss or atrophy of 20% or greater, consult with your physician for exercise clearance and restrictions. If you have slow progressive muscle loss or symptoms, resistance training may be appropriate. A manual muscle test performed by medical professionals can objectively assess strength in the affected muscle groups and will help determine the muscles that need strengthening and the appropriate exercise modes. Retesting can help you evaluate strength gains and program effectiveness.

Balance and trunk stability determine what mode of strengthening, free weights or machines, would be most appropriate and if you need external support to stabilize the upper and lower trunk during exercise. You may be able to perform overhead activities such as the shoulder press; however, you may require some form of support or assistance.

You must also assess your flexibility. Muscle weakness and imbalance, along with habitual postures, will lead to muscle tightness and contractures. Range of motion assessment helps identify which muscles need stretching.

A survey of your typical activity level can help you determine the appropriateness of exercise. Your daily activity level can indicate your tolerance to an exercise program—if you show high fatigue during low-level activities such as dressing, meal preparation, and wheelchair propulsion, you may not be able to exercise.

Exercise Modifications and Training Considerations

The level of fitness and trainability varies greatly among the different neuromuscular diseases according to the rate of disease progression and the degree of weakness secondary to muscle wasting (atrophy) and inactivity.

Depending on the remaining trunk musculature, there are several ways to assist sitting balance during exercise. The most common is

Table 8.4 Neuromuscular Disease Exercise Profiles	
Appropriate profile	Nonappropriate profile
Minimum degree of weakness	Severe weakness
Slow progression of disease	Fast progression of disease
Supervised exercise programs	Unsupervised exercise programs
Slow progression of exercise program (muscular endurance)	High-resistive fast progression of exercise program design
Concentric exercise	Eccentric exercise
Survey total daily physical activity level	Doesn't take daily physical activity into account

to wrap a binder or strap around you and the chair. If you have severely limited trunk muscles, you will require a firm binder or strap to safely perform an arm exercise. If you have only minimal muscle weakness or trunk balance difficulties, you can use an elastic binder with some "give."

If you have muscular weakness or wasting, you should maximize the strength of functioning muscles by splinting or using braces. For example, you can compensate for weak triceps muscles by using an elbow splint to maintain elbow extension, which allows you to perform shoulder exercises, such as shoulder front and side raises.

Progressive weakening and nonfunction of the muscles can lead to muscle tightness and contractures. To counteract contractures, include stretches in exercise routines. Because active stretches may be very physically demanding for people with significant muscle weakness, use rest periods judiciously during stretches or ask a family member or workout partner to perform the flexibility exercises for you (passive range of motion). In anyone with moderate to severe weakness, flexibility should be the primary or only exercise program focus.

The goal of a strengthening program is to maintain function in the working muscles. Resistance training is not appropriate for muscles that are unable to move against gravity; however, you may be able to use these muscles in gravity-eliminated active range-of-motion exercises. Active exercises can maintain range of motion and have positive psychological effects.

Be very careful when starting a resistance program, and ignore the overload principle. The initial program focus should consist of active range-of-motion exercises with few repetitions with minimal resistance. Use one set of 5 to 10 repetitions as tolerated and increase these parameters slowly.

If tolerated, perform multijoint exercises instead of single-joint exercises because they work more muscle groups, limiting the number of exercises needed to perform a balanced exercise program. This may help reduce or eliminate overfatigue. Use rest periods as needed.

Many neuromuscular diseases are progressive so you should be consistently monitored. If weakness appears to be increasing, stop the exercise program and consult with your physician before restarting the exercise program. When in doubt,

seek consultation. Overfatigue can cause permanent loss of muscle function.

Response to Exercise

People with neuromuscular diseases have significantly decreased maximum work capacities and oxygen consumption during submaximal and maximal exercise testing. The fact of decreased work capacity in neuromuscular disorders is well known, but the role and effects of exercise with this population have been controversial. The concept of overwork weakness has been well documented in ALS, poliomyelitis, and muscular dystrophies.

Overwork Weakness. This theory suggests that strenuous everyday activity accelerates weakness in the dystrophic muscles due to irreversible degeneration of the muscle fibers. Many of the studies involving Duchenne muscular dystrophy support the overwork weakness theory. Fowler et al. (1968) found excessively elevated muscular-derived enzymes in muscular dystrophy subjects compared to a normal control group following a strengthening program. Johnson and Braddom (1971) reported the occurrence of overwork weakness in a family with facioscapulohumeral muscular dystrophy. Their investigation showed asymmetrical weakness of the shoulder girdle on the dominant side, and they concluded that this decreased strength supported the overwork weakness theory.

Positive Exercise Response. Other studies show no definitive deleterious effects from strength training in slow progressive neuromuscular diseases, whereas they reported significant increases in muscle strength following exercise programs. Florence and Hagberg (1984) looked at subjects with slowly progressing neuromuscular disease and concluded that aerobic and anaerobic training adaptations may not differ from those in healthy subjects.

These studies suggest that exercise strength training is appropriate and beneficial for persons with neuromuscular disease if the degree of weakness is not severe and the progression of the disease is relatively slow. In people with severely weak muscles or significant muscle loss, as in Duchenne muscular dystrophy, resistive training is not recommended and may be counterproductive, accelerating further muscle weakness. Everyone with a neuromuscular disease must be considered individually in the design of an exercise program.

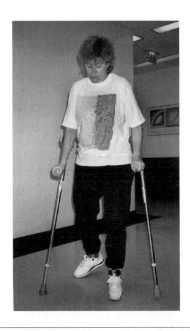

New weakness, presumably caused by the old polio conditions, can cause increased difficulties with walking.

NMD Exercise Precautions

- Receive medical clearance and restrictions before starting an exercise program.
- Avoid overfatigue. Take rest periods as needed.
- Keep exercise intensity low.
- Start with a low volume of exercise initially, one set of 5 to 10 repetitions as tolerated.
- Review your daily activity level before designing an exercise program.
- Use a slow and well-monitored exercise program progression.
- Modify or adjust the exercise program as needed according to your condition and capability. Gear the exercise program to you, not you to the program.

Your Next Move

Now that you have the background information, turn to page 153 to determine your classification. With your classification, you will be able to identify your training program.

Postpolio Syndrome

The polio virus causes damage or changes to the motor neurons resulting in muscle weakness, paralysis, and in some cases death. Poliomyelitis survivors often show significant recovery in strength following the acute or early illness, which has been attributed to the reinnervation of muscle fibers by collateral sprouting from the remaining motor neurons. Refer to chapter 6 for more specifics on polio. Vaccines have decreased the number of cases of paralytic polio in the United States from 28,000 cases in 1955 to an average of 10 cases per year. However, many polio survivors show significant decreases in muscle function, as well as weakness, pain, and fatigue approximately 30 years after the initial bout of the disease.

These new conditions, presumably caused by old polio conditions, are called postpolio syndrome. Studies estimate that 16% to 40% of polio survivors will experience one or more of the postpolio symptoms, with muscle weakness and fatigue being the most prevalent. Other identified late complications of polio include joint pain, joint instability, muscle fasiculations, muscle cramps, shortness of breath, and long bone fractures.

Late Changes of the Motor Unit Following Acute Poliomyelitis

In acute **poliomyelitis**, the virus directly attacks the motor neurons (anterior horn cells). These cells may die or recover with time. If a cell dies, the degeneration will progress down the axon and result in denervation of the muscle fibers. This means that the muscle fibers no longer have connections or input from the nervous system— the muscle has been "unplugged." The muscle can be "plugged in" again if new axons sprout from neighboring motor neurons which can lead to reinnervation of the denervated muscle fibers. The new parent motor neuron now has to nourish and innervate more muscle fibers than it did previously. Consequently, these motor units become very large with large cross-sectional areas of muscle fibers. Their size is the result of the natural adaptation to decades of impaired neuromuscular function. Studies have shown that over years these large motor units become unstable in individuals with polio.

Associated Conditions

Muscle weakness, fatigue, and joint and muscle pain may occur with postpolio syndrome.

Muscle Weakness.   Weakness is usually prominent in the muscles previously affected by the polio virus; however, new weakness has been reported in muscles that were apparently unaffected by the acute polio virus. Early studies used manual muscle testing for grading muscle function; when muscle strength was measured quantitatively, the average knee extensor strength in polio survivors graded "normal" by manual testing was actually 50% of normal. This indicates that the early studies overestimated strength from functioning motor units that were probably affected by the acute virus.

Most investigations indicate that changes in the motor unit, which is the motor neuron and all the muscle fibers that it innervates, are the primary reason for problems occurring some 30 years after the onset of polio. Some theories for these changes include reactivation of the poliomyelitis, the normal aging process in previously damaged motor neurons, musculoskeletal disuse, and overwork weakness.

The controversy about the appropriateness of exercise for individuals with postpolio syndrome stems from the overwork weakness theory, which states that remaining unstable motor neurons work under an increased metabolic load that eventually results in neurological dysfunction (muscle weakness). The instability may be due to delayed reinnervation of muscle, the inability of the motor neuron to sustain reinnervation in too large a muscle area, and limited metabolic capacity of the motor neuron. Studies suggest that the giant motor neurons may not be able to keep up with the metabolic demands of all their sprouts, resulting in slow deterioration. Weakness occurs progressively as more and more muscle fibers are lost. The loss of a large motor unit that innervates a significant amount of muscle fibers has a much greater functional impact than the loss of a single motor unit in a normal muscle.

You may show a high level of physical function following acute polio symptoms, which illustrates the ability to compensate for muscle weakness by using the spared functioning muscle groups. Late-onset muscle weakness can disrupt this compensation, severely decreasing your function and lifestyle. For example, you may have been walking independently with the use of an assistive device and leg brace for many years, and now you may progressively show less endurance with walking, driving, and dressing, and need more time to recover from these activities.

Fatigue.   Fatigue is a common but partly unexplained complaint present in 60% to 90% of polio patients. Fatigue may occur as a feeling of overwhelming exhaustion, a low level of energy and endurance, and sometimes a decrease in mental alertness. These feelings may be a combination of central fatigue—the failure of the central nervous system, the brain, and the spinal cord to consistently activate the muscles (decreased neural drive)—and peripheral fatigue—the failure of the motor unit, the motor neurons outside the spinal cord, and all the muscle fibers they innervate to maintain a given force during repeated contractions such as those needed in walking or wheelchair propulsion. Some studies have postulated that peripheral fatigue is the mechanism for a new onset of muscle weakness. When fatigue occurs, you must stop, rest, and pace your activity level.

One investigation reports that symptomatic postpolio subjects show much slower strength recovery time at the same relative force levels following exhausting isometric activity than asymptomatic postpolio subjects and nonpolio control subjects. This indicates the importance of pacing activities if you show symptomatic postpolio signs. Agre and Rodriguez (1991) found that postpolio individuals have the appropriate sensations to allow them to pace their activities and that they should avoid overfatigue.

Investigations of postpolio emphasize the importance of being active within the limits of safety and comfort for both physical and psychological reasons. Remember that cardiorespiratory and musculoskeletal deconditioning result from inactivity.

Joint and Muscle Pain.   Complaints of muscle and joint pain are common with polio. Joint pains are typically associated with specific weight-bearing activities such as walking, but they usually do not include swelling or inflammation. Muscle pains are also typically aggravated by activity and cold temperatures. In many cases, studies indicate that the weight-bearing joints are unstable and not adequately supported by orthosis or bracing. One investigation indicated that an appropriate orthotic prescription significantly improved the ability to walk, increased perceived walking safety, and reduced knee and overall pain in 36 polio survivors. Conservative treatments such as lowering activity levels, increasing support of the unstable joints, and improving biomechanics during daily activities are often recommended for pain management.

Exercise Readiness Assessment

Before beginning your exercise program, assess the following areas:

- Your medical screening
- Muscle strength
- Range of motion
- Your daily activities

You should have a medical screening and physician's clearance for exercise before starting an exercise program. Exercise restrictions and precautions should be recorded on the medical form. The following are questions that you should ask yourself:

- Have I experienced a recent onset of new muscle weakness? If so, in which muscles?
- Is the new weakness present in muscles initially affected by the polio virus, or are different muscles now weak?
- What is my daily activity level?

A muscle strength assessment will help determine which muscles are appropriate for exercise. EMG studies and isokinetic machines are excellent tools for objective strength assessment. Exercise is appropriate for the muscles that were not affected by the polio virus. Muscles that were initially affected but have not shown any signs of pain or new onset of muscle weakness may benefit from a short-term customized exercise program. Exercising symptomatic muscles or muscles that are experiencing pain or a new onset of muscle weakness is contraindicated. Exercising those muscles can potentially increase the symptoms of weakness and pain. See Table 8.5 for exercise guidelines.

Range of motion assessment can help identify movement limitations. Muscles affected by the polio virus are hypotonic and generally not limited in range of motion. The stronger muscles opposing the hypotonic muscles may get tight. This may set you up for a muscle imbalance that may eventually cause pain.

A personal survey of your typical daily activity level can help you determine the appropriateness of exercise. Your exercise program should coincide with your normal activities to avoid periods of fatigue. If your exercise program causes

Table 8.5 General Exercise Guidelines for Postpolio Syndrome	
Condition	Exercise Guidelines
Unaffected (normal) muscles	EMG studies can assist in the diagnosis of unaffected muscles. No restrictions for unaffected muscles. Slow progression of exercise program design. Emphasize endurance and pacing. Flexibility exercises should be included in all programs.
Asymptomatic affected muscles (no indication of new muscle weakness)	Follow physician's recommendations and guidelines. Supervised, slow progression of exercise program design. Training load should be kept at a submaximal level with emphasis on endurance. Limit resistance training period to 1 to 2 months to allow for strength gains and perform cycles to maintain gains. After completion of training period, progress to endurance activities or generally increased daily activities.
Symptomatic affected muscles (new onset of weak muscles)	Resistance training contraindicated. Emphasize body alignment and energy conservation.

excessive fatigue that interferes with your normal activities, stop and reassess the appropriateness of the exercise.

Exercise Modifications, Training Considerations, and Response

Next we'll review aerobic and resistance training as they apply to postpolio syndrome to help you set up your exercise program.

Aerobic Training. Despite concerns about overwork weakness, many researchers stress the importance of being physically active. The role, response, and mode of exercise for postpolio, however, varies greatly and relates to the amount of functioning muscle mass and the presence or absence of conditions such as new weakness, pain, fatigue, and the like. An exercise program can range from gentle, active stretches to more vigorous aerobic and resistance exercises. Studies have indicated that despite a compromised neuromuscular status, individuals with postpolio can show significant increases in cardiovascular fitness through exercise. Jones et al. (1989) recommend a day of rest between exercise sessions and a series of minirests between exercise bursts. For example, you can perform 2 to 3 min of exercise on a stationary bicycle with a 1-min rest between bouts. These authors conclude that the interval approach may allow postpolio individuals to increase cardiorespiratory endurance while minimizing chances of neuromuscular damage by allowing sufficient recovery time. Swimming, aquatic exercise, use of exercise bicycles, and other exercises that don't require weight bearing may be appropriate because they decrease microtrauma and joint overuse. More studies are needed on the long-term effects of aerobic exercise in the postpolio population. Those with symptomatic postpolio with symptoms of fatigue and pain, however, may be limited to general active stretching; aerobic exercise may be counterproductive for them.

Resistance Training.   Resistance training programs for postpolio have produced increases in strength and function without discomfort or negative effects on the neuromuscular system. Neural factors probably play a key role in strength gains in this population by increasing the activation of prime movers in a specific movement.

According to the overwork weakness theory, long-term resistance training may lead to new muscle weakness and decreased function. Because of the uncertainty of the effects of long-term resistance training, we recommend long-term resistance training only for people whose muscles show no clinical or EMG evidence of prior polio involvement. Polio-affected muscles used for daily activities may show muscle hypertrophy as an adaptation from long-term stresses, and further increases in load may be deleterious.

Some researchers have recommended short resistance training periods of 1 to 2 months for asymptomatic muscles affected by the initial polio virus to increase strength for general activity and possibly to enhance training programs. Training should be kept at a submaximal level with emphasis on endurance. Antigravity muscles should be strengthened including the knee extensors, hip extensors, and lower back muscles. Weakness in these postural muscles can decrease the ability to walk by demanding more effort from muscles, which causes a faster onset of fatigue. Symptomatic muscle groups, those having weakness, pain, or fatigue, should not be exercised. Further research is needed concerning the adaptations, limitation, and long-term training effects of resistance exercise programs.

All resistance programs should be closely supervised. You should start with low-intensity workouts and gradually increase the resistance tolerated under supervision. Continually monitor for symptoms of fatigue. The feeling of weakness and discomfort several hours following exercise is a sign of excessive activity—overtraining. If new muscle weakness, pain, or excessive fatigue occurs, stop the exercise program and consult your physician. Your physician should be notified before starting an exercise program.

 Note: These guidelines are to assist in prescribing safe exercise routines and may not strictly apply to everyone. Consult your physician for your individual restrictions and guidelines.

Postpolio Precautions and Guidelines

- Receive a physician's clearance and restrictions before starting an exercise program.
- Exercise asymptomatic muscles that were affected by polio carefully. Customize intentional exercise and perform the program cautiously.
- Do not exercise to exhaustion. It is important to pace all of your activities. Use intervals of work and rest rather than continuous activity if appropriate.
- Keep training loads at submaximal levels.
- Avoid long-term resistance training for asymptomatic muscles that were affected by polio. Keep periods of resistance training short and cycled (1-2 months), and progress to endurance activities or a general increase in daily activity.
- Resistance training for symptomatic muscles (which show a new onset of muscle weakness) is contraindicated.

- All exercise programs require supervision and monitoring.
- Keep the progression of your exercise program slow.
- Do not exercise if you have pain.

Your Next Move

Now that you have the background information, turn to page 153 to determine your classification. With your classification, you will be able to identify your training program.

Dwarfism

Dwarfism is defined as decreased physical growth that is greater than three standard deviations from the mean for the age group. The Dwarf Athletic Association (DAA), founded in 1985, provides people of short stature an opportunity to participate in fitness and athletic events. The DAA recognizes its membership as individuals under 5 ft tall.

Achondroplasia is the most common and best-known form of dwarfism; however, many other distinct forms of short-limbed dwarfism have been described. Achondroplasia may be inherited as an autosomal dominant trait; however, 80% to 90% of affected children are from new mutations present at birth. These findings contrast with the misconception that most growth retardation is the result of dysfunction of the endocrine system.

Most achondroplastic individuals are healthy and have normal intelligence with normal life expectancy. Some children may require surgery

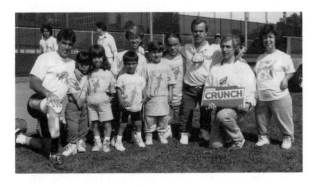

With strength training it's important to maintain muscular balance and emphasize full active range of motion, especially at the elbow due to the short extremities.

for deafness, but the need for other surgical procedures is rare. The most obvious clinical feature of achondroplasia is shortness of the extremities. The body or trunk may also appear smaller due to severe lumbar **lordosis**, which is excessive curvature of the low back. People with achondroplasia may have well-developed musculature and therefore appear to have greater than average strength.

Many of the problems associated with achondroplasia tend to be orthopedic, including bow legs, lax ligaments, spinal stenosis, and occasional paraplegia in adolescence.

Role of Exercise

Due to your overall short stature and short extremities, you may be more susceptible to weight gain and decreased range of motion. Emphasize muscle balance and flexibility in a resistance program to avoid range of motion or movement restrictions, especially of the elbow joints. Use aerobic activities and sport for weight management and to promote a healthier lifestyle.

Your Next Move

Now that you have the background information, turn to page 153 to determine your classification. With your classification, you will be able to identify your training program.

Osteogenesis Imperfecta

Osteogenesis imperfecta (OI), also known as brittle bone disease, is a disorder of collagen synthesis that results in weakness and fragility of all the bones in the body. The underlying cause of this inherited disease is unknown.

Sillence et al. (1979) identified four types of osteogenesis imperfecta based on genetic, clinical, and radiological features. The most commonly used classification divides this condition into two types—congenital, or present at birth, and tarda, later onset. The congenital type is severe and often fatal in childhood. Osteogenesis imperfecta tarda is much less severe and shows characteristically mild features. The most common of them are increased susceptibility to fractures (most typically of the lower limb), short stature, generalized joint laxity,

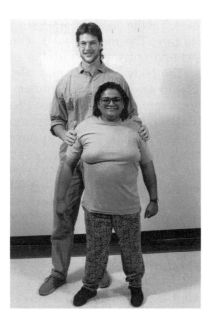

1991 World Champion female bench presser for the National Wheelchair Athletic Association with osteogenesis imperfecta. Note her short stature and bowed extremities, common characteristics of OI.

possible limb and spine deformities, and deafness in middle age.

Role of Exercise

The bones in people with OI seem to become stronger after puberty, and adults with the disorder have less frequent fractures; however, the fragility never completely disappears. Remain active to avoid disuse osteoporosis in the already-weak bones and the other ravages of inactivity (obesity, cardiovascular risks, etc.). The muscles and ligaments appear to be relatively stronger than the bones to which they are attached. Because of the typical joint instability or abnormal joint elasticity, resistance training is recommended to increase muscular strength around the joints, which promotes joint stability. Be cautious when starting an exercise program—begin with a lower initial load or intensity and progress slowly. Although uncommon, cases of tendon ruptures have been reported in jumping and sports activities. Avoid fast, ballistic, and closed kinetic exercises that move over a fixed limb due to the possibility of overstressing weakened tendons and lax joints. A physical with the physician's clearance and restrictions for exercise should be obtained before starting an exercise program.

Your Next Move

Now that you have the background information, turn to page 153 of this chapter to determine your classification. With your classification, you will be able to identify your training program.

Arthrogryposis

Arthrogryposis is not a specific disease but rather a descriptive term for significant limitations of movement and rigid joints at birth. Over 150 different conditions characterized by congenital contractures are classified as arthrogryposis. Their exact causes are not known; however, theories include decreased movement or immobility of the fetus, genetic defects, prenatal exposure to environmental agents, and maternal infection. Arthrogryposis is nonprogressive and occurs in 0.03% of the general population.

Arthrogryposis can be classified as neuropathic (originating in the nervous system), myopathic (originating in the muscles), or mixed. Neuropathic arthrogryposis is the most common, occurring in 90% of all cases.

Arthrogryposis severely limits range of motion, leaving only a few degrees of active or passive pain-free motion. Affected extremities are small and the joints quite large in comparison. Other features characteristic of arthrogryposis include weak, atrophied, or absent muscle groups, multiple joint dislocations, and fixed or rigid extremities. Extremities can be fixed in any position but there are familiar patterns, which are described in Table 8.6. The muscles of the head are typically spared.

Aggressive range of motion exercise during adulthood will not increase movement of stiff, deformed joints; however, the joints can be positioned in more functional positions early in life. Much of the medical management of arthrogryposis involves orthopedic procedures during infancy and early childhood such as range of motion training, surgical procedures, and positioning. Despite severe physical joint limitations, people with the condition often show great dexterity with good functional results. Adaptability in performing specific functions quite commonly makes surgical intervention unnecessary. Most people with arthrogryposis have normal intelligence and lead full, productive lives with the use of adaptive devices.

Table 8.6
Common Contractures Seen in Arthrogryposis

Joint	Position
Shoulder	Adduction, internal rotation
Elbow	Extension (flexion less common)
Wrist	Flexion, pronation, and ulnar deviation
Hip	Flexion, abduction, and external rotation
Knee	Flexion
Ankle	Equinovarus (club feet)

Role of Exercise

Assess your available active range of motion initially to identify what movements you can use for exercise. Then you can maintain these movements by simple active range-of-motion exercises without resistance.

Also assess your strength of available movements by using a manual muscle test to identify the antigravity and reduced gravity strength of the available joint movements. If joint movements are functional, try to strengthen the ones that are unable to move against gravity. Use simple active range-of-motion exercises to maintain the strength of the antigravity movements. You can use resistance if you need more strength for functional tasks such as reaching, eating, and so on.

Precautions

Due to changes in joint biomechanics and muscle imbalances, synovitis can occur. Synovitis is an inflammation of the synovial tissue in the joint, which appears as swollen, reddened, warm, and locally tender. Alert your physician if this occurs so that proper medical management can take place.

Your Next Move

Now that you have the background information, determine your classification so you will be able to identify your training program.

Classification and Exercise Guidelines

It is time to identify your classification and to locate the corresponding exercise program. Because of the great variability in all of the Les Autres disability groups, the classification system uses nine functional profiles (see Table 8.7). To use the following exercise programs and the exercise index, decide on the class that is appropriate for you using the following charts. Once you have found the appropriate class, photocopied the following training log, identified your training program, and made the necessary modifications to it, you can learn about the specific exercises you will perform during your workout. Part III provides explanations and photographs of these exercises.

Table 8.7
Les Autres Classification

Class	Description
LX	• Severe spasticity, athetosis, and/or deformity in all four extremities • Less than fair muscle strength and poor sitting balance • Requires a power wheelchair for daily living
L1	• Severe spasticity, athetosis, and/or deformity in all four extremities • Moderately reduced muscle strength, range of motion, and/or spasticity in throwing arm • Poor sitting balance • Requires a manual wheelchair for daily living
L2	• Moderate spasticity, athetosis, and/or deformity in throwing arm • Poor sitting balance • Requires a manual wheelchair for daily living
L3	• Normal function in throwing arm with poor to moderate reduction in sitting balance or minimal to moderate spasticity, athetosis, and/or deformity in throwing arm with good sitting balance • Requires a manual wheelchair for daily living
L4	• Normal function in throwing arm with good sitting balance
L5	• Walks with severe involvement (spasticity, athetosis, deformity) in function of lower extremities or with decreased balance together with minimally decreased function in throwing arm • Can ambulate with an assistive device (e.g., crutches)
L6	• Walks with moderate involvement (spasticity, athetosis, deformity) of lower extremities or with decreased standing balance • Throwing arm is normal • Does not use an assistive device for walking
L7	• Walks with minimal to moderate involvement (spasticity, athetosis, deformity) in lower extremities • Minimal standing balance and coordination difficulties with minimally decreased function in throwing arm
L8	• Walks with minimal trunk and lower extremity involvement • Normal function in throwing arm and reduced function in nonthrowing arm

Note. The above exercise protocols per class are general guidelines only and may not be exclusively appropriate for each les autres individual. Refer to the disability-specific sections to see if an exercise protocol is applicable to the individual.

Other Disabilities

Weight					Date	Sets/reps	Exercises	Notes

LA CLASS LX AND 1 EXERCISE GUIDELINES

Due to differences in coordination and associated conditions within these classes, prescribing a single routine for everyone is not possible. Each of you in these classes must have a customized program. Refer to the following guidelines when designing your program.

POSITION All exercises will be performed from your wheelchair—this is the optimal position to allow you adequate balance and support. Strapping may be useful to maintain your balance. Refer to the information about positioning and strapping on pages 26 to 29.

EXERCISE OPTIONS Suggesting specific exercises for this class is not appropriate because each of you will have control over different muscle groups or movements. Your exercise options will be limited to these movements. Choose movements that are, or can be, functional for you. Most of your exercises will focus on your arms, although some Class 1 individuals may have some purposeful movements in the legs that they can also emphasize. You typically will not have the coordination or the hand grasp function to allow the use of conventional exercise equipment, so your exercise options include manually guided resistance from a workout partner. You can use wraparound weights for movements you can safely perform independently with adequate strength and control. Despite limited exercise choices for these two classes, exercise training can enhance sports performance (i.e., boccie, slalom) and can have a positive psychological effect.

EXERCISE VARIABLES When coordination is poor, exercise intensity or resistance is less important. Emphasize reinforcing smooth, isolated movements. A workout partner can guide your arm through the exercise range of motion rather than you directly resisting the movement.

Apply resistance in planes perpendicular to the desired movement. This technique is sometimes helpful to decrease extraneous movements out of the desired exercise pattern. If you achieve better control of the exercise movement, you can decrease or eliminate the perpendicular resistance.

LA CLASS 2 EXERCISE GUIDELINES

| POSITION | You may exercise in your wheelchair, on a bench, or on a mat. You may be able to exercise on your stomach, but this must be determined individually. Scoliosis may limit your positions. Check with your physician regarding any precautions. People in this class typically have increased tone in the legs, especially with extreme effort using the arms. When performing arm exercises on your back or on your stomach, stretch your legs before positioning yourself on the bench or mat. Then position the legs with some slack in the muscles, keeping a small bend in the hips or knees. This position is less likely to predispose you to abnormal increases in muscle tone. Strapping may be beneficial for many of you, especially if you are performing heavy lifts such as on the bench press. Some of you in this class may have a history of hip dislocations or other hip disorders. If so, strapping should be at or above the waist level rather than directly on the hips. Refer to the information about positioning and strapping on pages 26 to 29.

| EXERCISE OPTIONS | You may be able to perform all upper extremity exercises with free weights or conventional exercise machines. If you have decreased coordination in your arms, you will have to determine whether you can safely control free weights with proper technique. Otherwise, use exercise machines for the movements you have difficulty controlling. Typically these are over-the-head exercises such as the shoulder press. Lower extremity exercises will be limited because of spasticity, so you'll have to individualize your lower extremity exercise program according to your abilities. Your emphasis may be stretching, but if you do have active, controllable movements in your legs, you should work these muscle groups. Throughout the exercise program emphasize the muscles that oppose the spastic ones. The following are suggested exercises for your class, but keep in mind that your exercise program needs to be customized to your abilities.

Upper Extremity
Bench press   p. 176
Straight-arm back raise   p. 187
Shoulder overhead press   p. 164
Lat pull-downs   p. 178

Lower Extremity
Leg side raises   p. 214
Leg back raises   p. 216
Knee extensions   p. 218
Leg curls   p. 212
Straight leg raise   p. 213

| EXERCISE VARIABLES | Your exercise intensity should start out low. Make sure that you have selected the appropriate exercise mode, free weights or machines, and that you perform the exercises with proper technique prior to adding more resistance.

LA CLASSES 3, 4, AND 5 EXERCISE GUIDELINES

POSITION You may exercise sitting in your wheelchair, on your stomach, or on your back. Position and secure yourself in the desired position. Your lower extremity muscle tone and range of motion usually do not limit your upper extremity exercise.

EXERCISE OPTIONS You should be able to perform most upper extremity exercises with free weights. The type of equipment available to you will be the only limiting factor in selecting the mode of your upper extremity exercises. Your lower extremity exercises will be limited secondary by spasticity and should be chosen according to your individual abilities. Your lower extremity emphasis should include stretching for your spastic muscles, emphasizing the muscle groups that oppose the spastic ones. Suggested exercises for your class follow, but keep in mind that you should customize your exercise program to your abilities.

Upper Extremity
Bench press   p. 176
Straight-arm back raise   p. 187
Shoulder overhead press   p. 164
Lat pull-downs   p. 178

Lower Extremity
Leg side raises   p. 214
Leg back raises   p. 216
Knee extensions   p. 218
Leg curls   p. 212
Straight leg raise   p. 213

LA CLASSES 6 AND 7 EXERCISE GUIDELINES

POSITION   You may exercise sitting in your wheelchair, on your stomach, on your back, or possibly standing if your balance allows. Position and secure yourself in the desired position. Your lower extremity muscle tone and range of motion usually do not limit your upper extremity exercise.

EXERCISE OPTIONS   You should be able to perform most upper extremity exercises with free weights. The type of equipment available to you will be the only limiting factor in selecting the mode of your upper extremity exercises. Your lower extremity exercises will be limited by spasticity and should be chosen according to your individual abilities. Your lower extremity emphasis should include stretching for your spastic muscles, emphasizing the muscle groups that oppose the spastic ones. Suggested exercises for your class follow, but keep in mind that you should customize your exercise program to your abilities.

Upper Extremity
Bench press   p. 176
Straight-arm back raise   p. 187
Shoulder overhead press   p. 164
Lat pull-downs   p. 178

Lower Extremity
Leg side raises   p. 214
Leg back raises   p. 216
Knee extensions   p. 218
Leg curls   p. 212
Straight leg raise   p. 213

LA CLASS 8 EXERCISE GUIDELINES

POSITION You have no limitations and can assume all positions; strapping for balance is rarely required.

EXERCISE OPTIONS No limitations. You can use free weights with all exercises. Initial supervision may be required. Your exercise routine should reflect your muscular balance. The following are suggested exercises for your class.

Upper Extremity
Bench press   p. 176
Bent-over rows   p. 174
Straight-arm back raise   p. 187
Shoulder overhead press   p. 164
Lat pull-downs   p. 178
Dips   p. 173
Triceps extensions   p. 188
Biceps curl   p. 191

Lower Extremity
Squats   p. 210
Lunges   p. 211
Leg curls   p. 212
Knee extensions   p. 218
Ankle curls   p. 219
Heel raises   p. 220

PART III

Conditioning Exercises and Classes

This section of the manual presents the exercises you will perform and information on how to organize and select an exercise class. The exercises listed offer options and different set-ups to work all your major muscle groups.

Although this part of the book offers a comprehensive exercise index, it is not all-inclusive. You may have additional exercise options based on the equipment available to you. Use the following exercises as a guide and pay attention to the line of pull in each so you are actually working the muscles that you set out to work.

The exercises are grouped by sections of the body. The order of exercises is as follows:

- Chapter 9, "Upper Extremity Exercises"
- Chapter 10, "Abdominal and Trunk Exercises"
- Chapter 11, "Lower Extremity Exercises"
- Chapter 12, "Elements of a Good Exercise Class"

A full menu of the exercises presented is listed at the beginning of each exercise chapter.

CHAPTER 9

Upper Extremity Exercises

The following exercises are found on the pages indicated.

UPPER EXTREMITY MULTIJOINT

UPPER EXTREMITY SINGLE JOINT

SHOULDER OVERHEAD PRESS

MUSCLES STRENGTHENED

Deltoids

Pectoralis major (clavicular)

Serratus anterior

Supraspinatus

Triceps

Upper and middle trapezius

BARBELL

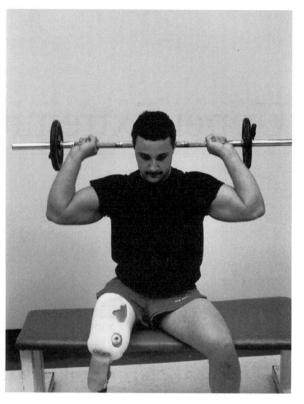

STARTING POSITION
Grip bar with palms facing forward (pronated) and hands slightly wider than shoulders. Hold barbell at shoulder level, keeping back straight and head level.

MOVEMENT
1. Press barbell overhead until elbows are completely extended and barbell is positioned above shoulders.
2. Slowly return barbell to starting position before starting next repetition.

ALTERNATE
For more emphasis on anterior musculature, perform same exercise lowering bar in front of head to upper chest.

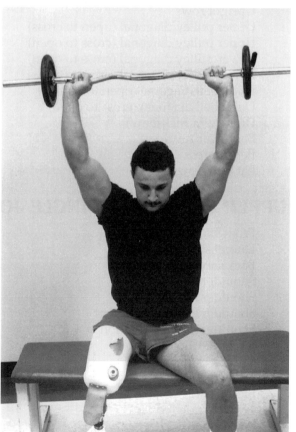

DUMBBELL

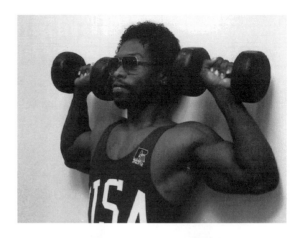

STARTING POSITION
Grasp dumbbells with palms facing forward (pronated). Hold dumbbells at shoulder level, keeping back straight and head level.

MOVEMENT
Use the movement described for the barbell.

TIPS
This is appropriate for mid- to high-paraplegic individuals. Keep shoulders square and body movement minimal. Lifter can lean against a wall or sit in a high-backed chair for greater trunk balance.

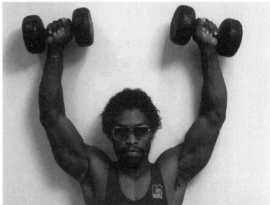

UNIVERSAL

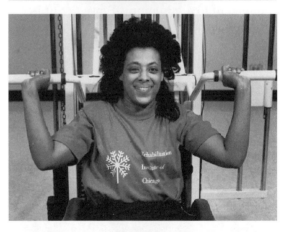

STARTING POSITION
Use the position described when using a barbell.

MOVEMENT
Use the movement described for the barbell.

TIPS
Machine exercises are the preferred mode for exercisers with decreased trunk balance or coordination. To avoid impingement syndromes, over-the-head exercises should not be performed until you have adequate scapular stability.

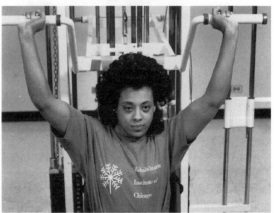

UPRIGHT ROWS

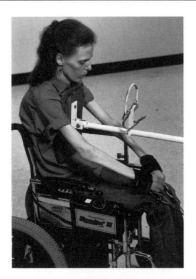

MUSCLES STRENGTHENED

Biceps brachii

Brachialis

Brachioradialis

Posterior and middle deltoid

Pronator teres

Upper and middle trapezius

STARTING POSITION

Start with arms extended, palms facing body (pronated), and cables crossed.

MOVEMENT

1. Pull arms up and back, with elbows pointed upward through full range of motion.
2. Hold at top position.
3. Slowly return to starting position.

TIPS

Keep cables, barbells, or dumbbells close to body throughout exercise. Stay erect. Keep body movement to a minimum. Tense the upper back muscles at the top position.

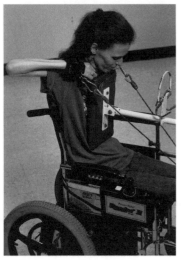

VARIATIONS AND ALTERNATE SET-UPS

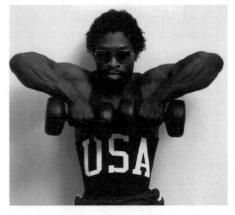

Dumbbell Upright Rows—Hold dumbbells close together and close to body. Raise arms with elbows pointed upward.

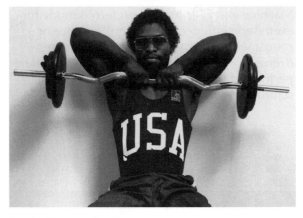

Barbell Upright Rows—Grip bar with hands 6 in. or closer together. Raise arms with elbows pointed up.

UPPER PULLEY DIAGONAL (Open to Cross)

MUSCLES STRENGTHENED

Anterior deltoid

Biceps brachii

Brachialis

Brachioradialis

Pectoralis major

Pronator quadratus

Pronator teres

Subscapularis

STARTING POSITION

Stand or sit perpendicular to pulley system with arm up and out to side, shoulder externally rotated, elbow extended, and palm facing forward (supination).

MOVEMENT

1. Turn palm in and down.
2. Bend elbow to bring arm across body until hand is down on outside of opposite hip with palm facing backward (pronation).

TIPS

Move only upper extremity, keeping upper trunk erect and stationary. Diagonal patterns are sport- and movement-specific. If you have decreased standing or trunk balance, perform in a sitting position.

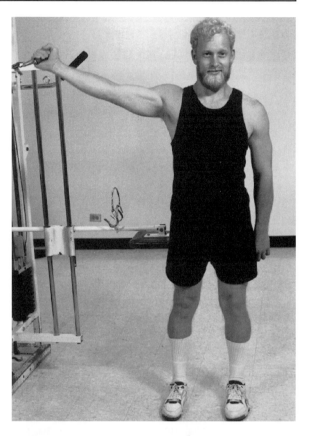

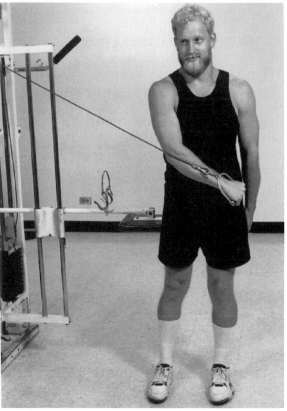

UPPER PULLEY DIAGONAL (Cross to Open)

MUSCLES STRENGTHENED

Infraspinatus

Latissimus dorsi

Middle trapezius

Posterior deltoid

Pronator quadratus

Pronator teres

Rhomboids

Teres major

Teres minor

Triceps

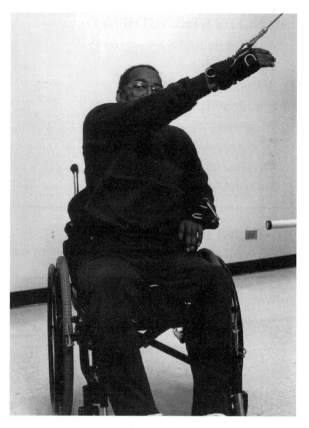

STARTING POSITION

Stand or sit perpendicular to pulley system with arm across body, shoulder externally rotated, elbow slightly flexed, and palm facing body (supination) above opposite shoulder.

MOVEMENT

1. Turn forearm in (pronation) as elbow and shoulder extend.
2. Move arm downward across body until palm is facing backward with extended arm away from body.
3. Slowly return to starting position.

TIPS

Move only upper extremity, keeping upper trunk erect and stationary. Diagonal patterns are more sport- and movement-specific. If balance allows, perform in standing position.

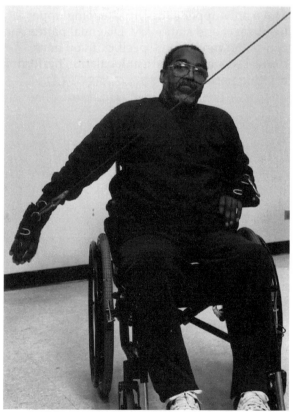

LOWER PULLEY DIAGONAL (Cross to Open)

MUSCLES STRENGTHENED

Infraspinatus

Latissimus dorsi

Middle trapezius

Posterior deltoid

Rhomboids

Supinator

Teres major

Teres minor

Triceps

STARTING POSITION

Stand or sit perpendicular to pulley system with arm across body, shoulder internally rotated, elbow slightly flexed, palm of hand facing backward (pronation) and on outside of opposite hip.

MOVEMENT

1. Turn palm forward and up (supination).
2. Extended elbow and shoulder move upward away from the body until hand faces forward with arm fully extended and above shoulder level.
3. Slowly return to starting position.

TIPS

Move only upper extremity, keeping upper trunk erect and stationary. Diagonal patterns are more sport- and movement-specific. If balance allows, perform in standing position.

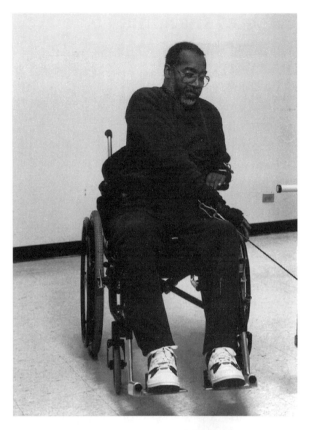

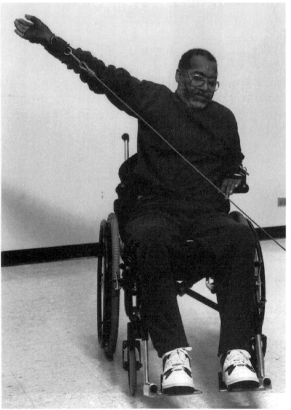

LOWER PULLEY DIAGONAL (Open to Cross)

MUSCLES STRENGTHENED

Anterior deltoid

Biceps brachii

Brachialis

Brachioradialis

Pectoralis major

Pronator quadratus

Pronator teres

Subscapularis

Supinator

STARTING POSITION

Stand or sit perpendicular to pulley system with palm of hand facing forward (supination), elbow extended, and shoulder externally rotated with arm out to the side of the body.

MOVEMENT

1. Turn palm forward and toward body.
2. Bring arm up and across body.
3. Flex elbow and shoulder joint until hand is over the opposite shoulder with palm facing backward (pronation).
4. Slowly return to starting position.

TIPS

Move only upper extremity, keeping upper trunk erect and stationary. Diagonal patterns are more sport- and movement-specific. Perform in sitting position if you have decreased standing or trunk balance.

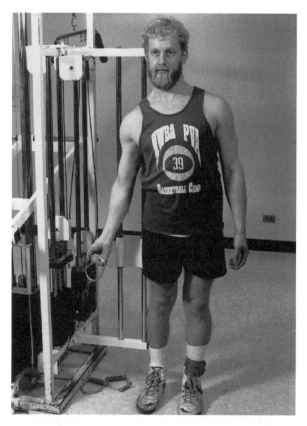

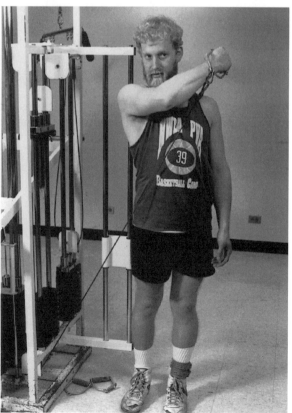

DUMBBELL DIAGONAL (Open to Cross)

MUSCLES STRENGTHENED

Anterior deltoid

Biceps

Brachialis

Brachii

Brachioradialis

Pectoralis major

Pronator quadratus

Pronator teres

Subscapularis

Supinator

STARTING POSITION

Stand or sit with arms extended and down to side. Use palms-up grip (supination) on the dumbbells.

MOVEMENT

1. Turn palms inward and up toward body (pronation).
2. Bring arms across body.
3. Flex elbows and shoulder joints until hands are over opposite shoulders with palms facing backward.
4. Slowly return to starting position.

TIPS

Move only upper extremities, keeping upper trunk erect and stationary. Bilateral activities emphasize trunk muscles by requiring trunk stabilization during arm movements. Use strapping if you have decreased upper trunk balance or coordination.

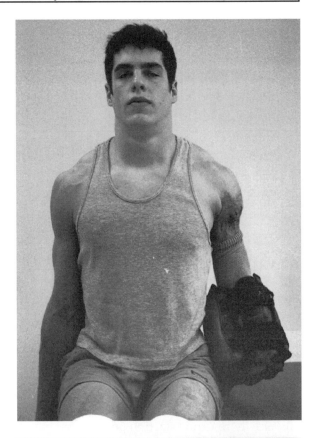

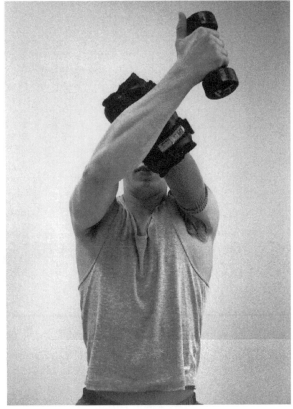

DUMBBELL DIAGONAL (Cross to Open)

MUSCLES STRENGTHENED

Infraspinatus

Latissimus dorsi

Middle trapezius

Posterior deltoid

Rhomboids

Supinator

Triceps

Teres major

Teres minor

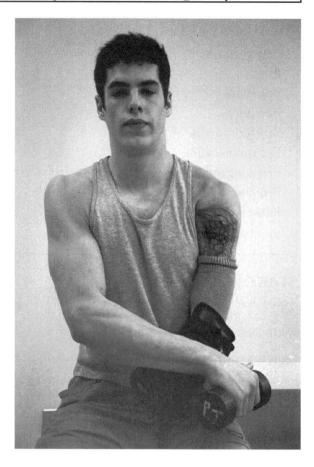

STARTING POSITION

Stand or sit with arms crossed, hands over opposite hips with palm-down grip (pronation) on the dumbbells.

MOVEMENT

1. Turn palm up (supination).
2. Elbows and shoulders extend upward away from body until hands are facing forward with arms fully extended above shoulder level.
3. Slowly return to starting position.

TIPS

Move only upper extremities, keeping upper trunk erect and stationary. Bilateral activities emphasize trunk muscles by requiring trunk stabilization during arm movement. Use strapping if you have decreased upper trunk balance or coordination.

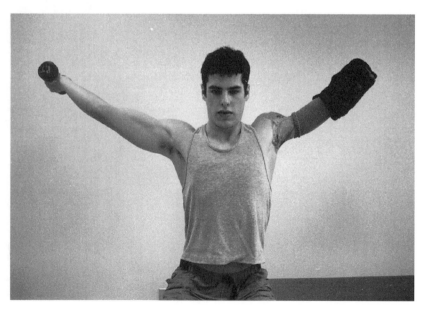

DIPS

MUSCLES STRENGTHENED

Latissimus dorsi

Lower trapezius

Pectoralis major (sternal)

Pectoralis minor

Rhomboids

Subclavius

Teres major

Triceps

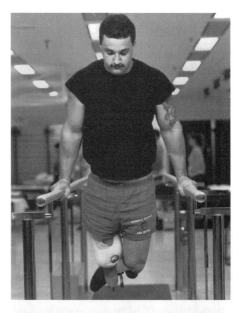

STARTING POSITION
Grip bar with palms facing body, elbows extended, shoulders depressed, and chin tucked.

MOVEMENT
1. Slowly lower body or weight until elbows are completely flexed and shoulders are shrugged up as high as ears.
2. Press body up completely, extending elbows and depressing shoulders.

TIPS
Be sure to fully depress shoulders at the start and finish of the exercise (shoulders should not be at ear level). The Rickshaw exercise can help strengthen the shoulder muscles used to perform pressure reliefs and transfers.

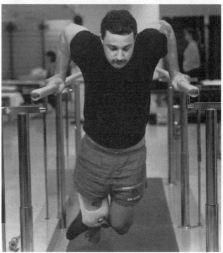

RICKSHAW

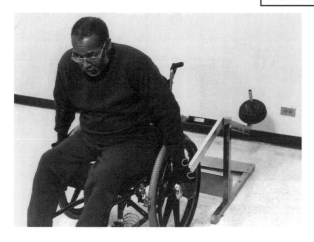

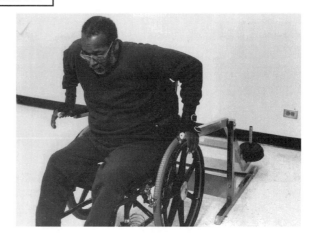

BENT-OVER ROWS

MUSCLES STRENGTHENED

Infraspinatus

Latissimus dorsi

Middle trapezius

Posterior deltoid

Rhomboids

Teres major

Teres minor

BARBELL

STARTING POSITION

Use a pronated grip slightly wider than shoulder width, bend forward at waist, keep back straight with elbows extended.

MOVEMENT

1. Pull weight to chest.
2. Slowly return to starting position.

TIPS

Keep body stationary while working arms. On the up movement, allow elbows to flex but do not forcefully flex them. Do not let bar drop on downward movement; this could cause low back injuries or weaken the shoulder joint.

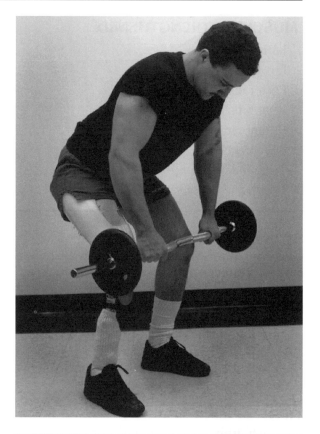

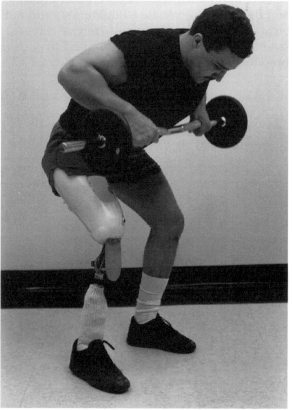

ONE-ARM PULLEY

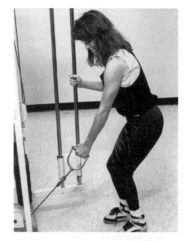

STARTING POSITION

Bend forward at waist, keeping back straight with elbow extended.

MOVEMENT

Use the movement described for the barbell.

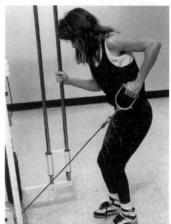

ONE-ARM DUMBBELL

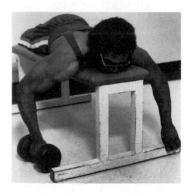

STARTING POSITION

Lay prone on bench, grip dumbbell with palm facing in and arm down to floor.

MOVEMENT

Pull the weight up and elbow back as far as possible.

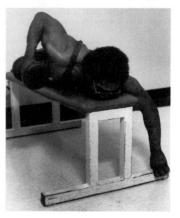

BENCH PRESS

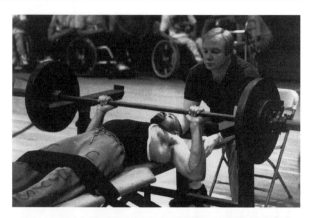

MUSCLES STRENGTHENED
Anterior deltoid
Coracobrachialis and serratus anterior
Pectoralis major
Pectoralis minor
Subscapularis
Triceps

STARTING POSITION
Lie flat on the bench with knees flexed and feet flat on the floor. Keep buttocks and shoulder blades flat on the bench with head and neck in a neutral position (in the middle). Hold the bar with arms fully extended.

MOVEMENT
1. Lower bar to chest.
2. Press upward and slightly back so the bar is approximately over the neck with elbows fully extended.

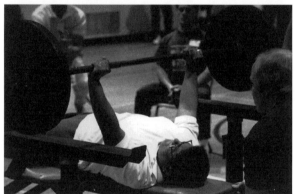

TIPS
Grip—The spacing of the hands determines how much the exercise affects triceps and pectoralis major. The closer grip puts more emphasis on the triceps and the wider grip puts more emphasis on the pectoralis major.

Serratus anterior—To focus on this muscle, use lighter resistance to allow you to fully protract your scapulas by rounding your shoulders off the mat with elbows extended.

Do not arch back excessively, which can cause potential injury. Do not bounce the bar off chest—this can damage the sternum and soft tissues (including the heart). If you do not have full use of legs and trunk muscles (abdominals and back), you may have to strap your legs to allow for balance during the exercise. If you still have difficulty with balance, use the machine bench press.

The machine bench press is also a safer mode if you do not have good hand function or safety racks for free weights. You should have a spotter for the free-weight bench press.

ALTERNATE SET-UP

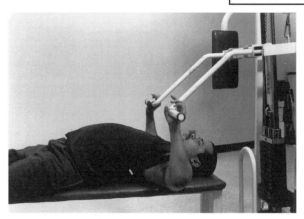 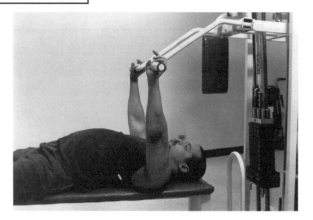

Universal Bench Press—Start with elbows bent and a shoulder-width grip.

Press bar up until elbows are fully extended. Slowly lower the bar back down to starting position.

LAT PULL-DOWNS

MUSCLES STRENGTHENED

Latissimus dorsi

Pectoralis major (sternal portion)

Pectoralis minor

Posterior deltoid

Rhomboids

Teres major

STARTING POSITION

Extend arms with hands out and above shoulders. Use a wide, palm-down grip (pronated) on lat-bar or tubing.

MOVEMENT

1. Pull bar, springs, or rubber tubing down as far as possible or until bar is in front of or behind the base of the neck.
2. Slowly return to starting position.

TIPS

Keep upper body straight; do not jerk or raise body to assist the movement.

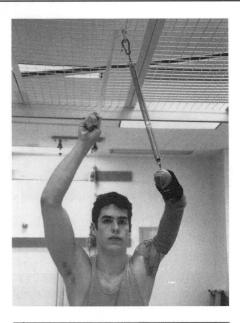

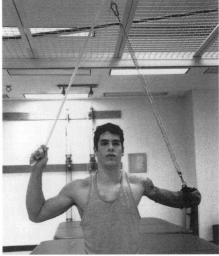

VARIATIONS AND ALTERNATE SET-UPS

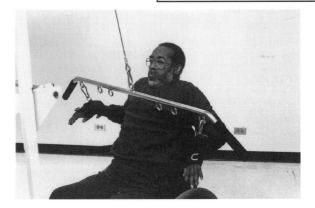

Front Pull-Down

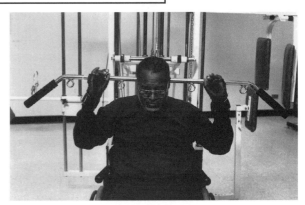

Back Pull-Down

FRONT SHOULDER RAISE

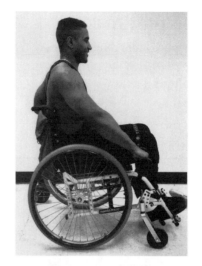

MUSCLES STRENGTHENED
Anterior deltoid

Clavicular pectoralis major

Coracobrachialis

STARTING POSITION
Sit or stand with palms facing down (pronated), elbows extended, and arms down at sides.

MOVEMENT
1. With palms facing down and elbows extended, raise arm slightly above shoulders.
2. Slowly lower weight to starting position.
3. Start next repetition.

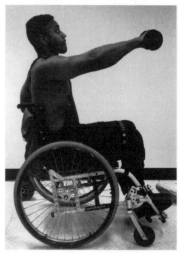

TIPS
Keep body stationary during entire exercise. Do not swing the weight. Use shoulder muscles, not your body's momentum. You can perform exercises with one arm and use opposite arm for balance if needed. You can also perform exercise with both arms (bilaterally) if balance allows, to provide a greater emphasis on trunk muscles as stabilizers. Upper extremity amputees may require more resistance on the residual limb due to the decreased lever arm.

VARIATIONS AND ALTERNATE SET-UPS

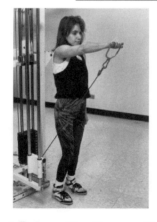

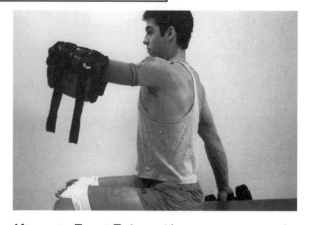

Pulley Front Raise—Standing parallel to cable, pull cable up toward front of body with palm-down grip (pronated) until hand is slightly above shoulder. Slowly lower to starting position.

Alternate Front Raise—Alternate arms on each raise. Keep body swing to a minimum.

LATERAL SHOULDER RAISE

MUSCLES STRENGTHENED

Clavicular pectoralis major (arms above
    horizontal)

Middle deltoid

Supraspinatus

Upper and lower trapezius

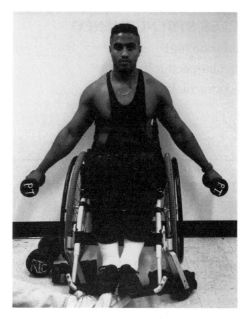

STARTING POSITION

Sit or stand with palms facing in toward body,
elbows extended, and arms down by side.

MOVEMENT

1. With palms facing down and elbows extended, raise arms up sideways (laterally) to slightly above shoulders.
2. Slowly lower weight to starting position.
3. Begin next repetition.

TIPS

Keep body stationary during entire exercise. You
can perform exercise one arm at a time if you
need opposite arm to balance body or trunk.
Keep palms facing down. Individuals with weak
triceps may turn palm up using gravity and
weight (resistance) to maintain arms straight.
This position puts less emphasis on middle
deltoid and more emphasis on the anterior
deltoid and biceps.

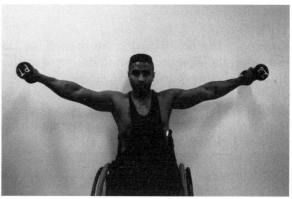

VARIATIONS AND ALTERNATE SET-UPS

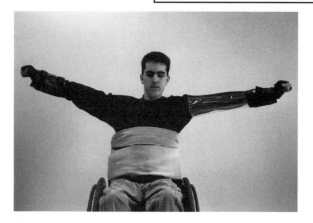

Elbow Splint—Air cast or elbow splint maintains
elbow extension with palms down to avoid
muscle substitution. Straps around upper body
and wheelchair can aid in balance during exercise.

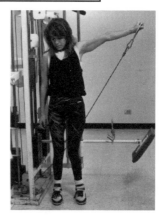

Lateral Pulley Raise—Standing perpendicular
to cable, pull cable with a palm-down grip until
hand is slightly above shoulder.

BACK SHOULDER RAISE

MUSCLES STRENGTHENED

Latissimus dorsi

Posterior deltoid

Teres major

Triceps brachii

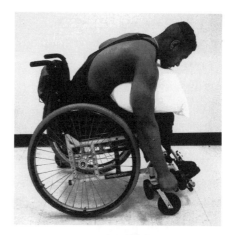

STARTING POSITION

Lie prone (on stomach) on bench or sit bent over in chair with arm hanging down perpendicular to floor and elbow extended.

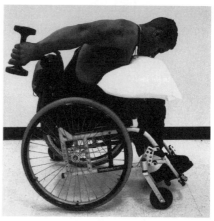

MOVEMENT

1. With elbow extended, move arm back as far as possible.
2. Slowly lower weight to starting position.
3. Begin next repetition.

TIPS

Keep body stationary during entire exercise. Do not swing the weight. Use shoulder, not your body's momentum. Individuals bending over in a chair to perform the exercise can use a pillow in the lap if needed to help support trunk.

VARIATIONS AND ALTERNATE SET-UPS

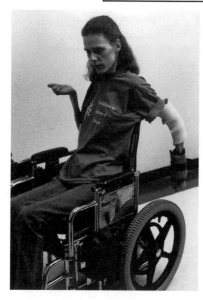

Seated Elbow Splint Raises—Elbow splint or air cast maintains elbow in extension to isolate shoulder muscles.

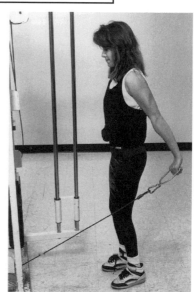

Pulley Back Raise—Pull arm back with elbow extended. Slowly return to starting position.

SHOULDER DEPRESSORS

MUSCLES STRENGTHENED

Latissimus dorsi

Lower trapezius

Pectoralis minor

Subclavius

Teres major

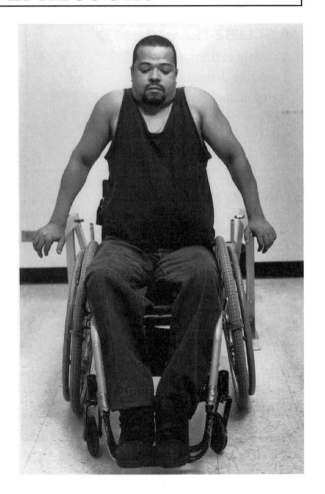

STARTING POSITION

With elbows locked into extension, elevate and externally rotate shoulders.

MOVEMENT

1. Press shoulders down, keeping elbows locked in extension.
2. Slowly return to starting position.

TIPS

This exercise is most useful for wheelchair users with weak triceps because it helps strengthen the shoulder muscles used to perform transfers and pressure reliefs. Positioning the shoulders in external rotation with elbows straight assists the weak triceps to maintain elbow extension. Elbow splints can be used to maintain elbow extension for individuals who have very weak or absent triceps.

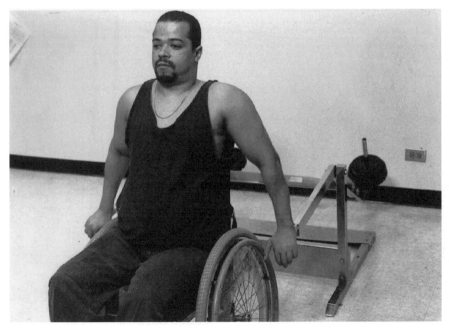

SHOULDER SHRUGS

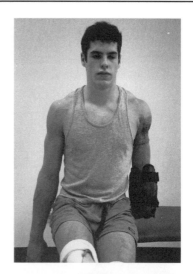

MUSCLES STRENGTHENED

Levator scapulae

Upper trapezius

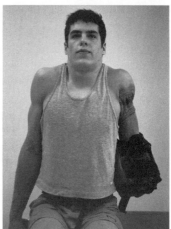

STARTING POSITION

Sit with shoulders relaxed, arms at sides, and elbows extended, with dumbbell in hand or strap-on weights attached to forearm.

MOVEMENT

1. Elevate the shoulder girdle by shrugging shoulders toward ears.
2. Hold end position and slowly relax shoulders to starting position.
3. Begin next repetition.

VARIATIONS

May be performed with barbell or standing.

ALTERNATE SET-UP

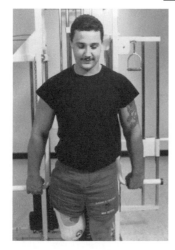

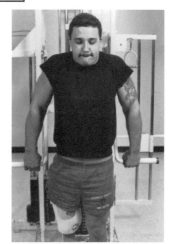

Exercise Machine Shoulder Shrugs—Start with back to machine and palms to the back (pronated).

Elevate shoulder girdle and slowly lower back down to starting position.

SHOULDER EXTERNAL ROTATION

MUSCLES STRENGTHENED

Infraspinatus

Posterior deltoid

Rhomboids

Teres minor

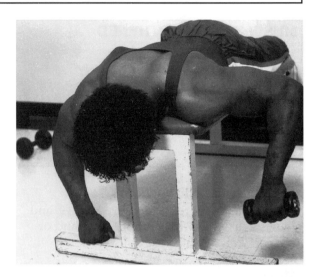

STARTING POSITION

Lie prone (on stomach) on bench with upper arm (humerus) perpendicular to body, elbow flexed to 90°, forearm perpendicular to floor, and palm facing backward.

MOVEMENT

1. Maintain body position while rotating dumbbell upward (toward head) as far as possible.
2. Slowly return to starting position.

TIPS

This exercise is beneficial to counteract the muscle imbalance of tight shoulder interval rotators often found in wheelchair users.

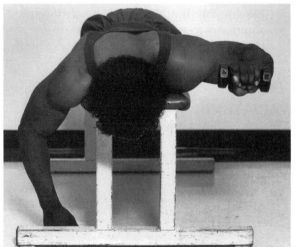

ADDITIONAL VARIATIONS

MUSCLES STRENGTHENED

Infraspinatus

Middle trapezius

Posterior deltoid

Rhomboids

Teres minor

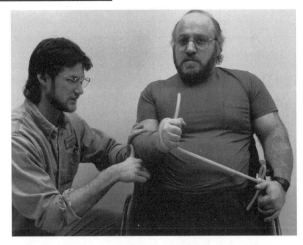

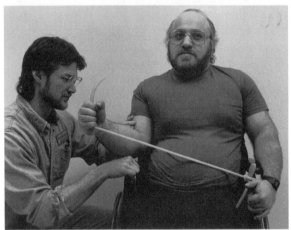

STARTING POSITION

Sit with upper arm (humerus) positioned vertically downward, elbow flexed to 90° and next to side, and palm internally rotated toward body (facing body and shoulder).

MOVEMENT

1. Keep elbow next to body.
2. Pull (rotate) resistance (wall pulley, Theraband, etc.) away from the body as far as possible.
3. Slowly return to starting position.

ALTERNATE SET-UP

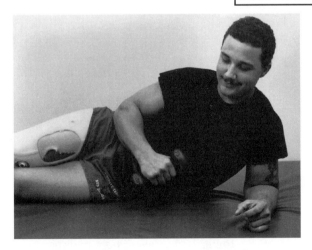

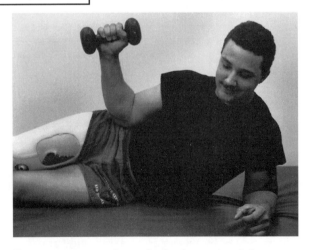

Lie on side with top arm next to body, elbow flexed to 90° with shoulder internally rotated toward body, and dumbbell in hand.

Rotate arm away from the body, maintaining elbow flexion 90° with elbow next to side. Slowly return to starting position.

SHOULDER INTERNAL ROTATION

MUSCLES STRENGTHENED

Latissimus dorsi

Pectoralis major

Serratus anterior

Subscapularis

Teres major

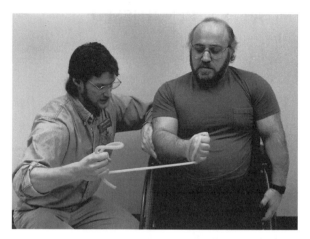

STARTING POSITION

Sit with upper arm (humerus) positioned vertically downward, elbow flexed to 90° and next to body, and palm facing body.

MOVEMENT

1. Keep elbow next to side of body.
2. Pull (rotate) resistance (wall pulley, Theraband, etc.) toward midline of body.
3. Slowly return to starting position.

VARIATION

Lie supine (on back) with upper arm parallel to the trunk, elbow flexed to 90°, and back of forearm against mat. Rotate dumbbell up until forearm is perpendicular to mat. Slowly return to starting position.

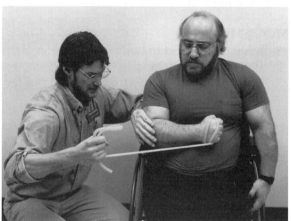

VARIATION AND ALTERNATE SET-UP

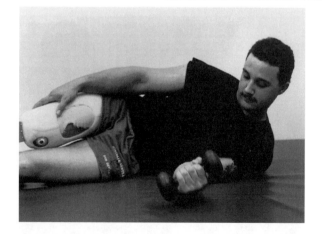

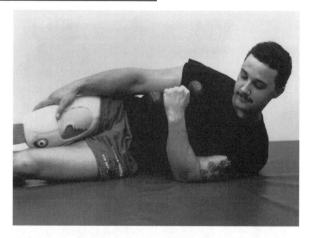

Lie on side with bottom arm next to body and elbow flexed to 90°, with back of forearm against mat and palm facing up.

Rotate arm toward midline of body, maintaining 90° of elbow flexion with elbow next to side. Slowly return to starting position.

STRAIGHT-ARM BACK RAISE

MUSCLES STRENGTHENED

Posterior deltoid

Rhomboids

Triceps brachii

Upper, middle, and lower trapezius

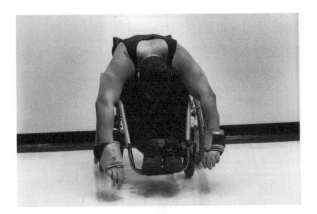

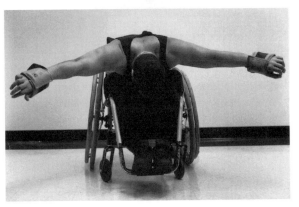

NOTE

If you do the exercise with shoulder internally rotated, it emphasizes the rhomboids, whereas externally rotating shoulder emphasizes the middle and lower trapezius. Performing the exercise with shoulder positioned at 90° emphasizes the middle trapezius, and with shoulder positioned at 120° emphasizes the lower trapezius.

STARTING POSITION

Lie on stomach (prone) or bent over in chair with arms extended and resting down in front of body.

MOVEMENT

1. Raise shoulders straight up and back as far as possible with elbows extended.
2. Pinch shoulder blades together.
3. Slowly return to starting position.

TIPS

If you do the exercise bending over in a chair, use a pillow in the lap if needed to help support the trunk. If you have rods or other spine stabilizing devices, bending may be contraindicated.

TRICEPS EXTENSIONS

MUSCLES STRENGTHENED

Anconeus

Triceps brachii

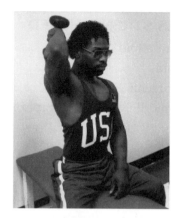

DUMBBELL

STARTING POSITION

Stand or sit with elbow flexed and pointing forward so hand with dumbbell drops behind head.

MOVEMENT

1. Extend elbow and raise dumbbell above head while keeping the upper arm upright.
2. Lower weight slowly until elbow is completely flexed.
3. Start next repetition.

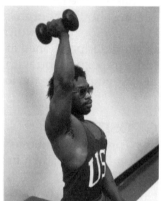

BARBELL

STARTING POSITION

Use same position as for basic triceps extension.

MOVEMENT

Again, use same movement as for basic triceps extension.

GRIP

Use overhand (pronated) grip with hands 12 in. apart or closer.

TIPS

Do not allow elbows to flare out to the sides, which decreases resistance on the triceps. Restrict the movement of upper arms.

ALTERNATE POSITION

Lie flat on bench with knees bent and feet flat on the floor.

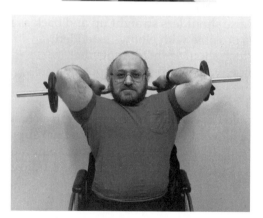

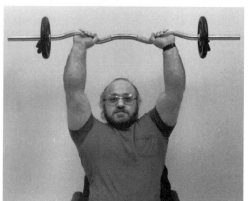

UPPER PULLEY (Exercise Machine)

STARTING POSITION
Stand or sit at machine with elbow bent at side and with hand in a palm-down (pronated) grip.

MOVEMENT
1. Extend elbow until completely straight.

TIPS
Keep body and upper arm stationary. Elbow should remain at side.

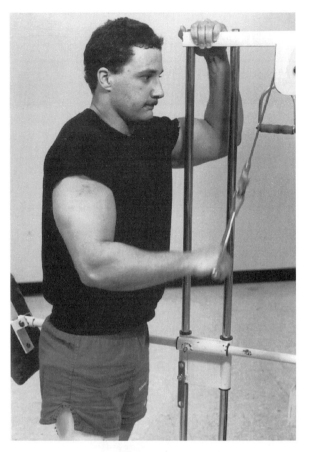

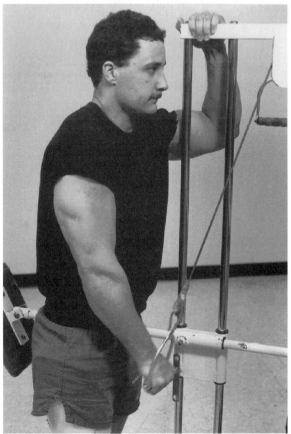

CHEST FLYS

MUSCLES STRENGTHENED

Anterior deltoid

Pectoralis major

Pectoralis minor

Serratus anterior

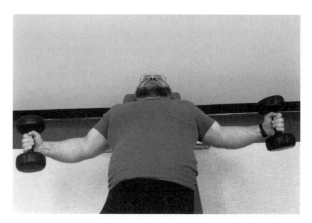

STARTING POSITION

Lie supine (on back) on a bench with elbows slightly flexed and arms parallel to floor and perpendicular to the body.

MOVEMENT

1. Pull dumbbells up and in toward each other.
2. Continue until arms are above the chest with elbows extended and palms facing each other.
3. Slowly return to starting position.

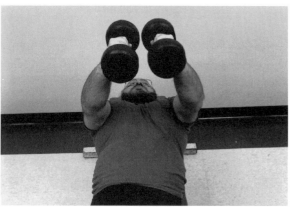

TIPS

To decrease stress on low back and abnormal muscle tone in legs, position hips in flexion by keeping a small bend in knees or by placing a pillow or bolster under knees.

VARIATION AND ALTERNATE SET-UP

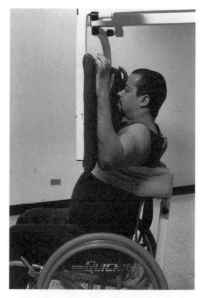

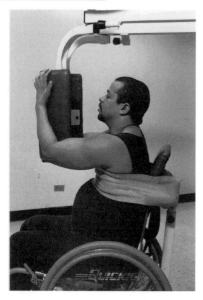

Seated Chest Press—Start with elbows flexed at 90°, upper arm at shoulder level, and forearms and palms flush against pads.

Press pads together and slowly return to starting position.

BICEPS CURL

MUSCLES STRENGTHENED

Biceps brachii
Brachialis
Brachioradialis
Pronator teres

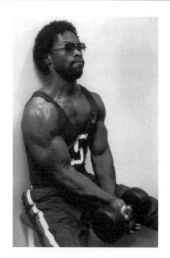

STARTING POSITION

Stand or sit with palm facing up and elbow nearly extended and close to body. If sitting, support back against wall and brace the opposite arm on inside of legs.

MOVEMENT

1. Flex elbow bringing dumbbell to the shoulder.
2. Lower weight slowly until elbow is completely extended.
3. Begin next repetition.

TIPS

Keep elbow close to body. Use a smooth, even motion; do not jerk or use unnecessary movement. Use control, not momentum.

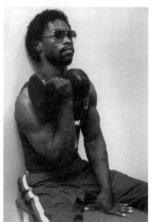

VARIATIONS AND ALTERNATE SET-UPS

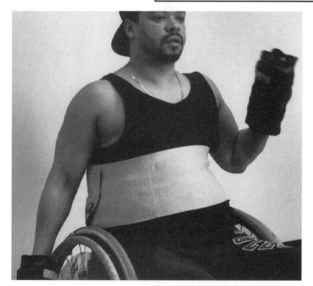

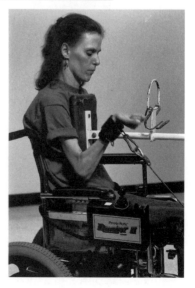

Alternate Arm Curls—Alternate arms on each curl. Keep shoulder and body swing to a minimum.

Low-Pulley Curls (Exercise Machine)—Keep elbow next to side and bring palm to shoulder.

WRIST FLEXION (Curls)

MUSCLES STRENGTHENED

Flexor carpi radialis

Flexor carpi ulnaris

Flexor digitorum superficialis

Palmaris longus

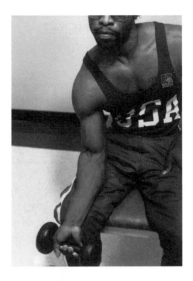

STARTING POSITION

Grasp dumbbell or barbell with a palm-up grip, supporting the forearm on the thigh, and extend hand beyond the knee.

MOVEMENT

1. Curl weight upward as high as possible, without moving forearm.
2. Return to starting position.

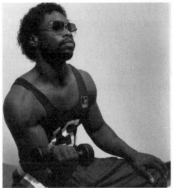

ALTERNATE SET-UP

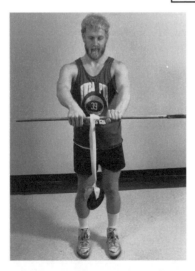

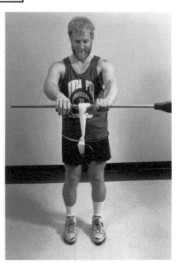

Wrist Rollers—Grasp bar with palm-down grip (pronated) with hands approximately 8 in. apart to use the wrist roller, a weight attached to a bar by a rope. Keep arms extended and parallel to the floor.

Rotate hands around the bar clockwise until rope is wrapped about the bar. Return to starting position.

WRIST EXTENSION (Reverse Curls)

MUSCLES STRENGTHENED
Extensor carpi radialis brevis

Extensor carpi radialis longus

Extensor carpi ulnaris

Extensor digitorium

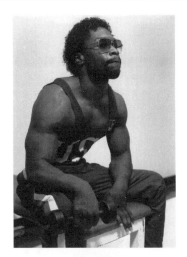

STARTING POSITION
Grasp dumbbell or barbell with a palm-down grip (pronated) and support forearm on thigh with hand extended beyond knee. Relax muscles so wrist is flexed as much as possible.

MOVEMENT
1. Lift weight upward, as high as possible, without moving the forearm.

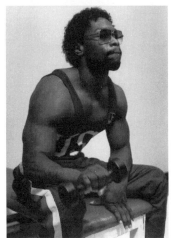

ALTERNATE SET-UP

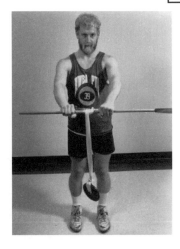

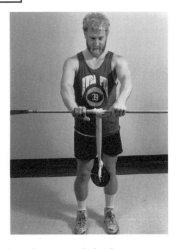

Wrist Rollers (Counterclockwise)—Grasp bar with palm-down grip (pronated) with hands approximately 8 in. apart to use the wrist roller, a weight attached to a bar by a rope. Keep arms extended and parallel to the floor.

Rotate the hands around the bar counterclockwise until rope is wrapped around the bar.

CHAPTER 10

Abdominal and Trunk Exercises

The following exercises are found on the pages indicated.

POSTERIOR PELVIC TILT—HOOK LYING

MUSCLES STRENGTHENED

External oblique abdominis

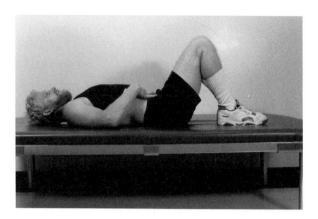

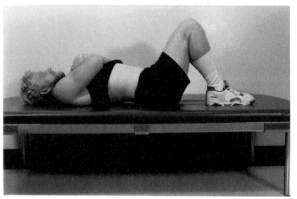

STARTING POSITION

Lie supine (on back) with knees flexed and feet flat on the mat. Rest hands on lower abdominals just above the pelvis.

MOVEMENT

1. Tighten abdominal muscles (suck in the stomach).
2. Push the back flat on the mat—you'll feel the muscles tighten.
3. Hold for 5 sec.
4. Return to starting position by relaxing lower abdominals, begin next repetition. Remember, do not hold your breath.

POSTERIOR PELVIC TILT—LEGS STRAIGHT

MUSCLES STRENGTHENED

External oblique abdominis

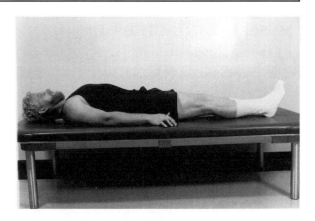

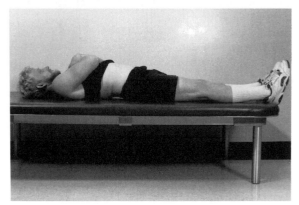

STARTING POSITION

Lie supine (on back) with legs fully extended and arms relaxed next to body.

MOVEMENT

1. Tighten lower abdominals (suck in stomach) to flatten lower back on the mat.
2. Hold for 5 sec, but do not hold your breath; breathe naturally.
3. Relax between each exercise.

LOWER ABDOMINALS—SINGLE LEG SLIDES #1

MUSCLES STRENGTHENED

External oblique abdominis

Iliopsoas (hip flexor)

Rectus abdominis

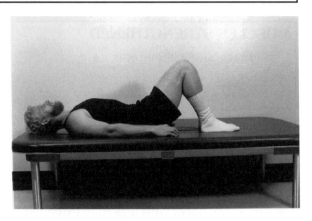

STARTING POSITION

Lie supine (on back) with hips and knees flexed and feet flat on the mat. Flatten back against the mat (posterior pelvic tilt).

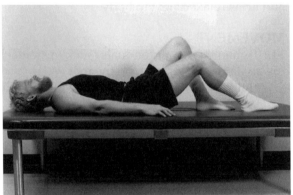

MOVEMENT

1. Slide one heel on the mat while straightening leg to an extended position.
2. Keep back flat against exercise mat.
3. Slide leg back to starting position.
4. Repeat with other leg.

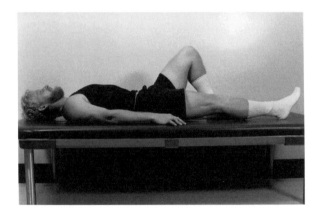

LOWER ABDOMINALS—SINGLE LEG SLIDES #2

MUSCLES STRENGTHENED

External oblique abdominis

Iliopsoas (hip flexor)

Rectus abdominis

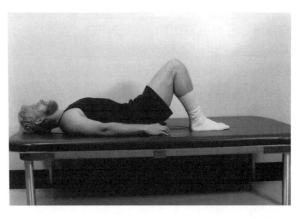

STARTING POSITION

Lie supine (on back) with hips and knees flexed and feet flat on the mat. Flatten back against the mat (posterior pelvic tilt).

MOVEMENT

1. Lift heel of one leg off the mat by flexing hip and knee to chest.
2. Straighten leg out to an extended position.
3. Slowly return leg to starting position; be sure to keep heel off mat during entire sequence.
4. Repeat with other leg.

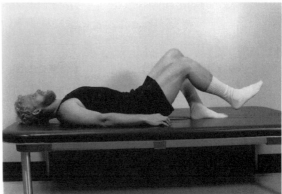

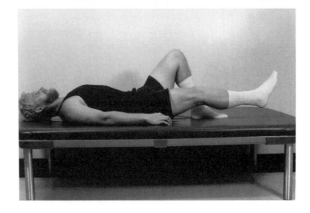

LOWER ABDOMINALS—DOUBLE LEG SLIDES #1

MUSCLES STRENGTHENED

External oblique abdominis

Iliopsoas (hip flexor)

Rectus abdominis

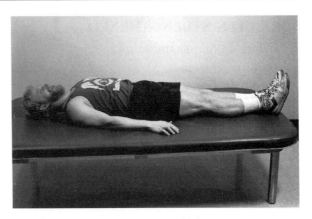

STARTING POSITION

Lie supine (on back) with legs fully extended. Flatten back against the mat (posterior pelvic tilt).

MOVEMENT

1. Slide both legs with heels on mat to bring both knees toward chest.
2. Stop when hips are flexed to 90° or perpendicular to mat and feet off the mat.
3. Lower feet to mat, keeping stomach and back flat.
4. Slide feet along the mat back to the starting position.

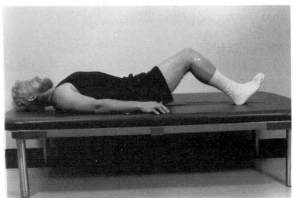

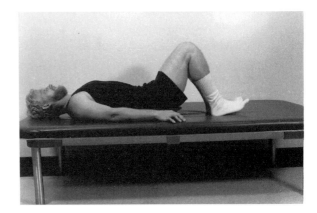

LOWER ABDOMINALS—DOUBLE LEG SLIDES #2

MUSCLES STRENGTHENED

External oblique abdominis

Iliopsoas (hip flexors)

Rectus abdominis

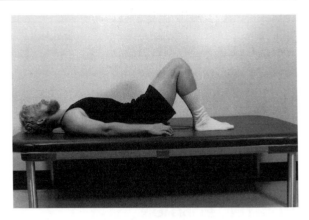

STARTING POSITION

Lie supine (on back) with knees flexed and feet flat on the mat. Flatten back against the mat (posterior pelvic tilt).

MOVEMENT

1. Lift heels off mat by flexing hips and knees.
2. Bring knees to chest.
3. Straighten both knees as you return to starting position; be sure to keep heels off the mat.
4. Keep your back flat on the mat at all times.

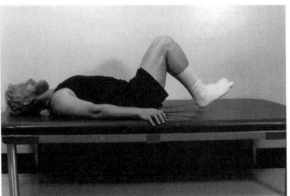

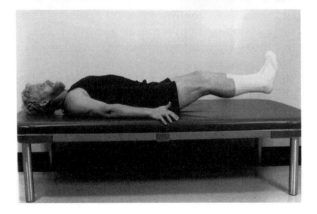

UPPER ABDOMINALS— ABDOMINAL CRUNCHES #1

MUSCLES STRENGTHENED

External oblique abdominis

Internal oblique abdominis

Rectus abdominis

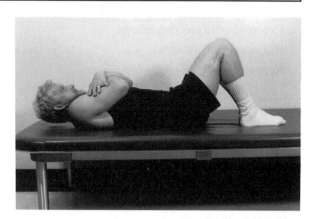

STARTING POSITION

Lie supine (on back) with knees flexed and feet flat on mat. Knees and feet should be hip-width apart. Rest arms on chest in a crossed position. Flatten back against the mat (posterior pelvic tilt).

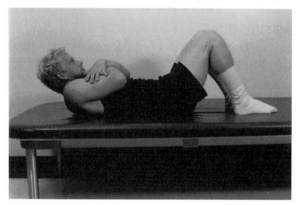

MOVEMENT

1. Raise neck and shoulders off the mat toward the ceiling.
2. Hold for 3 sec.
3. Slowly return to starting position.

TIPS

Individuals with lower extremity paralysis who have abdominal musculature may perform exercise with legs supported on a stool or chair. Lower extremity amputees may find more stability by placing leg and stump on a stool or chair during exercise.

UPPER ABDOMINALS— ABDOMINAL CRUNCHES #2

MUSCLES STRENGTHENED

External oblique abdominis

Internal oblique abdominis

Rectus abdominis

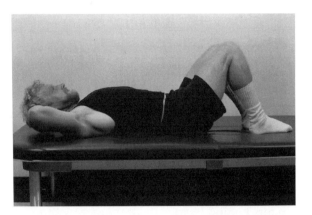

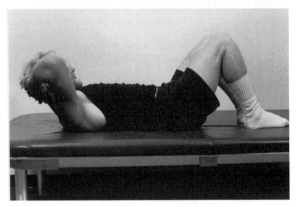

STARTING POSITION

Lie supine (on back) with knees flexed and feet flat on mat. Knees and feet should be hip-width apart. Clasp fingers behind your head. Flatten your back against the mat (posterior pelvic tilt).

MOVEMENT

1. Raise head and shoulders off the mat toward the ceiling.
2. Hold for 3 sec.
3. Slowly return to starting position.

TIPS

Individuals with lower extremity paralysis who have abdominal musculature may perform exercise with legs supported on a stool or chair. Lower extremity amputees may find more stability by placing leg and stump on a stool or chair during exercise.

LATERAL ABDOMINAL CRUNCH

MUSCLES STRENGTHENED

External oblique abdominis

Internal oblique abdominis

Rectus abdominis

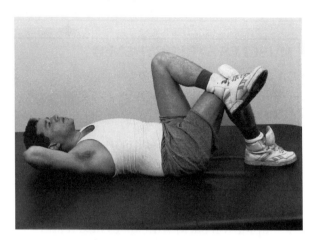

STARTING POSITION

Lie supine (on back) with both knees flexed. Cross one leg with ankle on opposite knee. Clasp fingers behind head.

MOVEMENT

1. Curl shoulders off mat while twisting to move elbow toward opposite knee.
2. Return slowly to starting position.
3. Repeat with alternate elbow and knee.

TIPS

Individuals with lower extremity paralysis who have abdominal musculature may perform exercise with legs supported on a stool or chair. Lower extremity amputees may find more stability by placing leg and stump on a stool or chair during exercise.

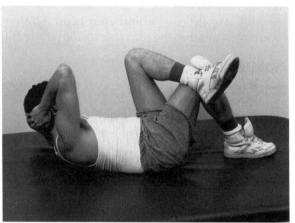

UPPER BACK EXTENSION #1

MUSCLES STRENGTHENED

Erector spinae muscle group

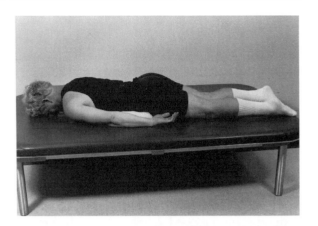

STARTING POSITION

Lie prone (face down) with chin tucked, legs extended, and arms relaxed next to body.

MOVEMENT

1. Raise head and shoulders off the mat.
2. Hold for 3 sec.
3. Slowly return to starting position.

TIPS

Keep hips, legs, and feet on the mat—lift only upper trunk.

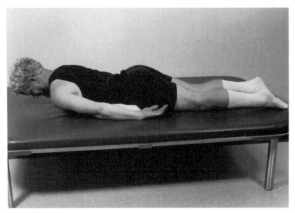

UPPER BACK EXTENSION #2

MUSCLES STRENGTHENED

Erector spinae muscle group

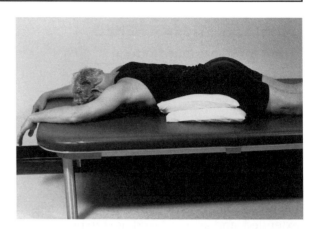

STARTING POSITION

Lie prone (face down) with chin tucked, legs extended, and extended arms above the head.

MOVEMENT

1. Raise head and shoulders off the mat.
2. Hold for 3 sec.
3. Slowly return to starting position.

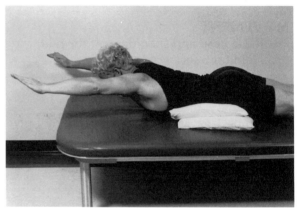

UPPER TRUNK ROTATION

MUSCLES STRENGTHENED

External oblique abdominis

Internal oblique abdominis

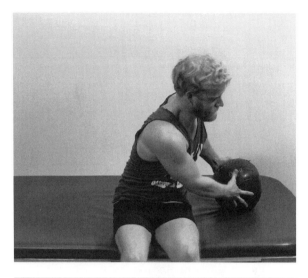

STARTING POSITION

Sit or stand with trunk rotated to one side and grip a medicine ball or dumbbell with both hands.

MOVEMENT

1. Rotate trunk, bringing medicine ball or dumbbell to opposite side while keeping arms stiff.
2. Return to opposite side.

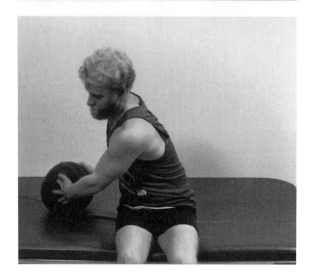

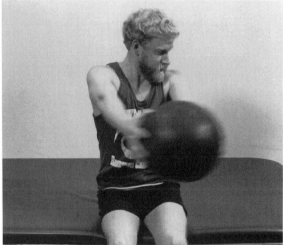

CHAPTER 11

Lower Extremity Exercises

The following exercises are found on the pages indicated.

SQUATS

MUSCLES STRENGTHENED

Gluteus maximus and gastrocnemius

Hamstrings

Quadriceps

Supporting muscles of the abdomen

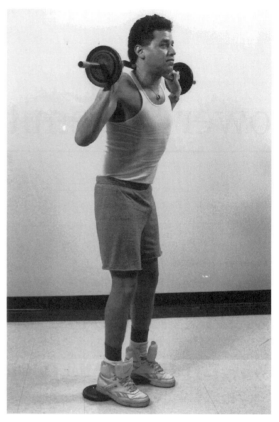

STARTING POSITION

Stand with feet shoulder-width apart and rotated outward at a 35° to 45° angle. Place the bar across shoulders and behind neck. (Dumbbells can also be used for resistance with arms extended and held next to body.)

MOVEMENT

1. Maintaining upper trunk in a fixed erect posture, lower buttocks until thigh is parallel to the floor.
2. Return to starting position.

TIPS

Keep head forward and slightly up to help maintain the upper trunk in proper position. If you have difficulty keeping heels on the floor during the movement, place a two-by-four board or barbell plates underneath heels.

PRECAUTIONS

Do not lower hips below the knees or bounce at the bottom of the squat because this can place excessive stress on knee ligaments and lower back. Do not bend over waist; keep bar in line with feet.

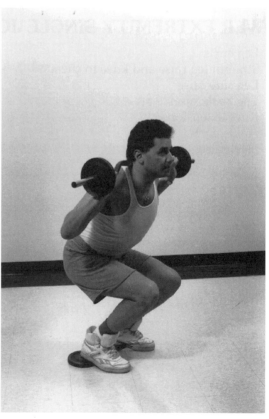

LUNGES

MUSCLES STRENGTHENED

Down phase:

Abdominals

Ankle dorsiflexors (tibialis anterior, extensor digitorum longus, peroneus tertius)

Hip flexors (psoas major, iliacus)

Hamstrings

Up phase:

Abdominals

Gastrocnemius

Gluteus maximus

Quadriceps femoris

Spinal extensors

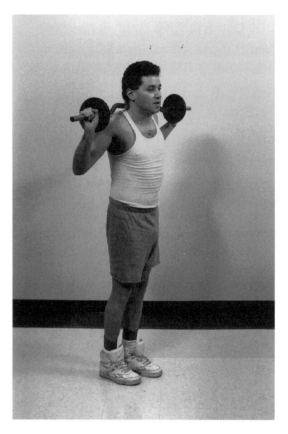

STARTING POSITION

Hold barbell on shoulders behind head or hold dumbbells with arms fully extended and next to body. Stand with feet less than shoulder-width apart and keep plenty of room in front.

MOVEMENT

1. Stride forward with one leg until foot is in a good stride position. The knee should not extend past the foot.
2. Lower body forward, until knee is over ankle of front leg. Front hip should be as low or lower than front knee, and rear leg nearly extended.
3. Push back with front leg.
4. Direct upper body back to the erect starting position.
5. Change legs and repeat the movement. Count the two movements as one repetition.

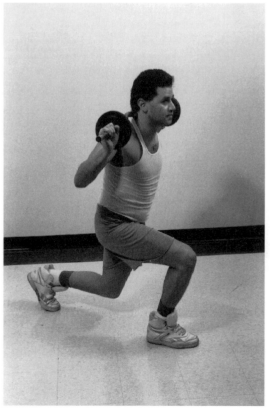

LEG CURLS

MUSCLES STRENGTHENED

Hamstring muscle group (semitendinosus, semimembranosus, biceps femoris)

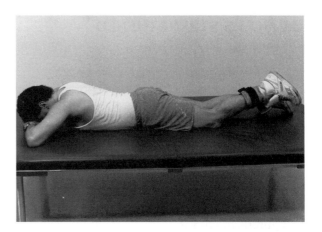

STARTING POSITION

Lie on stomach (prone) with legs straight.

MOVEMENT

1. Bend one knee, raising heel up to buttocks while keeping hips down.
2. Slowly return leg to starting position.

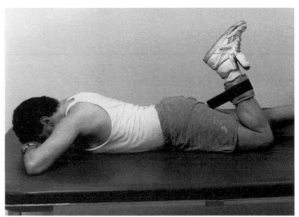

ALTERNATE SET-UP

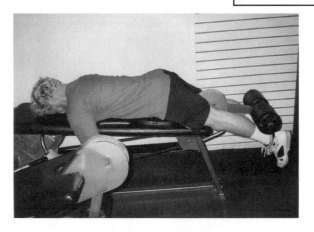

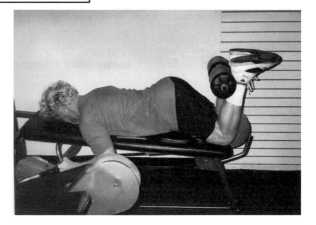

STRAIGHT LEG RAISE AND KNEE TO CHEST

MUSCLES STRENGTHENED

Iliacus

Psoas major

Quadriceps

Sartorius

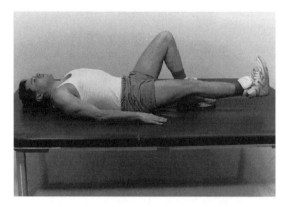

STARTING POSITION

Lie supine (on back) on mat with one knee flexed so foot is flat on mat and opposite leg is extended.

MOVEMENT

1. Raise straight leg up, to the height of flexed knee, keeping knee extended.
2. Slowly return to starting position.

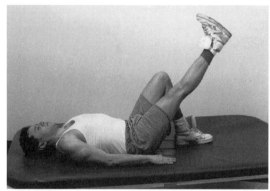

KNEE TO CHEST

MUSCLES STRENGTHENED

Iliacus

Psoas major

Quadriceps

Sartorius

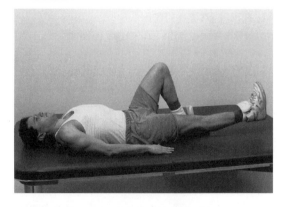

STARTING POSITION

Lie supine (on back) on mat with one knee flexed so foot is flat on mat and opposite leg is extended.

MOVEMENT

1. Raise knee up toward chest while flexing knee and keeping foot off the mat.
2. Slowly return to starting position.

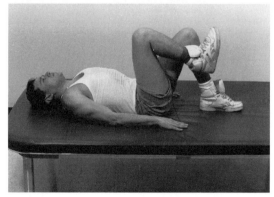

LEG SIDE RAISES

MUSCLES STRENGTHENED

Gluteus medius

Gluteus minimus

Tensor fascia latae

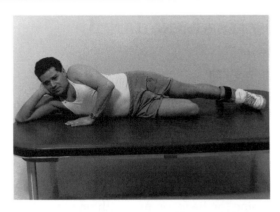

STARTING POSITION

Lie on side with bottom knee flexed and top leg extended.

MOVEMENT

1. Keeping top leg extended, slowly raise leg straight up as far as possible. Stay on your side and do not let hips rotate forward or back. Be sure to keep foot horizontal—do not point the toes.
2. Slowly lower to starting position.

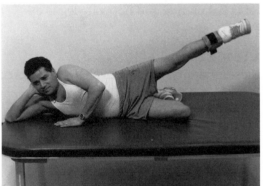

STRETCH BANDS

STARTING POSITION

Lie supine (on back) with knees flexed and together and feet flat on mat. Place Theraband ring around both knees.

MOVEMENT

1. Keep feet on mat while slowly spreading knees apart as far as possible so Theraband is taut.
2. Slowly return to starting position.

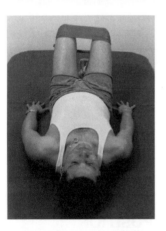

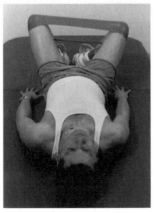

UNIVERSAL

STARTING POSITION
Stand perpendicular to machine or wall with legs and back straight.

MOVEMENT
1. Keeping back straight, slowly move leg out to side as far as possible.
2. Slowly return to starting position.

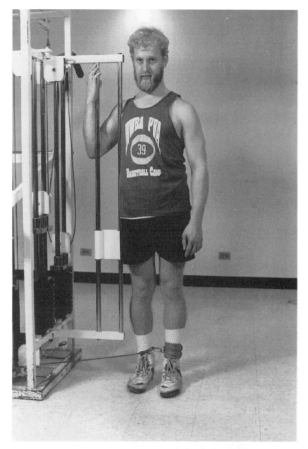

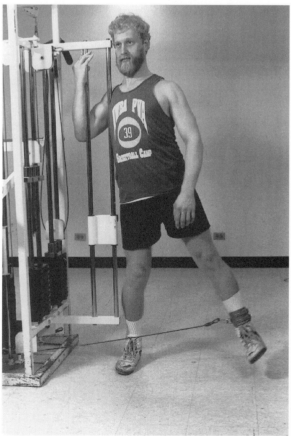

LEG BACK RAISES

MUSCLES STRENGTHENED

Gluteus maximus

Hamstring muscles

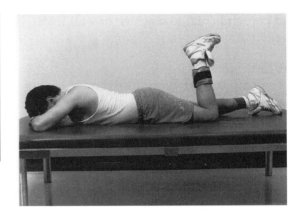

STARTING POSITION

Lie prone (on stomach) with knee flexed.

MOVEMENT

1. Raise thigh upward off the mat, keeping knee flexed and pelvis flat on mat.
2. Slowly return to starting position.

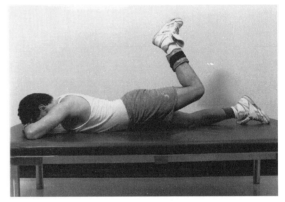

VARIATION

STARTING POSITION

Lie prone (on stomach) with knees extended.

MOVEMENT

1. Raise leg upward off mat, keeping knee extended and pelvis flat on mat.
2. Slowly return to starting position.

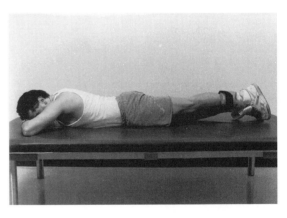

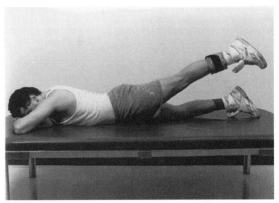

UNIVERSAL

STARTING POSITION
Stand facing machine or wall.

MOVEMENT
1. Move leg backward, keeping knee and back straight.
2. Slowly return to starting position.

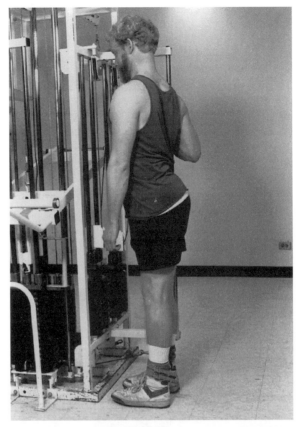

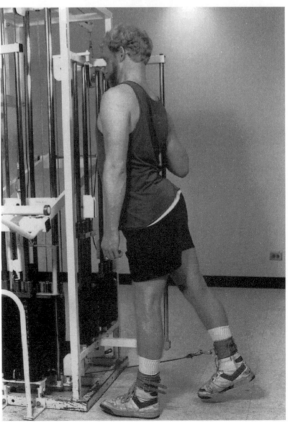

KNEE EXTENSIONS

MUSCLES STRENGTHENED

Quadriceps muscle group (vastus intermedius, vastus medialis, vastus lateralis, rectus femoris)

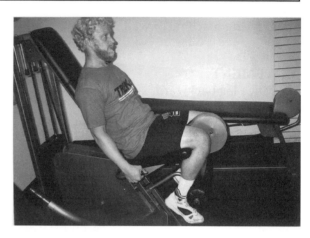

STARTING POSITION

Seated with knees flexed (stretching quadriceps).

MOVEMENT

1. Extend legs until knees are straight.
2. Pause, and then control weight back down to starting position. (This exercise also can be performed one leg at a time.)

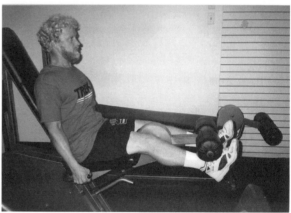

ALTERNATE SET-UP

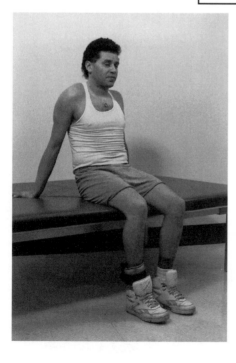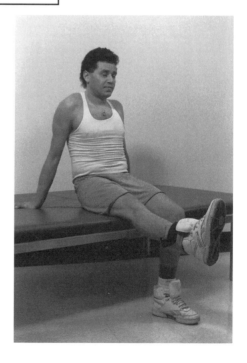

ANKLE CURLS

MUSCLES STRENGTHENED

Anterior compartment: tibialis anterior, extensor digitorum longus, peroneus tertius, and extensor hallucus longus

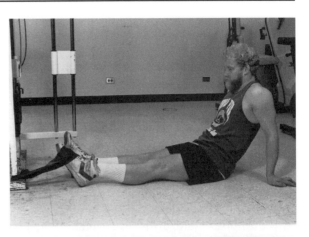

STARTING POSITION

Seated with knee in full extension, attach one end of elastic tubing or band to a stationary object at foot level in front of body. Wrap the other end around the foot so resistance pulls foot into plantar flexion (ankle extension).

MOVEMENT

1. Bend ankle, bringing forefoot and toes toward body.
2. Slowly return to starting position.

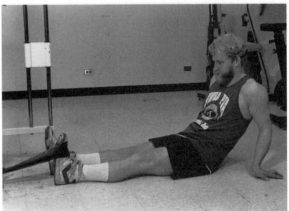

HEEL RAISES

MUSCLES STRENGTHENED

Posterior compartment: gastrocnemius, soleus, tibialis posterior, flexor digitorum longus, and flexor hallucus longus

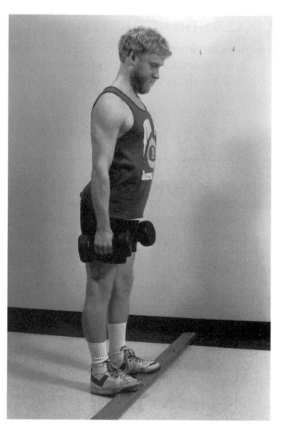

STARTING POSITION

Place barbell across shoulders behind head or grip dumbbells with arms extended and next to body. Standing erect, point feet straight ahead approximately 8 to 12 in. apart.

MOVEMENT

1. Raise up on forefoot and toes, lifting heels as high as possible.
2. Slowly return to starting position.

TIPS

Keep body erect and knees straight during the exercise. To avoid muscle tightness, stretch this muscle group following the exercise to maintain flexibility and good range of motion.

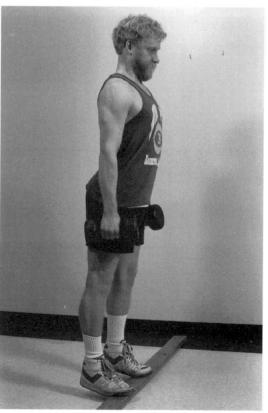

CHAPTER 12

Elements of a Good Exercise Class

To maximize space, time, staff, and equipment, exercise classes may be more appropriate than one-on-one personal training. We advise one-on-one attention when you start an exercise program, but after identifying special set-ups you'll need for exercises and introducing the exercises and techniques, group exercise classes can be fun. Group exercising may also increase compliance and motivation.

Although this chapter is directed to exercise instructors and exercise facilities that are starting to have individuals with physical disabilities in their classes, it is a good chapter for you to read, too. It is just as important for you to know what constitutes a good exercise class as it is for your instructor.

Exercise classes should be relatively small (no more than 10 to 12 participants) to ensure that the staff can watch for proper technique and body mechanics. If the group exercise leader is not aware of the exercise and medical history of each participant, the class is too big! If the class enrollment is high and increasing, beginning, intermediate, and advanced classes should be developed. Each class would be structured similarly, but would offer varying intensity and volume according to the capabilities of the class.

Beginning Class—Participants with moderate weakness or who are moderately deconditioned. Individuals with quadriplegia who have weak or absent triceps are appropriate. Athletes may require bracing or assistance to perform exercises.

Intermediate Class—Participants with full upper extremity function who are minimally to moderately weak, deconditioned, or both. Individuals with lower levels of paraplegia could participate here.

Advanced Class—Participants with full upper extremity function and good strength, for example, individuals with paraplegia or amputations.

Group Leader

A qualified exercise instructor should lead the class. The class leader's responsibilities should include planning exercise routines, correcting exercise technique and body mechanics, and helping determine appropriate weights or Theraband resistance. The instructor should also help chart the weights used and number of repetitions performed.

Exercise Guidelines

1. Exercise positions will vary depending on class focus and routine.

2. All routines should have warm-up exercises, strengthening exercises, cool-down exercises, and stretches.

3. Use rest periods as appropriate.

4. Encourage participants to pace themselves. They should feel free to stop and rest or decrease the exercise intensity. Participants should not push themselves too hard to keep pace with others.

5. Encourage participants to count the exercises out loud. This reminds the athletes to breathe, exhaling with exertion.

6. Weaker individuals may need slower counting or exercise pacing. Be sensitive to individuals who are deconditioned or working with limited muscle mass—they may need increased time to perform a repetition. Slower, controlled movements focus on muscle contractions (muscular control) and avoid using momentum to complete the exercise movements.

7. Emphasize quality of exercises, not quantity. Have participants concentrate on the muscles they are exercising.

8. Prone (on stomach) routines can be performed bent over in a wheelchair or lying face down on a mat.

9. Upright or sitting routines can be performed in a chair with a back or a wheelchair. Individuals with quadriplegia or higher levels of paraplegia may require a binder or strap around themselves and the wheelchair for trunk stability and balance during exercises.

10. If an individual's trunk control permits adequate balance independently or with a binder to assist, remove wheelchair armrests so that full range of motion with arms and trunk can be performed.

11. Use enough resistance to stress the muscle within the recommended number of sets and repetitions. If the athlete can easily complete the repetitions, the resistance (weight) should be increased. The last two repetitions should be challenging.

12. Theraband may be used in place of weights for variety. Theraband is fairly inexpensive and can be purchased in a variety of strengths or elasticity. The different colors represent different levels of resistance.

13. When using Theraband, be sure to assess whether the resistance works the muscles while maintaining proper body mechanics and exercise technique.

14. Allow approximately 1 to 2 min between sets when performing bilateral activities, or alternate arms by resting one side while the other is working.

Exercise Routines

1. *Muscle endurance upper extremity class (beginning/intermediate)*—Class should focus on increasing muscle endurance to perform activities of daily living (wheelchair propulsion, walking, dressing, bathing, etc.).

2. *Muscle strength upper extremity class (intermediate/advanced)*—Class should focus on increasing strength for more demanding activities such as wheelchair transfers, walking with assistive devices and braces, and the like.

Endurance class—2 sets of 10 to 12 repetitions, progressing to 3 sets

Strength class—2 sets of 4 to 8 repetitions, progressing to 3 sets

(Provide 1 to 2 min rest periods between sets. Use rest periods to educate class as a whole or for individual instruction.)

Instructor's Note: The following routines are examples that can be used when starting class programs; however, these routines should be varied to meet the needs of the class. Exercise routines will only be limited by the capabilities of the participants and by the creativity of the exercise group leader.

These programs emphasize multijoint exercises and postural musculature. Single-joint exercises and abdominal work may be used for variety.

ENDURANCE AND STRENGTH CLASS PROGRAMS FOR THE LOWER EXTREMITIES

SUPINE, SIDELYING, AND PRONE POSITIONS
(suggested—adapt as appropriate)

Warm-Up
Lower trunk rotation 10-20 reps.
Stretching—knees to chest and hold 10-20 sec.
(p. 57).

Supine Exercises
Knee to chest (p. 213)
Straight leg raise (p. 213)
Leg side raises (abduction) with
Theraband (p. 214)
Ankle curls with Theraband (p. 219)

Sidelying Exercises
Leg side raises (p. 214)

Prone Exercises
Leg curls (p. 212)
Leg back raises (p. 216)

Cool-Down
Adductor stretch (p. 60)
Knees to chest stretch (p. 57)
Calf stretch (p. 59)
Hamstring stretch (p. 59)

SITTING AND PRONE POSITIONS FOR THE UPPER EXTREMITIES
(suggested—adapt as appropriate)

Warm-Up
Do these exercises slowly, especially stretches, neck rotation, and side bending. The goal is to mildly stretch muscles and increase circulation to muscles and joints.
Shoulder circles: small, large, small forward and backward for a total of 1 min.
Stretch trunk and arms: full shoulder flexion (p. 55), anterior shoulder (p. 54), posterior shoulder (p. 56), triceps (p. 56).
Neck rotation and side bending

Sitting Exercises
Scapular depression (chair dips) (p. 173):
Hands on mat at sides or on wheelchair arm rests, push with arms and raise trunk
Shoulder shrugs (p. 183): Ears to shoulders
Open to cross: (p. 171)
Cross to open: (p. 172)
Shoulder overhead press: (p. 164)
Upright rows: (p. 166)

Prone Exercises (bent over in chair or lying on stomach)
Straight-arm back raise (supermans): (p. 187)
With shoulders abducted to 120° and thumbs up, squeeze scapula together to focus on lower trapezius.
Bent-over rows (p. 174)

Cool-Down
May be done in supine position while waiting to transfer with assistance, or in chair.
Shoulder rolls—roll shoulders backward, then reverse for up to 1 min.
Stretch arms overhead as far as possible (p. 55).
Stretch one arm across the body and then the other (p. 56).

Additional Sitting Exercises
Lateral shoulder raise: (p. 180)
Front shoulder raise: (p. 179)
Back shoulder raise: (p. 181)
Triceps extensions: (p. 188)
Biceps curl: (p. 191)
Wrist extension: (p. 193)

SUPINE AND SIDELYING POSITIONS
FOR THE UPPER EXTREMITIES
AND TRUNK
(suggested—adapt as appropriate)

Warm-Up
Do these slowly with good stretch to shoulders and trunk.

Stretch trunk and arms: Full shoulder flexion (p. 55), anterior shoulder (p. 54), posterior shoulder (p. 56), triceps (p. 56).
Deep breathing.
Neck rotation and side bending.

Supine (lying on back) Exercises
Chest flys (p. 190): Pretend you are hugging a tree, then open arms, keeping elbows slightly flexed.
Bench press (p. 176): Start with hands next to shoulders, push weights to ceiling (pretend you are holding a cane in your hands).
Cross to open: (p. 172)
Open to cross: (p. 171)

Side-Lying Exercises
Shoulder external rotation: (p. 184)
Shoulder internal rotation: (p. 186)

Cool-Down
May be done supine or in a chair.
Repeat warm-up exercises.

Additional Single-Joint Exercises
Supine
Triceps extensions: (p. 188)
Biceps curl: (p. 191)
Front shoulder raise: (p. 179)
Wrist extension: (p. 193)
Wrist flexion: (p. 192)
Sidelying
Back shoulder raise: (p. 181)
Lateral shoulder raise: (p. 180)

Abdominal Exercises:
In hook-lying, do not anchor feet. Cross arms over chest with hands resting over opposite shoulders. Breathe throughout exercise (p. 202).

Progression:
Posterior pelvic tilt (p. 196): Tuck chin and isometrically contract abdominals.
Abdominal crunches #1 (p. 202): Tuck chin and lift head off mat with abdominal muscles tightened. Return slowly.
Abdominal crunches #2 (p. 203): Tuck chin, tighten abdominals, lift head and shoulders off mat. Return slowly.

APPENDIX A

Accessible Exercise Equipment

Most fitness centers and gyms do not have specialized equipment for people with physical disabilities. Depending on your disability, you may be able to use standard weightlifting equipment found in most health clubs. Many gyms can be made accessible by using wrist cuffs with hooks to access existing pulley systems at the facility (p. 101). Lat pull-down bars can be made accessible to individuals with quadriplegia by using welded rings attached to the bar (refer to p. 178).

Speciality equipment is also available for community health clubs, home exercise, and disability sport programs. One of the most functional exercises for wheelchair users is the Rickshaw exerciser, which can be used to perform modified dips in a wheelchair. It strengthens the triceps and shoulder depressors needed to move body weight for transfers and pressure reliefs, and helps when walking with assistive devices such as forearm crutches.

The Rickshaw exerciser is not typically available in community fitness centers and is not readily available to the general public. But it is a simple one-arm lever that can be built as a community project by a disabled sports or fitness program. Component dimensions and assembly instructions for a Rickshaw-type machine follow. Rickshaw exerciser machines may also be purchased directly from the manufacturer or through some medical equipment vendors. You can meet your exercise

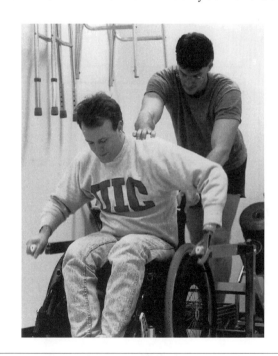

The Rickshaw exerciser is an excellent machine for developing the upper body.

Component Dimensions (in inches)

A (2) Bases: 2 × 4 × 24
B (2) Legs: 2 × 4 × 28
C (4) Leg supports, short: 2 × 4 × 17
  (ends cut to 45 degrees)
D (1) Base brace: 2 × 4 × 33
E (2) Leg supports, long: 2 × 4 × 21
  (ends crosscut to 45 degrees)
F (1) Lower hinged beam: 2 × 4 × 36
G (2) Handles: 2 × 4 × 60
H (1) Upper hinged beam: 2 × 4 × 36
I (1) Weight support beam: 2 × 4 × 36
J (2) Floor stands: 2 × 4 × 36
K (1) Floor stand brace: 2 × 4 × 36

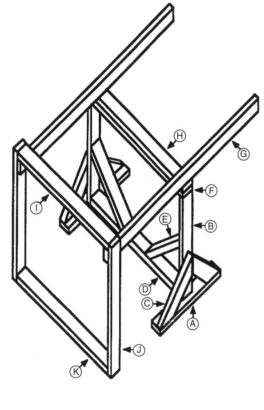

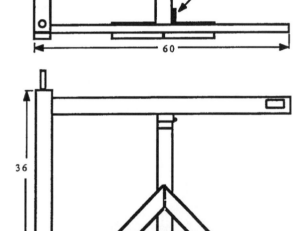

Door Hinges (3)
(attach with bolts)

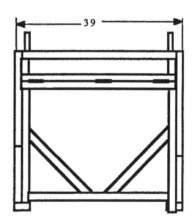

Assembly

Drywall screws or flathead wood screws, #8 x 2 1/2 inches long, can be used for assembly. A 5/64 drill bit should be used for wood screw pilot holes.

1. Assemble 2 sets of bases, legs, and short leg supports.
2. Join leg assemblies together with base brace, long leg supports, and lower hinged beam.
3. Attach 3 door hinges to upper and lower hinged beams with bolts and locknuts.
4. Attach handles to upper hinged beam.
5. Attach weight support beam to floor stands.

6. Attach floor stand to handles.
7. Attach floor stand brace to floor stands.

Rods to stack weights on may be mounted on weight support beam or on floor stand brace, to allow easiest loading and unloading of weights.

Floor stands and floor stand brace may be replaced by a table of suitable height under the weight beam or handles.

The handles may be modified with holes, as shown in the side view, for easier gripping and hand position.

Note. Original drawing by David Casement, rehabilitation engineer, Rehabilitation Institute of Chicago. Reprinted by permission.

> **KEY**
> a. Individual exercise units
> b. Multistation exercise units
> c. Wheelchair rollers
> d. Upper body ergometers (table-top bikes)
> e. Arm-driven tricycles
> f. Hand-pedal attachment for manual wheelchair
> g. Wrist cuffs with hooks
> h. Hand mitts (quadriplegic gloves)

needs through these specialized exercise equipment manufacturers:

Access to Recreation, Incorporated (a)
2509 E. Thousand Oaks Blvd., Ste. 430
Thousand Oaks, CA 91367
800-634-4351
805-498-7535

Accessible Fitness Systems (a, b, c, d)
925 Harbor Lake Dr., Ste. B
Safety Harbor, FL 34695
813-725-9180
813-725-9063 FAX

Cleo Living Aids (a, d, g)
3987 Mayfield Rd.
Cleveland, OH 44121
800-321-0595
800-537-9880 FAX

G.E. Miller, Inc. (a, d, g)
484 S. Broadway
P.O. Box 266
Yonkers, NY 10705
800-431-2924
914-969-4036
212-549-4850 (in New York)

GPK Design & Manufacturing (a, b)
7942 Calle Posada
Carlsbad, CA 92009
800-468-8679
619-436-6095

Helm Distributing, Inc. (a, b)
911 Kings Point Rd.
Polson, MT 59860
406-883-2147

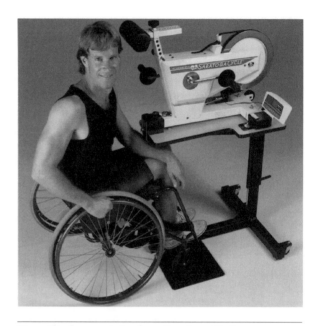

Upper body ergometer from Saratoga Cycle.

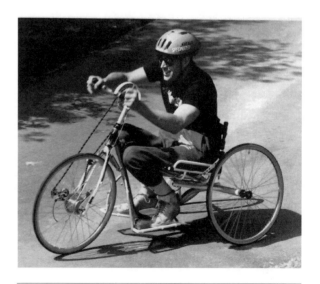

Mach 3 hand-powered sports vehicle from Magic in Motion.

IDEA (c, h)
1393 Meadowcreek Dr.
Pewaukee, WI 53072
414-691-4248

Kustom Built Athletic Equipment, Inc. (b)
North 409 Dyer Rd.
Spokane, WA 99212
800-537-5539
509-534-4680

Magic in Motion (c, e, f)
20604 84th Ave. South
Kent, WA 98032
800-342-1579
206-872-0722
206-872-0741 FAX

McLain Cycle Products (c)
1718 106th Ave.
Ostego, MI 49078
616-694-9704

Nautilus Sports/Medical Industries, Inc. (b)
P.O. Box 809014
Dallas, TX 75380-9014
800-874-8941
214-490-9155

Olympic Enterprises, Inc. (b, g)
2323 West Encanto Blvd.
Phoenix, AZ 85009
602-271-4931

ParaMed Exercise Equipment (a, b)
P.O. Box 6469
Jackson, MS 39282-6469
601-354-2211
601-354-2239 FAX

Patton Medical Glove (h)
P.O. Box 7100
Jacksonville, FL 32210

Saratoga Access & Fitness, Inc. (d, h)
P.O. Box 1427
Fort Collins, CO 80522-1427
303-484-4010

Special Concepts Integrated, Inc. (b)
16835 Algonquin Ave., Ste. 627
Huntington Beach, CA 92649
310-493-0231

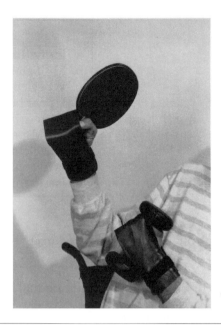

An exercise hand mitt from IDEA.

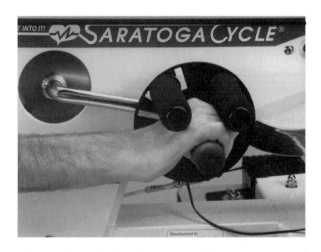

Saratoga's limited-grasp handgrip.

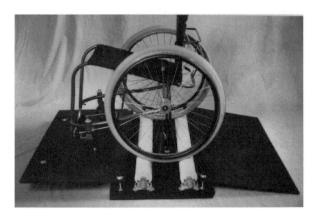

A wheelchair roller from IDEA.

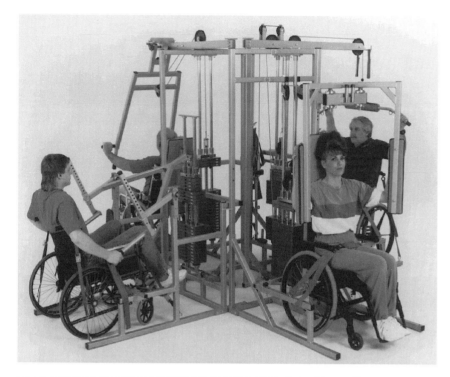

Toro Co. (a)
Fitness Equipment Division
8111 Lyndale Ave., South
Minneapolis, MN 55420

Total Tone (b)
P.O. Box 188
Hackensack, NJ 56452

TRI KING Corp. (e)
10 Drake Terrace
Prospect Heights, IL 60070
708-537-6032

A multistation unit by ParaMed Exercise Equipment.

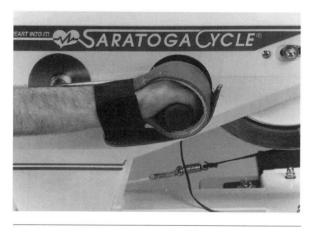

Saratoga's grip cuffs.

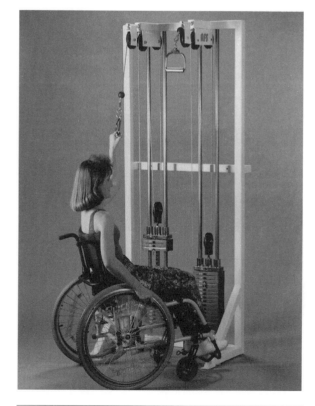

An individual exercise unit from Accessible Fitness
Systems.

APPENDIX B

Fitness and Sports Associations

ARCHERY

American Wheelchair Archers
Chuck Focht
RD #2, Box 2043
West Sunbury, PA 16061
412-735-4359

BASKETBALL

National Wheelchair Basketball Association
Stan Labanowich
110 Seaton Building
University of Kentucky
Lexington, KY 40506
606-257-1623

BOWLING

American Wheelchair Bowling Association
Daryl Pfister
N54 W15858 Larkspur Lane
Menomonee Falls, WI 53051
414-781-6876

FLYING

Freedom's Wings International
1832 Lake Ave.
Scotch Plains, NJ 07076
908-232-6354

International Wheelchair Aviators
John Earle, President
Bill Blackwood, Secretary
1117 Rising Hill
Escondido, CA 92029
619-746-5018

MULTISPORT

Canadian Wheelchair Sports Association
1600 James Naismith Dr.
Gloucester, Ontario K1B 5N4, Canada
613-748-5685
613-748-5722 FAX

Eastern Amputee Athletic Association
Jack Graff, President
Mike Donals, Vice President
2080 Ennabrock Rd.
North Bellmore, NY 11710
516-826-8340

National Handicapped Sports
Kirk Bauer, Executive Director
451 Hungerford Dr., Ste 100
Rockville, MD 20850
301-217-0960

National Wheelchair Athletic Association
3595 East Foundation Blvd., Ste. L-1
Colorado Springs, CO 80910
719-574-1150

United States Cerebral Palsy Athletic Association
Jerry McCole
3810 W. Northwest Highway, Ste. 205
Dallas, TX 75220
214-352-4100
214-352-1477 FAX

Les Autres Athletic Association
Dave Stephenson
1475 West Gray St., Ste 166
Houston, TX 77019
713-521-3737

QUAD SPORTS

United States Quad Rugby Association
Brad Mikkelsen
2418 West Fallcreek Ct.
Grand Forks, ND 58201
701-772-1961

RACQUET SPORTS

International Foundation for Wheelchair Tennis
Peter Burwash
2203 Timberloch Pl., Ste. 126
The Woodlands, TX 77380
713-363-4707

International Wheelchair Tennis Federation
Ellen De Lange
Palliser Road, Barons Ct.
London W14 9EN, England
011-44-71-610-1264 FAX

National Federation of Wheelchair Tennis
Brad Parks, Director
940 Calle Amanecer, Ste. B
San Clemente, CA 92672
714-361-6811

National Wheelchair Racquetball Association
Joe Hagar
535 Kensington Rd., #4
Lancaster, PA 17603
717-394-2111

RECREATION

*National Association of Handicapped Outdoor
    Sportsmen, Inc.*
R.R. 6, Box 25
Centralia, IL 62801
618-532-4565

ROADRACING

International Wheelchair Roadracers Club, Inc.
Joseph M. Dowling, President
30 Myano Lane
Stamford, CT 06902
203-967-2231

SHOOTING

National Wheelchair Shooting Federation
Deanna Greene, President
505 Tish Circle #401
Arlington, TX 76006
817-261-1737

SKIING

National Handicapped Sports
Kirk Bauer, Executive Director
451 Hungerford Dr., Ste. 100
Rockville, MD 20850
301-217-0960

Ski for Light, Inc.
Jeff Pagels, Mobility Impaired Coordinator
1400 Carole Lane
Green Bay, WI 54313
414-494-5572

SOFTBALL

National Wheelchair Softball Association
Jon Speake, Commissioner
1616 Todd Ct.
Hastings, MN 55033
612-437-1792

TABLE TENNIS

American Wheelchair Table Tennis Association
Jennifer Johnson
23 Parker St.
Port Chester, NY 10573
914-937-3932

TRACK & FIELD

Wheelchair Athletics of the USA
Judy Einbinder
1475 West Gray St., #161
Houston, TX 77019
713-522-9769

WATER SPORTS/RECREATION

Access to Sailing
19744 Beach Blvd., Ste. 340
Huntington Beach, CA 92648
714-722-5371

American Canoe Association
7432 Alban Station Blvd., Ste. B-226
Springfield, VA 22150
703-451-0141
703-451-2245 FAX

American Water Ski Association
Phil Martin, Aquatics Director
Disabled Ski Committee
Camp ASCCA
P.O. Box 21
Jackson Gap, AL 36861
205-825-9226

Handicapped Scuba Association
Jim Gatacre
1104 El Prado
San Clemente, CA 92672
714-498-6128

US Association of Disabled Sailors
Southern California Chapter
Mike Watson
P.O. Box 15245
Newport Beach, CA 92659
714-534-5717

US Rowing Association
Adaptive Rowing Committee
Richard Tobin
11 Hall Pl.
Exeter, NH 03833
603-778-0315

US Wheelchair Swimming
Larry Quintiliani
229 Miller St.
Middleboro, MA 02346
508-946-1964

WEIGHTLIFTING & FITNESS

United States Wheelchair Weightlifting Federation
Bill Hens
39 Michael Pl.
Levittown, PA 19057
215-945-1964

National Strength & Conditioning Association
P.O. Box 81410
Lincoln, NE 68501

Glossary

adolescent—A person in the period of life beginning with the appearance of secondary sex characteristics and ending with the cessation of body growth. Roughly the ages from 11 to 19 years.

aerobic—Dependent on oxygen; aerobic fitness implies an enhanced ability to deliver oxygen to the working tissues.

aerobic capacity—A measure of cardiovascular fitness (VO_2max).

anaerobic—Without oxygen. Anaerobic exercise is limited to short duration activities that rely on quick energy sources, i.e., muscle glycogen versus oxygen.

ankylosis—Stiffness or fixation of a joint.

aphasia—Impairment of the ability to communicate through speech, writing, or signs after brain damage.

apraxia—The inability to perform a purposeful movement despite the ability to perform the movement components.

arthrogryposis—A persistent contracture of a joint.

associated reaction—An involuntary movement consisting of increased stiffness in the arms or legs with effort.

asymmetrical—When one side of the body differs from the other in size, strength, or shape.

ataxia—Loss of muscular coordination in the trunk or limbs resulting from damage to the cerebellum.

atherosclerosis—Infiltration of the arterial wall by lipids, with secondary degenerative changes, resulting in a localized narrowing of the vessel with a relative ischemia of distal tissues.

athetosis—Uncontrolled, purposeless writhing movements.

atrophy—Reduction in size and bulk of an organ due to disuse or degeneration.

autism—Self-centered mental state marked by disturbances of speech and repetitious, purposeless movements. Autistic people usually have normal intelligence.

autonomic hyperreflexia or dysreflexia—Condition that can occur in anyone with a spinal cord injury with a complete or incomplete lesion above T6 that produces an exaggerated autonomic response to irritating stimuli to the skin and viscera below the level of the spinal cord damage. (Please see p. 94 for description.)

autonomic nervous system—Maintains the internal environment of the body at an optimal level (homeostasis). A regulatory control system that governs involuntary visceral function (cardiac muscle, smooth muscle, and glands).

bilateral—Involving two sides of the body (e.g., reaching with both hands).

brain stem—Part of the central nervous system that contains the nerve centers of the head and centers for breathing and heart control; connects the cerebrum to the spinal cord.

235

cardiac output—The volume of blood pumped from the heart to the peripheral circulation in a given amount of time. Cardiac output is equal to stroke volume times heart rate.

catheter—Tube used to drain urine from the bladder.

central nervous system—The brain, brain stem, cerebellum, and spinal cord.

cerebellum—The part of the brain that coordinates motor movement.

cerebrospinal fluid (CSF)—Clear fluid surrounding the brain and spinal cord that acts as a shock absorber to protect them.

congenital—A condition that has existed since birth but is not necessarily hereditary.

continence—The ability to control urination and defication.

contracture—Shortening of muscle or other connective tissue that prevents a joint or muscle from moving through its full range of motion.

contralateral—The opposite side of the body.

deep vein thrombosis (DVT)—A blood clot in the veins. People who have had a stroke, a traumatic spinal cord injury, and the like, show a predisposition to developing DVTs in the lower extremities, which can develop into a pulmonary embolism.

dysarthria—Slurred speech.

edema—Local or generalized condition in which body tissues contain excessive fluid.

embolus—A mass of undissolved matter floating freely in the blood vessels or vascular system. Lodged emboli can occlude blood vessels.

ergometer (bicycle)—An apparatus for measuring the muscular, metabolic, and respiratory effects of exercise.

exacerbation—The flaring of clinical symptoms.

exercise hypotension—A drop in blood pressure during exercise attributed to a dysfunctional autonomic nervous system and blood pooling in paralyzed lower extremities. Most often seen in people who have quadriplegia because of a spinal cord injury.

flaccid (hypotonic)—Absence of muscle tone.

hemiplegia—Motor impairment on one side of the body.

heterotopic ossification—The excessive laying down of bone in tissues across joints.

hydrocephalus—Excessive accumulation of cerebrospinal fluid in the ventricles of the brain due to blocked fluid circulation. Results in compression of the brain and eventually head enlargement.

hyperplasia—Increase in the number of muscle fibers, for example, in response to long-term, heavy training.

hypertension—Pathological increase of resting blood pressure, commonly a systolic reading of more than 160 mmHg or a diastolic reading of more than 90 to 95 mmHg.

hypertrophy—Increase in size, for example, of individual muscle fibers.

innervation—Connection and stimulation to a muscle through nerve action.

les autres—Heterogeneous category of disabled sports competitors other than those who are paraplegics, amputees, blind, deaf, or cerebral palsied.

ligaments—Connective tissue that connects bone to bone.

lordosis—The anterior concavity in the curvature of the lumbar and cervical spine as viewed from the side. Refers to abnormally increased curvature (swayback) and normal curvature (normal lordosis).

meningocele—Protrusion of the protective covering of the spinal cord (the meninges) through an opening in the spinal column forming a sac. If the spinal cord and nerves remain intact, there tends to be no neurological deficit after surgical removal of the sac.

muscular dystrophy—A familial disease characterized by progressive wasting of muscles with eventual loss of ambulation ability and respiratory involvement. Onset is usually at an early age.

myelin—A fatty substance surrounding certain nerves that allows faster, more efficient electrical transmission.

myelomeningocele—Protrusion of the meninges and a portion of the spinal cord through an opening in the spine to form a sac. The spinal cord and nerves are usually damaged, resulting in a neurological deficit.

neglect—Not attending to, recognizing, or acknowledging the affected side of the body.

nerves—Body structures that allow electrical stimulation of muscles and glands.

nystagmus—Rhythmical oscillation of the eyeballs, either horizontal, vertical, or rotary.

orthosis—A device used to correct a deformity, support the body, or control involuntary movements. Orthopedic appliances can include shoe inserts, splints, and braces.

orthostatic hypotension—An intolerance to an upright position because one is not able to adjust to the body's position and not enough blood reaches the brain when the blood pressure drops.

osteoporosis—Progressive decrease in the internal content of the bone, seen as a consequence of lack of weight-bearing activity that predisposes the affected body part to fractures.

overload principle—Stressing or overloading a muscle that increases muscle strength, size, or both.

paralysis—Loss of voluntary muscle use due to damage of the neural or muscular mechanism.

paraplegia—Neurological impairment to lower extremity that may also involve part of the trunk, although the person retains full use of the upper extremity, including the hand. Paraplegia can be complete or incomplete depending on the extent of spinal cord damage.

parasympathetic nervous system—Part of the autonomic nervous system that is partially responsible for automatic functions, such as the heart beating, blood pressure, bladder and bowel functions, and sexual responses; centered in the head and sacral spinal region. Some effects of the parasympathetic nervous system include slowing the heart rate and increasing gland secretion (except sweat glands) to help the body's internal environment return to a normal level after a stressful event has occurred.

passive stretching—The movement of a person's muscles to a stretched position by someone else.

poliomyelitis—More properly, anterior poliomyelitis; a viral infection that localizes in the anterior horn cells of the spinal cord and causes paralysis of the affected motor units.

power—Maximal strength-producing capacity of an individual expressed relative to time.

$$\frac{(Force \times Distance)}{Time}$$

preadolescent—The period of life before the completion of the pubertal changes.

prepubescent—The period of life before puberty.

pressure sores—A breakdown of skin and other tissues from continuous sitting or reclining.

proprioception—Appreciation of body or limb position.

prosthesis—Artificial body part; in the present context, an artificial limb.

pubescent—Arrived, or arriving, at puberty.

pulmonary embolism—A circulating clot in the blood stream that lodges and obstructs blood flow in the pulmonary artery of the lungs.

quadriplegia—Neurological impairment in all four extremities and the trunk with complete or incomplete damage to the spinal cord.

reciprocal inhibition—A process within the nervous system that inhibits or relaxes an antagonist muscle while simultaneously stimulating the agonist muscle, for example, contraction of the biceps and relaxation of the triceps during a biceps curl.

reflexes—Involuntary postures and movements excited in response to a stimulus applied to the periphery and transmitted to the nervous centers in the brain or spinal cord.

remission—The stabilization of a disease process clinically; lessening of symptoms.

sensory—Relating to perception by the senses (touch, taste, smell, sight, hearing).

scoliosis—A large lateral deviation in the normally straight vertical line of the spine as viewed from the back; it may be accompanied by varying degrees of abnormal rotation of the spinal column.

shunt—Flexible tube surgically inserted from the ventricles to the heart (ventriculoatrial shunt) or the abdominal cavity (ventriculoperitoneal shunt) to drain excess cerebrospinal fluid from the brain.

spasm—Sudden tightening of muscles, increase in spasticity.

spasticity—An abnormal, velocity-dependent increase in muscle tone (hypertonia).

spina bifida—Congenital spine malformation characterized by failure of the vertebrae to fuse.

spinal cord—The part of the central nervous system that connects the brain and its related structures to the peripheral nervous system.

stroke volume—Blood pumped out of the heart with each beat.

submaximal workload—Workload less than a single maximum effort. Involves lower intensities to maintain work for longer durations.

symmetrical—When both sides of the body are the same in size, strength, or shape.

sympathetic nervous system—Part of the autonomic nervous system that is partially responsible for many automatic functions such as sweating, heart beating, sexual activity, and bowel and bladder functions; centered in the thoracic and lumbar back region. It functions to help maintain homeostasis during rest and to prepare the body for stressful events.

synergistic muscles—Muscle groups that contract together to perform a specific movement.

tendon—Connective tissue that connects muscle to bone.

tenodesis—Using wrist extension to passively pull the fingers into flexion. It can be used by someone who does not have working muscles in the hand for a functional grasp.

thermoregulation—Regulating the temperature of the body.

thrombosis—Development of a blood clot (thrombus) within the vascular system.

trunk—The body distinct from the limbs.

vasomotor tone—Muscular tone of the blood vessels.

ventricles—Cavities deep within the brain that secrete cerebrospinal fluid.

vertebrae—Bones that link together to form the spinal column.

vital capacity—Volume of air that can be exhaled following full inspiration.

work—Product of force times the distance through which force is exerted (often expressed in joules).

Sources

Chapter 1

American Academy of Pediatrics. (1983). Weight training and weight lifting: Information for the pediatrician. *Physician and Sportsmedicine,* **11**(3), 157-161.

American Academy of Pediatrics. (1991). Guidelines for teens. *Better health through fitness.* (Brochure)

American College of Sports Medicine (1991). *Guidelines for graded exercise testing and exercise prescription.* Philadelphia: Lea & Febiger.

Avers, D., & Wharton, M. (1991). Improving exercise adherence: Instructional strategies. *Topics in Geriatric Rehabilitation,* **6**(3), 62-73.

Bar-Or, O. (1989). Trainability of the prepubescent child. *Physician and Sports-medicine,* **17**(5), 65-82.

Berg, K. (1970). Effect of physiological training of school children with cerebral palsy. *ACTA Paediatrica Scandinavica (Supplement),* 27-52.

Bernard, B., Creswell, J., Erikson, V., Ivey, J., Johnston, B., & Alexander, L. (1981). Exercise for children with physical disabilities. *Issues in Comprehensive Pediatric Nursing,* **5,** 99-107.

Bohannon, R.W. (1983). Results of resistance exercise on a patient with amyotrophic lateral sclerosis. *Physical Therapy,* **63,** 965-968.

Brady, T., Cahill, B., & Bodnar, L. (1982). Weight training related injuries in the high school athlete. *American Journal of Sports Medicine,* **10,** 1-5.

Brown, E., & Kimball, R. (1983). Medical history associated with adolescent powerlifting. *Pediatrics,* **72,** 636-644.

Brunnstrom, S. (1941). Muscle group testing. *Physiotherapy Review,* **21,** 3-21.

Cahill, B. (Ed.) (1988). *Proceedings of the conference on strength training and the prepubescent* (pp. 1-14). Chicago: American Orthopaedic Society for Sports Medicine..

Daniels, L., & Worthingham, C. (1986). *Manual muscle testing: Techniques of manual examination.* Philadelphia: Saunders.

Duda, M. (1986). Prepubescent strength training gains support. *Physician and Sportsmedicine,* **14**(2), 157-161.

Dyment, P. (1989). Controversies in pediatric sports medicine. *Physician and Sportsmedicine,* **17**(7), 57-71.

Einarsson, G. (1991). Muscle conditioning in late poliomyelitis. *Archives of Physical Medicine and Rehabilitation,* **72,** 11-14.

Fillyaw, M.J., & Ades, P.A. (1989). Endurance exercise training in Friedreichs ataxia. *Archives of Physical Medicine and Rehabilitation,* **70,** 787-788.

Florence, J.M., & Hagberg, J.M. (1984). Effect of training on the exercise responses of neuromuscular disease patients. *Medicine in Science, Sports and Exercise,* **16,** 460-465.

Fowler, W.M., & Taylor, M. (1982). Rehabilitation management of muscular dystrophy and related disorders: The role of exercise. *Archives of Physical Medicine and Rehabilitation*, **63**, 319-321.

Fox, M., & Atwood, J. (1955). Results testing Iowa school children for health and fitness. *Journal of Health, Physical Education and Recreation*, **26**, 20-21.

Grimby, G. (1988). Physical activity and the effects of muscle training in the elderly. *Annals of Clinical Research*, **20**, 62-66.

Gumbs, V., Segal, D., Halligan, J., & Lower, G. (1982). Bilateral distal radius and ulnar fractures in adolescent weight lifters. *American Journal of Sports Medicine*, **10**, 375-379.

Hartley-O'Brien, S.J. (1980). Six mobilization exercises for active range of hip flexion. *Research Quarterly for Exercise and Sport*, **51**, 625-635.

Hedrick, B., & Morse, M. (1992, March/April). Preventing burnout in junior athletes: Training tips. *Sports 'N Spokes*, pp. 64-66.

Heyward, V.H. (1984). *Designs for fitness: A guide to physical fitness appraisal and exercise prescription*. New York: Macmillan.

Hjeltnes, N. (1982). Capacity for physical work and training after spinal injuries and strokes. *Scandinavian Journal of Socialized Medicine (Supplement)*, **29**, 245-251.

Holland, L.J., & Steadward, R.D. (1990, Summer). Effects of resistance and flexibility training and strength, spasticity muscle tone and range of motion of elite athletes with cerebral palsy. *Palaestra*, pp. 27-31.

Inaba, M., Edberg, E., Montgomery, J., & Gillis, K.M. (1973). Effectiveness of function training, active exercise and resistive exercise for patients with hemiplegia. *Physical Therapy*, **54**, 28-35.

Jesse, J. (1977). Olympic lifting movements endanger adolescents. *Physician and Sportsmedicine*, **5**(9), 61-67.

Koebel, C., Swank, A., & Shelburne, L. (1992). Fitness testing in children: A comparison between PCPFS and AAHPERD standards. *Journal of Applied Sport Science Research*, **6**(2), 107-114.

Larson, C., & McMahan, R. (1966). The epiphyses and the childhood athlete. *Journal of the American Medical Association*, **196**(7), 99-104.

Legwold, G. (1982). Does lifting weights harm a prepubescent athlete? *Physician and Sportsmedicine*, **10**(7), 141-144.

Lewis, C. (1991, August). Experts urge exercise for osteoarthritis. *Physical Therapy Bulletin*, p. 2.

Malina, R. (1988). The average child deserves more fitness programs. *Physician and Sportsmedicine*, **16**(10), 39.

Micheli, L. (1983). Overuse injuries in children's sports: The growth factor. *Orthopedic Clinics of North America*, **14**(2), 337-359.

Milner-Brown, H.S., & Miller, R.G. (1988). Muscle strengthening through high-resistance weight training in patients with neuromuscular disorders. *Archives of Physical Medicine and Rehabilitation*, **69**, 14-19.

Monga, T.N., Deforge, D.A., Williams, J., & Wolfe, L.A. (1988). Cardiovascular responses to acute exercise in patients with cerebrovascular accidents. *Archives of Physical Medicine and Rehabilitation*, **69**, 937-940.

Moskwa, C., & Nichols, J. (1989). Musculoskeletal risk factors in the young athlete. *Physician and Sportsmedicine*, **17**(11), 49-59.

Naso, F., Carner, E., Blankfort-Doyle, W., & Coughey, K. (1990). Endurance training in the elderly nursing home patient. *Archives of Physical Medicine and Rehabilitation*, **71**, 241-243.

National Strength and Conditioning Association. (1985). Position statement on prepubescent strength training. *National Strength and Conditioning Association Journal*, **7**, 27-31.

Nelson, M. (1991). Developmental skills and children's sports. *Physician and Sportsmedicine*, **19**(2), 67-79.

Palmer, S.S., Mortimer, J.A., Webster, D.D., Bistevins, R., & Dickinson, G.L. (1986). Exercise therapy for Parkinson's disease. *Archives of Physical Medicine and Rehabilitation*, **67**, 741-745.

Pearl, B., & Moran, G. (1986). *Getting stronger: Weight training for men and women*. Bolinas, CA: Shelter.

Raithel, K. (1987). Are girls less fit than boys? *Physician and Sportsmedicine*, **15**(11), 157-162.

Raithel, K. (1988). Are American children really unfit? (Part 1 of 2): *Physician and Sportsmedicine*, **16**(10), 146-154.

Rimmer, J. (1993). *Exercise and aging*. Chicago: Rehabilitation Institute of Chicago course material from "Aging and Rehabilitation: Exercise and Exercise Programming for Elderly Populations."

Sailors, M., & Berg, K. (1987). Comparison of responses to weight training in prepubescent boys and men. *Journal of Sports Medicine*, **27**, 30-37.

Sawaka, M., Glaser, R., Loubach, L., Al-Samakari, O., & Suryaprasad, A. (1981). Wheelchair exercise performance of the young, middle aged and elderly. *Journal of Applied Physiology: Respiratory Environmental Exercise Physiology*, **50**, 824-828.

Sewall, L., & Micheli, L. (1986). Strength training for children. *Journal of Pediatric Orthopedics*, **6**(2), 143-146.

Sherrill, C. (1993). *Adapted physical activity, recreation and sport: Crossdisciplinary and lifespan.* Dubuque, IA: Brown and Benchmark.

Terbizan, D.J. (1992). Body composition management: What can we use in the conditioning facility? *National Strength and Conditioning Association Journal*, **14**, 30-34.

Wilkins, K. (1980). The uniqueness of the young athlete: Musculoskeletal injuries. *American Journal of Sports Medicine*, **8**, 377-382.

Additional Readings

Kraemer, W.J., & Fleck, S.J. (1993). *Strength training for young athletes.* Champaign, IL: Human Kinetics.

Winnick, J.P., & Short, F.X. (1985). *Physical fitness testing of the disabled (Project Unique).* Champaign, IL: Human Kinetics.

Winnick, J.P. (1990). *Adapted physical education and sport.* Champaign, IL: Human Kinetics.

Chapter 2

Abraham, W.M. (1977). Factors in delayed muscle soreness. *Medicine and Science in Sports*, **9**, 11-20.

Adrian, M., & O'Connor, J. (1992). Pumping safety. *Training and Conditioning*, **2**(4), 21-23.

American College of Sports Medicine. (1988). *Musculoskeletal injury: Risks, prevention, and first aid* (pp. 285-294). Philadelphia: Lea & Febiger.

Armitage-Johnson, S. (1990). Maintenance and safety: Emergency procedures. *National Strength and Conditioning Association Journal*, **12**(4), 39-43.

Armstrong, R.B. (1986). Muscle damage and endurance events. *Sports Medicine*, **3**, 370-381.

Asmussen, E. (1953). Positive and negative muscular work. *Acta Physiologica Scandinavia*, **28**, 364-382.

Asmussen, E. (1956). Observations on experimental muscle soreness. *Acta Rheum. Scandinavia*, **2**, 109-116.

Bennet, R.L., & Knowlton, G.C. (1958). Overwork weakness in partially denervated skeletal muscle. *Clinical Orthopaedics*, **12**, 22-29.

Berger, R.A. (1965). Effect of varied weight training programs on strength. *Research Quarterly*, **33**, 44-54.

Bigland-Ritchie, B., & Woods, J.J. (1976). Integrated electromyogram and oxygen uptake during positive and negative work. *Journal of Physiological Conditioning*, **250**, 267-277.

Bilcheck, H., Marech, C., & Kraemer, W. (1992). Muscular fatigue: A brief overview. *National Strength and Conditioning Association Journal*, **14**(6), 9-15.

Bompa, T. (1990). Periodization of strength: The most effective methodology of strength training. *National Strength and Conditioning Association Journal*, **12**, 49-52.

Borselen, F., Vos, N., Fry, A., & Kraemer, W. (1992). The role of anaerobic exercise in overtraining. *National Strength and Conditioning Association Journal*, **14**(3), 74-79.

Burgener, M. (1991). How to properly miss with a barbell. *National Strength and Conditioning Association Journal*, **13**(3), 24-25.

Cantu, R. (1981). The prevention of athletic head and spine injuries. In *Health maintenance through physical conditioning* (pp. 123-159). Littleton, MA: PSG.

Carr, J.H., & Shepard, R.B. (1980). Hypertonus in physiotherapy. In *Physiotherapy in disorders of the brain.* London: William Heinemann Medical Books.

Curtis, K. (1981, May/June). Part I: Basics of exercise physiology. *Sports 'N Spokes*, pp. 26-28.

Curtis, K. (1982, January/February). Part IV: Athletic injuries. *Sports 'N Spokes*, pp. 20-24.

Delorme, T.L., & Watkins, A.L. (1948). Techniques of progressive resistance exercise. *Archives of Physical Medicine*, **29**, 263-271.

DeVries, H.A. (1966). Quantitative electromy investigation of the spasm theory of muscle pain. *American Journal of Physical Medicine*, **45**, 119-134.

DeVries, H.A. (1980). *Physiology of exercise for physical education and athletics.* Dubuque, IA: Brown.

Drachman, D.B., Murphy, S.R., Nigam, M.P., & Hills, J.R. (1967). Myopathic changes in chronically denervated muscle. *Archives of Neurology*, **16**, 14-24.

Ebbeling, C.B., & Clarkson, P.M. (1989). Exercise induced muscle damage and adaptation. *Sports Medicine*, **7**, 207-233.

Einarsson, G. (1991). Muscle conditioning in late poliomyelitis. *Archives of Physical Medicine and Rehabilitation, 72,* 11-14.

Feldman, R.M. (1985). The use of strengthening exercises in post polio sequelae. *Orthopaedics, 8,* 889-890.

Figoni, S., Morse, M., & Hedrick, B. (1993). Overtraining in wheelchair sports. *Sports 'N Spokes, 18*(5), 43-48.

Fillyaw, M.J., & Andes, P.A. (1989). Endurance exercise training in Friedreich's ataxia. *Archives of Physical Medicine and Rehabilitation, 70,* 786-788.

Fleck, S.J. (1983). Interval training—physiological basis. *National Strength and Conditioning Association Journal, 5*(5), 40.

Fleck, S.J., & Flalkel, J.E. (1986). Value or resistance training for the reduction of sports injuries. *Sports Medicine, 3,* 61-68.

Florence, J.M., & Hagberg, J.M. (1984). Effect of training on the exercise responses of neuromuscular disease patients. *Medicine and Science in Sports and Exercise, 16,* 460-465.

Fowler, M. (Ed.) (1988). Management of musculoskeletal complications in neuromuscular diseases: Weakness and the role of exercise. *Physical Medicine and Rehabilitation: State of the Art Reviews.* Philadelphia: Honely & Blefus.

Fox, E.L., & Mathews, D.K. (1981). *The physiological basis of physical education and athletics* (3rd ed.). Philadelphia: W.B. Saunders.

Gambetta, V. (1991). Concept and application of periodization. *National Strength and Conditioning Association Journal, 13,* 64-66.

Gardner, G.W. (1963). Specificity of strength changes of the exercised and nonexercised limb following isometric training. *Research Quarterly, 34,* 98.

Gettman, L.R., & Pollock, M.L. (1981). Circuit weight training: A critical review of its physiological benefits. *Physician and Sports Medicine, 9,* 44-60.

Gonyea, W.J. (1981). Muscle fiber splitting in trained and untrained animals. In R.S. Hutton & D.I. Miller (Eds.), *Exercise and Sports Sciences Reviews* (Vol. 9). Philadelphia: Franklin Institution Press.

Gonyea, W.J., Sale, D.G., Gonyea, F.B., Mikesky, A. (1986). Exercise induced increases in muscle fiber number. *European Journal of Applied Physiology and Occupational Physiology, 55,* 137-141.

Hakkinen, K., & Komi, P. (1982). Specificity of training: Induced changes in strength performance considering the integrative functions of the neuromuscular system. *World Weightlifting, 3,* 44-46.

Hakkinen, K. (1989). Neuromuscular and hormonal adaptations during strength and power training. *Journal of Sports Medicine and Physical Fitness, 29,* 9-26.

Harman, E., & Frykman, P. (1990). The effects of knee wraps on weightlifting performance and injury. *National Strength and Conditioning Association Journal, 12*(5), 30-35.

Herbison, G.J., Jawed, M.M., Ditanno, J.F., & Scott, C.M. (1973). Effects of overwork during reinnervation of rat muscle. *Experimental Neurology, 41,* 1-14.

Heyward, V.H. (1984). *Designs for fitness: A guide to physical fitness appraisal and exercise prescription.* New York: Macmillan.

Hjelthes, N. (1982). Capacity for physical work and training after spinal injuries and strokes. *Scandinavian Journal of Socialized Medicine (Supplementum), 29,* 245-251.

Holland, L.J., & Steward, R.D. (1990, Summer). Effects of resistance and flexibility training on strength, spasticity, muscle tone, and range of motion of elite athletes with cerebral palsy. *Palaestra,* pp. 27-31.

Hoskins, T.A. (1975). Physiologic responses to known exercise loads in hemiparetic patients. *Archives of Physical Medicine and Rehabilitation, 56,* 544.

Inaba, M., Edberg, E., Montgomery, J., & Gillis, K.M. (1973). Effectiveness of functional training, active exercise, and resistive exercise for patients with hemiplegia. *Physical Therapy, 53,* 28-35.

Johnson, E.W., & Braddom, R. (1971). Overwork weakness in facioscapulohumeral muscular distrophy. *Archives of Physical Medicine and Rehabilitation, 52,* 333-336.

Jones, J.A. (Ed.) (1988). *Training guide to cerebral palsy sports* (3rd ed.). Champaign, IL: Human Kinetics.

Komi, P.V., & Buskirk, E.R. (1972). The effect of eccentric and concentric muscle activity on tension and electrical activity of human muscle. *Ergonometrics, 15,* 417-434.

Kraemer, W.J. (1982). Weight training: What you don't know will hurt you. *Journal of Health, Physical Education, Recreation and Dance, 5,* 8.

Kraemer, W.J. (1984/1985). Exercise prescription series. *National Strength and Conditioning Association Journal, 6*(1) to *7*(3).

Kraemer, W.J. (1990a). Anaerobic exercise program prescription guidelines. *National Strength and Conditioning Association Symposium.* San Diego, pp. 99-104.

Kraemer, W.J. (1990b). Training responses and adaptations. *National Strength and Conditioning Association Symposium* (pp. 22-27). San Diego, CA.

Kraemer, W.J., & Fleck, S.J. (1982). Anaerobic metabolism and its evaluation. *National Strength and Conditioning Association Journal,* **4**(2), 20.

Kultury, T., Filin, A., & Rubin, V. (1990). Load and periodization of the training process of young athletes during individual phases of multi-year preparation in cyclical endurance sports. *National Strength and Conditioning Association Journal,* **25**, 133-135.

Lenman, J.A. (1959). A clinical and experimental study of the effects of exercise on motor weakness in neurological diseases. *Journal of Neurological Neurosurgery and Psychiatry,* **22**, 144-182.

McCartney, N., Moroz, D., Garner, S.H., & McComes, A.J. (1988). The effects of strength training in patients with selected neuromuscular disorders. *Medicine and Science in Sports and Exercise,* **20**, 362-368.

Miller-Brown, H.S., & Miller, R.G. (1988). Muscle strengthening through high-resistance weight training in patients with neuromuscular disorders. *Archives of Physical Medicine and Rehabilitation,* **69**, 14-19.

Millikan, T., Morse, M., Hart, A., & Hedrick, B. (1993). Injury treatment in wheelchair athletics. *Sports 'N Spokes,* **18**(6), 85-88.

Morgan, W., Costill, D., Flynn, M., Raglin, J., & O'Conner, P. (1988). Mood disturbance following increased training in swimmers. *Medicine and Science in Sports and Exercise,* **20**, 408-414.

Moritani, T., & DeVries, H.A. (1979). Neural factors versus hypertrophy in the time course of muscle strength gain. *American Journal of Physical Medicine,* **58**, 115-130.

Nygard, E., & Nielsen, E. (1978). Skeletal muscle fiber composition with extreme endurance training in man. *Swimming Medicine.* Baltimore: University Park Press.

Olgiati, R., Burgunder, J.M., & Mumenthaler, M. (1988). Increased energy cost of walking in multiple sclerosis: Effects of spasticity, ataxia and weakness. *Archives of Physical Medicine and Rehabilitation,* **69**, 846-849.

Pauletto, B. (1986). Let's talk training. Series #1: Sets and reps; #2: Intensity; #3: Choice and order of exercise. *National Strength and Conditioning Association Journal,* **7**(6), 67; **8**(1), 33IT; **8**(2), 71IT.

Peach, P.E. (1990). Overwork weakness with evidence of muscle damage in patients with residual paralysis from polio. *Archives of Physical Medicine and Rehabilitation,* **71**, 248-250.

Pearl, B., & Moran, G. (1986). *Getting stronger: Weight training for men and women* (pp. 354-357). Bolinas, CA: Shelter.

Poliquin, C. (1984, July-September). Theory and methodology of strength training. *Sports Coach,* pp. 25-27.

Pollack, M.L., Ward, A., & Ayers, J.J. (1977). Cardiorespiratory fitness: Response to differing intensities and durations of training. *Archives of Physical Medicine and Rehabilitation,* **58**, 467.

Round Table. (1983). Overtraining of athletes: A round table. *Physician and Sports Medicine,* **11**, 92-110.

Roy, S., & Irvin, R. (1983). *Sports medicine: Prevention, evaluation, management and rehabilitation* (p. 361). Englewood Cliffs, NJ: Prentice-Hall.

Russell, W.R. (1947). Poliomyelitis: The preparalytic stage and the effect of physical activity on the severity of paralysis. *British Medical Journal,* **2**, 1023-1028.

Sale, D.G. (1988). Neural adaptation to resistance training. *Medicine and Science in Sports and Exercise (Supplement),* **20**, 135-145.

Shellock, F. (1986). Physiological, psychological and injury prevention aspects of warm-up. *National Strength and Conditioning Association Journal,* pp. 12-14.

Sherrill, C. (1993). *Adapted physical activity, recreation and sport: Crossdisciplinary and lifespan.* Dubuque, IA: Brown and Benchmark.

Skerker, R.S. (1991). Review and update: The aerobic exercise prescription: Critical reviews. *Physical Rehabilitation and Medicine,* **2**, 257-271.

Smith, L.L. (1992). Causes of delayed onset muscle soreness and the impact in athlete performance: A review. *Journal of Applied Sports Science Research,* **6**(3), 135-141.

Southmayd, W., & Hoffman, M. (1981). *Sports health: The complete book of athletic injuries* (pp. 53-69). New York: Perigree Books.

Stauber, W.T., Clarkson, P.M., Fritz, V.K., & Evans, W.J. (1990). Extracellular matrix disruption and pain after eccentric muscle action. *Journal of Applied Physiology*, **69**(3), 868-874.

Stone, M.H., O'Bryant, H., Grahammer, J., McMillan, J., & Rozenek, R. (1982). A theoretical model of strength training. *National Strength and Conditioning Association Journal*, **4**, 4.

Stone, M.H. (1983). Cardiovascular responses to short term Olympic style weight training in young men. *Journal of Applied Sport Science*, **8**, 134-139.

Stone, M.H. (1988). Implications for connective tissue and bone alterations resulting from resistance exercise training. *Medicine and Science in Sports and Exercise*, **20**, 5162-5168.

Stone, M., Keith, R., Kearney, J., Fleck, S., Wilson, G., & Triplett, N. (1991). Overtraining: A review of the signs, symptoms and possible causes. *Journal of Applied Sport Science Research*, **5**(1), 35-50.

Stotts, K.M. (1986). Health maintenance: Paraplegic athletes and nonathletes. *Archives of Physical Medicine and Rehabilitation*, **67**, 104-114.

Talag, T.S. (1973). Residual muscle soreness as influenced by concentric, eccentric and static contractions. *Research Quarterly*, 458-469.

Tesch, P.A., & Karlsson, J. (1983). Muscle fiber type characteristics of deltoids in wheelchair athletes: Comparison with other trained athletes. *American Journal of Physical Medicine*, **62**, 239-243.

Tesch, P.A., & Karlsson, J. (1985). Muscle fiber types and size in trained and untrained muscles of elite athletes. *Journal of Applied Physiology*, **59**, 1716-1720.

Tesch, P.A. (1988). Skeletal muscle adaptations consequent to long term heavy resistance exercise. *Medicine and Science in Sports and Exercise*, **20**, 5132-5134.

Tschiene, P. (1978). The distinction of training structure in different stages of the preparation of athletes. Paper presented at the International Congress of Sports Sciences, Edmonton, Alberta, Canada, July 25-29.

Verma, S., Mahindro, S., & Kansal, D. (1978). Effect of four weeks of hard physical training on certain physiological and morphological parameters of basketball players. *Journal of Sports Medicine and Physical Fitness*, **18**(4), 379-384.

Vogel, J.A. (1988). Introduction to the symposium: Physiological responses and adaptations to resistance exercise. *Medicine and Science in Sports and Exercise*, **20**, 5-31.

Vorobeyev, A. (1978). *Weightlifting* (W. Brice, Trans.). Budapest: International Weightlifting Federation (Medical Committee).

Willoughby, D. (1993). The effects of meso-cycle length weight training programs involving periodization and partially equated volumes on upper and lower body strength. *Journal of Strength and Conditioning Research (NSCA)*, **7**(1), 2-8.

Wolf, J. (1971). Mental characteristics: Staleness. In Larson and Herrmann (Eds.), *Encyclopedia of sport sciences and medicine* (pp. 1048-1050). New York: Macmillan.

Young, W. (1992). The planning of resistive training for power sports. *National Strength and Conditioning Association Journal*, **13**(4), 26-29.

Chapter 3

American College of Sports Medicine. (1991). *Guidelines for exercise testing and prescription* (pp. 16, 69, 100, 104, 105). Philadelphia: Lea & Febiger.

American Heart Association. (1990). *Exercise physiology in healthy adults (exercise handout/worksheet)*. Dallas: Author.

Åstrand, P.O., & Rodahl, K. (1977). *Textbook of work physiology*. New York: McGraw-Hill.

Bernhardt, D.B. (1985). Exercise testing and training for disabled populations: The state of the art. *Recreation for the Disabled Child* (pp. 13-25). Boston: Haworth Press.

Borg, G.A. (1982). Psychophysical bases of perceived exertion. *Medicine and Science in Sports and Exercise*, **14**(5), 377-381.

Cooper, R.A., & Baldini, F.D. (1991). What do VO_2max and body composition assessment mean to the wheelchair athlete? *National Wheelchair Athletic Association*, 4-5.

Cowell, L.L., Squires, W.G., & Raven, P.B. (1986). Benefits of aerobic exercise for the paraplegic: A brief review. *Medicine and Science in Sports and Exercise*, **18**(5), 501-508.

Curtis, K.A. (1981, May-June). Part 1: Basics of exercise physiology. *Sports 'N Spokes*, pp. 26-28.

Curtis, K.A. (1981, May-June). Part 2: Training. *Sports 'N Spokes*, pp. 26-28.

Davis, G.M., Shephard, R.J., & Jackson, R.W. (1981). Cardio-respiratory fitness and muscular strength in the lower-limb disabled.

Canadian Journal of Applied Sport Sciences,
6(4), 159-165.

DiCarlo, S.E. (1988). Effect of arm ergometry training on wheelchair propulsion endurance of individuals with quadriplegia. *Physical Therapy,* **68**(1), 40-44.

Einarsson, G. (1991). Muscle conditioning in late poliomyelitis. *Archives of Physical Medicine and Rehabilitation,* **72**, 11-14.

Eriksson, P., Lofstrom, L., & Ekblom, B. (1988). Aerobic power during maximal exercise in untrained and well-trained persons with quadriplegia and paraplegia. *Scandinavian Journal of Rehab Medicine,* **20**, 141-147.

Figoni, Stephen F. (1990). Perspectives on cardiovascular fitness and SCI. *Journal of the American Paraplegia Society,* **13**(4), 63-71.

Fillyaw, M.J., & Andes, P.A. (1989). Endurance exercise training in Friedreichs ataxia. *Archives of Physical Medicine and Rehabilitation,* **70**, 786-788.

Fleck, S.J. (1983). Interval training—physiological basis. *National Strength and Conditioning Association Journal,* **5**(5), 40.

Florence, J.M., & Hagberg, J.M. (1984). Effect of training on the exercise responses of neuromuscular disease patients. *Medicine and Science in Sports and Exercise,* **16**(4), 460-465.

Fowler, M. (Ed.) (1988). Management of musculoskeletal complications in neuromuscular diseases: Weakness and the role of exercise. *Physical Medicine and Rehabilitation: State of the Art Reviews.* Philadelphia: Honley & Belfus.

Fox, E.L., & Mathews, D.K. (1981). *The physiological basis of physical education and athletics* (3rd ed.). Philadelphia: W.B. Saunders.

Frankel, D., & Buxbaum, R. (1982). *Maximizing your health: A program of graded exercise and meditation for persons with multiple sclerosis.* New York: National Multiple Sclerosis Society.

Glaser, R.M., Sawka, M.N., Young, R.E., & Suryaprasad, A.G. (1980). Applied physiology for wheelchair design. *Journal of Applied Physiology,* **48**, 41-44.

Gorman, D., Brown, B., & Marty, P.J. (1984, February). The role of aerobic exercise in fat loss. *Paraplegia News,* pp. 25-28.

Hakkinen, K., Alen, M., & Komi, P.V. (1984). Neuromuscular anaerobic and aerobic performance characteristics of elite power athletes. *European Journal of Applied Physiology,* **53**, 47-105.

Hjelthes, N. (1982). Capacity for physical work and training after spinal injuries and strokes. *Scandinavian Journal of Social Medicine (Supplementum),* **29**, 245-251.

Hoskins, T.A. (1975). Physiologic responses to known exercise loads in hemiparetic patients. *Archives of Physical Medicine and Rehabilitation,* **56**, 544.

Hunter, G. (1990). Aerobic exercise prescription program guidelines. *Proceedings of the National Strength and Conditioning Association Symposium* (pp. 87-98). San Diego, CA.

Kraemer, W.J., & Fleck, S.J. (1982). Anaerobic metabolism and its evaluation. *National Strength and Conditioning Association Journal,* **4**(2), 20.

Kraemer, W.J. (1984/1985). Exercise prescription series. *National Strength and Conditioning Association Journal,* **6**(1) to **7**(3).

Kraemer, W.J. (1990). Anaerobic exercise program prescription guidelines. *Proceedings of the National Strength and Conditioning Association symposium* (pp. 99-104). San Diego, CA.

Kraemer, W.J. (1990). Training responses and adaptations. *Proceedings of the National Strength and Conditioning Association Symposium* (pp. 22-27). San Diego, CA.

Lenman, J.A. (1959). A clinical and experimental study of the effects of exercise on motor weakness in neurological diseases. *Journal of Neurology, Neurosurgery, and Psychiatry,* **22**, 144-182.

McCarthy, J.P., & Hunter, G.H. (1983). Blood pressure adaptations to training. *National Strength and Conditioning Association Journal,* **5**(6), 44.

McCartney, N., Moroz, D., Garner, S.H., & McComes, A.J. (1988). The effects of strength training in patients with selected neuromuscular disorders. *Medicine and Science in Sports and Exercise,* **20**(4), 362-368.

Micheo, W.F., & Frontera, W. (1989). Fitness and the disabled. *Boletin-Asociacion Medica de Puerto Rico (San Juan),* **81**(11), 447-450.

Noble, B.J. (1986). *Physiology of exercise and sport* (pp. 358, 369, 416). St. Louis: Times Mirror/Mosby College.

Nygard, E., & Nielsen, E. (1978). Skeletal muscle fiber composition with extreme endurance training in man. In B.O. Ericksson & B. Furberg (Eds.), *Swimming medicine* (pp. 282-293). Baltimore: University Park Press.

Pauletto, B. (1985/1986). Let's talk training. Series #1: Sets and repetitions; #2: Intensity; #3: Choice and order of exercises. *National Strength and Conditioning Association Journal*, **7**(6), 67; **8**(1), 33IT; **8**(2), 71IT.

Richard, D., & Birrer, R. (1988). Exercise stress testing. *Journal of Family Practice*, **26**, 425-435.

Rimmer, J.H. (1991). Exercise physiology in healthy adults. *Aging and Rehabilitation: Exercise and Exercise Programming in the Elderly Populations*. Chicago, IL: Course presentation at the Rehabilitation Institute of Chicago, September 12-13, 1992.

Russell, W.R. (1947). Poliomyelitis: The pre-paralytic stage and the effect of physical activity on the severity of paralysis. *British Medical Journal*, **2**, 1023-1028.

Sale, D.G. (1988). Neural adaptation to resistance training. *Medicine and Science in Sports and Exercise (Supplement)*, **20**, 135-145.

Skerker, R.S. (1991). Review and update: The aerobic exercise prescription. *Critical Reviews in Physical and Rehabilitation Medicine*, **2**(4), 257-271.

Stiggins, C. (1990). Testing and evaluation of athletes. *Proceedings of the National Strength and Conditioning Association National Symposium* (pp. 74-86). San Diego, CA.

Stone, M.H., O'Bryant, H., Garhammer, J., McMillan, J., & Rozenek, R. (1982). A theoretical model of strength training. *National Strength and Conditioning Association Journal*, **4**(4), 36.

Stone, M.H., Wilson, D., Rozenek, R., & Newton, H. (1983). Anaerobic capacity: Physiological basis. *National Strength and Conditioning Association Journal*, **5**(6), 40.

Stotts, K.M. (1986). Health maintenance: Paraplegic athletes and nonathletes. *Archives of Physical Medicine and Rehabilitation*, **67**, 104-114.

Tesch, P.A., & Karlssor, L.M. (1983). Muscle fiber type characteristics of deltoids in wheelchair athletes: Comparison with other trained athletes. *American Journal of Physical Medicine and Rehabilitation*, **62**, 239-243.

Tesch, P.A., & Karlson, J. (1985). Muscle fiber types and size in trained and untrained muscles of elite athletes. *Journal of Applied Physiology*, **59**, 1716-1720.

Thorstensson, A., Hulfen, B., Von Dobeln, W., & Karlson, J. (1976). Effect of strength training on enzyme activities and fiber characteristics in human skeletal muscle. *Acta Physiologica Scandinavica*, **96**, 342-398.

Vokac, Z., Bell, H., Bautz-Holter, E., & Rodahl, K. (1975). Oxygen uptake/heart rate relationship in leg and arm exercise, setting and standing. *Journal of Applied Physiology*, **39**, 54-59.

Young, A. (1984). Exercise against disease, disuse, and disability. *Update*, **29**, 531-538.

Chapter 4

American College of Sports Medicine (1991). *Guidelines for Exercise Testing and Prescription* (4th ed.) (pp. 50, 51, 111). Philadelphia: Lea & Febiger.

Anderson, B. (1980). *Stretching*. Bolinas, CA: Shelter.

Asmussen, E., & Bøje, O. (1945). Body temperature and capacity for work. *ACTA Physiologica Scandinavica*, **10**, 1-22.

Beedle, B., Jessee, C., & Stone, M.H. (1991). Flexibility characteristics among athletes who weight train. *Journal of Applied Sport Science Research*, **5**(3), 150-154.

Curtis, K.A. (1981, September-October). Part 3: Stretching routines. *Sports 'N Spokes*, pp. 1-4.

Curtis, K.A. (1982, January-February). Part 4: Athletic injuries. *Sports 'N Spokes*, pp. 20-24.

DeVries, H.A. (1966). Quantitative electromyographic investigation of the spasm theory of muscle pain. *The American Journal of Physical Medicine*, **45**, 119-134.

Flippin, R. (1990, September). The moves you've missed. *American Health*, pp. 57-63.

Fox, M., & Atwood, J. (1955). Results of testing Iowa school children for health and fitness. *Journal of Health, Physical Education and Recreation*, **26**, 20-21.

Gordon, G.A. (1982). Proprioceptive neuromuscular facilitation "The super stretch." *National Strength and Conditioning Association Journal*, **4**(2), 26.

Hartley-O'Brien, S.J. (1980). Six mobilization exercises for active range of hip flexion. *Research Quarterly for Exercise and Sport*, **51**, 625-635.

Heyward, V.H. (1986). *Designs for fitness: A guide to physical fitness appraisal and exercise prescription*. New York: Macmillan.

Holland, L.J., & Steadward, R.D. (1990, Summer). Effects of resistance training and flexibility training on strength, spasticity/muscle tone, and range of motion of elite athletes with cerebral palsy. *Palaestra*, pp. 27-31.

Karpovich, P.V., & Hale, C.J. (1956). Effect of warming-up upon physical performance. *Journal of the American Medical Association*, **162**(12), 1117-1119.

Knott, M., & Voss, D. (1977). *Proprioceptive Neuromuscular Facilitation*. London: Balliere, Tindall and Cassell.

Kraus, H., & Hirschland, R. (1954). Minimum muscular fitness tests in school children. *Research Quarterly*, **25**, 178-188.

Lauffenburger, S.K. (1992). Efficient warm ups: Creating a warm up that works. *Journal of Physical Education, Recreation and Dance*, 21-25.

Leighton, J. (1957). Flexibility characteristics of four specialized skill groups of college athletes. *Archives of Physical Medicine and Rehabilitation*, **38**(1), 24-28.

McAtee, R.E. (1993). *Facilitated stretching*. Champaign, IL: Human Kinetics.

Millikan, T., Morse, M., Hart, A., & Hedrick, B. (1993). Injury treatment in wheelchair athletics. *Sports 'N Spokes*, **18**(6), 85-88.

Pearl, B., & Moran, G.T. (1986). *Getting stronger: Weight training for men and women* (pp. 19, 58, 92, 97, 112). Bolinas, CA: Shelter.

Pink, M., & Jobe, R.W. (1991). Shoulder injuries in athletes. *Clinical Management*, **11**(6), 39-47.

Riddle, D.L., Rothstein, J.M., & Lamb, R.C. (1987). Goniometric reliability in a clinical setting: Shoulder measurements. *Physical Therapy*, **67**, 668-673.

Rusling, K. (1988). Flexibility. In J. Jones (Ed.), *Training guide to cerebral palsy sports* (pp. 61-70). Champaign, IL: Human Kinetics.

Schmid, L. (1947). Increasing bodily output by warming-up. *Casopis Lekaru Ceskych*, **86**, 950-958.

Shellock, F.G. (1986). Physiological, psychological and injury prevention aspects of warm up. *National Strength and Conditioning Association Journal*, October-November, 12-14.

Siff, M.C. (1991). Flexibility training: Modified PNF as a system of physical conditioning. *National Strength and Conditioning Association Journal*, **13**(4), 73-77.

Simonson, E., Teslenko, N., & Gorkin, M. (1936). Einfluss von Vorubungen auf die Leistung beim 100m - Lauf. *Arbeitsphysiologie*, **9**, 152-165.

Surburg, P.R. (1986). New perspectives for developing range of motion and flexibility for special populations. *Adapted Physical Activity Quarterly*, **3**, 227-235.

Winnick, J. (1990). *Adapted Physical Education and Sport* (pp. 302-303, 306, 310-312, 369-370). Champaign, IL: Human Kinetics.

Wright, V., & Johns, R.J. (1960). Physical factors concerned with the stiffness of normal and diseased joints. *Bulletin of Johns Hopkins Hospital*, **106**, 215-231.

Additional Readings

Evans, S., Housch, T., Johnson, G., Beaird, J., Housch, D., & Pepper, M. (1993). Age specific differences in the flexibility of high school wrestlers. *Journal of Strength and Conditioning Research*, **7**(1), 39-42.

Kennedy, S.O. (1988, January/February). Flexibility training for wheelchair athletes. *Sports 'N Spokes*, pp. 43-46.

Chapter 5

American Heart Association. (1988). *Stroke facts*. Dallas: Author.

American Heart Association. (1989). *How stroke affects behavior*. Dallas: Author.

Bach-y-Rita, P. (1980). *Recovery of functions: Theoretical considerations for brain injury rehabilitation*. Baltimore: University Park Press.

Car, O., Inbar, O., & Spira, R. (1976). Physical effects of a sports rehabilitation program on cerebral palsied and post-poliomyelitic adolescents. *Medicine and Science in Sports and Exercise*, **8**, 157-161.

Berg, K., & Bjure, J. (1970). Methods for evaluation of physical working capacity of school children with cerebral palsy. *Acta Paediatrica Scandinavia (Supplement)*, **204**, 15-26.

Berger, R.A., & Smith, K.J. (1991). Effects of the tonic neck reflex in the bench press. *Journal of Applied Sport Science Research*, **5**, 188-191.

Bleck, E.E., & Nagel, D. (Eds.) (1982). *Physically handicapped children: A medical atlas for teachers (2nd ed.)*. New York: Grune & Stratton.

Bobath, B. (1971). Motor development: Its effect on general development and application to the treatment of cerebral palsy. *Physiotherapy*, **57**, 526-532.

Brunnstrom, S. (1970). *Movement therapy in hemiplegia*. New York: Harper & Row.

Burke, W. (1988). *Head injury rehabilitation: An overview*. Houston: HDI.

Cailliet, R. (1980). *The shoulder in hemiplegia*. Philadelphia: Davis.

Carr, J.H., & Shepard, R. (1980). *Physiotherapy in disorders of the brain*. London: William Heinemann Medical Books.

Corcoran, P.J., Jebsen, R.H., & Brengelmann, G.L. (1970). Effects of plastic and metal leg braces in speed and energy cost of hemiparetic ambulation. *Archives of Physical Medicine and Rehabilitation, 51*, 64-77.

Craft, A.W. (1972). Head injuries in children. *British Medical Journal, 4*, 20.

Dickstein, R. (1986). Stroke rehabilitation: Three exercise therapy approaches. *Physical Therapy, 66*, 1233-1238.

Dickstein, R. (1989). Contemporary exercise therapy approaches in stroke rehabilitation. *Critical Reviews in Physical and Rehabilitative Medicine, 1*, 161-181.

Eames, P. (1988). *Rehabilitation of the physically disabled adults* (pp. 399-425). New York: Goodwill.

Fiorentino, M.R. (1972). *Normal and abnormal development: Influence of primitive reflexes on motor development*. Springfield, IL: Charles C Thomas.

Gersten, J.W., & Orr, J. (1971). External work of walking in hemiparetic patients. *Scandinavian Journal of Rehabilitative Medicine, 3*, 85-88.

Haas, A., & Pelosofish, M. (1967). Respiratory function in hemiplegic patients. *Archives of Physical Medicine and Rehabilitation, 48*, 174-179.

Halpern, D. (1984). Cerebral palsy therapeutic exercise (4th ed.). J.V. Basmajian (Ed.). Baltimore: Williams & Wilkins.

Hjeltnes, N. (1982). Capacity for physical training after spinal injuries and strokes. *Scandinavian Journal of Societal Medicine (Supplement), 29*, 245-251.

Holland, L.J., & Steadward, R.D. (1990, Summer). Effects of resistance and flexibility/training on strength, spasticity/muscle tone and range of motion of elite athletes with cerebral palsy. *Palaestra*, pp. 27-31.

Hoskins, T.A. (1975). Physiologic responses to known exercise loads in hemiparetic patients. *Archives of Physical Medicine and Rehabilitation, 56*, 544.

Inaba, M., Edberg, E., Montgomery, J., & Gillis, K.M. (1973). Effectiveness of functional training, active exercise, and resistive exercise for patients with hemiplegia. *Physical Therapy, 53*, 28-35.

Jankowski, L.W., & Sullivan, J.S. (1990). Aerobic and neuromuscular training: Effect of the capacity, efficiency and fatigability of patients with traumatic brain injuries. *Archives of Physical Medicine and Rehabilitation, 71*, 500-504.

Kottke, F., Stillwell, G.K., & Lehmann, J. (1982). *Krusens handbook of physical medicine and rehabilitation*. Philadelphia: W.B. Saunders.

Levine, M., Carey, W., Crocker, A., & Gross, R. (1983). *Developmental behavioral pediatrics*. Philadelphia: W.B. Saunders.

Logigian, M.D., Samuels, M.A., & Falcuoer, F.A. (1983). Clinical exercise trial for stroke patients. *Archives of Physical Medicine and Rehabilitation, 64*, 364-367.

Lundberg, A. (1975). Mechanical efficiency in bicycle ergometer work of young adults with cerebral palsy. *Developmental Medicine and Child Neurology, 17*, 434-439.

Lundberg, A. (1978). Maximal aerobic capacity of young people with spastic cerebral palsy. *Developmental Medicine and Child Neurology, 20*, 205-210.

McCubbin, J.A., & Shasby, G.B. (1985). Effects of isokinetic exercise on adolescents with cerebral palsy. *Adapted Physical Activity Quarterly, 2*, 56-64.

Molbech, S. (1966). Energy cost in level walking in subjects with an abnormal gait. In K. Evans & K.L. Anderson (Eds.), *Physical activity in health and disease*. Baltimore: Williams & Wilkins.

Molnar, G., & Taft, L. (1977). Cerebral palsy and spinal cord injuries. *Current Problems in Pediatrics, 7*, 28.

Monga, T.N. (1988). Cardiovascular responses to acute exercise in patients with cerebrovascular accidents. *Archives of Physical Medicine and Rehabilitation, 69*, 937-940.

Nelson, K.B., & Ellenberg, R.B. (1978). Epidemiology of cerebral palsy. In B.S. Schoenber (Ed.), *Advances in Neurology*. New York: Raven Press.

Odia, G.I. (1978). Spirometry in convalescent hemiplegic patients. *Archives of Physical Medicine and Rehabilitation, 59*, 314-321.

Olney, S.J., MacPhail, A., Hedden, D.M., & Boyce, W.F. (1990). Work and power in hemiplegic cerebral palsy gait. *Physical Therapy, 70*, 431-438.

Peganoff, S.A. (1984). The use of aquatics with cerebral palsied adolescents. *American Journal of Occupational Therapy, 38*, 467-473.

Perry, C. (1967). Principles and techniques of the Brunnstrom approach to the treatment of hemiplegia. *American Journal Physical Medicine*, **46**, 789-796.

Quinn, C.E. (1971). Observations on the effects of proprioceptive neuromuscular facilitation techniques in the treatment of hemiplegia. *Rheumatic Physical Medicine*, **11**, 186-192.

Richter, K.J. (1989). Seizures in athletes. *Journal of Osteopathic Sports Medicine*, **3**, 4, 19-22.

Richter, K.J., Adams-Mushett, C., Ferrara, M.S., & McCann, B.C. (1992). Integrated swimming classification: A faulted system. *Adapted Physical Activity Quarterly*, **9**, 5-13.

Robins, M., & Baum, H. (1981). The national survey of stroke. *Stroke*, **12**, 45-58.

Roth, E.J. (1988). The elderly stroke patient: Principles and practices of rehabilitation management. *Topics in Geriatric Rehabilitation*, **3**(4), 26-61.

Ryerson, S.J. (1985). Hemiplegia resulting from vascular insult or disease. In D.A. Umphred (Ed.), *Neurological rehabilitation* (pp. 474-514). St. Louis: Mosby.

Saltin, B., & Landin, S. (1975). Work capacity, muscle strength and SDH activity in both legs of hemiparetic patients and patients with Parkinson's disease. *Scandinavian Journal of Clinical Laboratory Investigation*, **35**, 531-538.

Scherzer, A.L., & Tscharauter, I. (1982). *Early diagnosis and therapy in cerebral palsy*. New York: Marcel Dekker.

Shephard, R.J. (1990). *Fitness in special populations*. Champaign, IL: Human Kinetics.

Sherrill, C., & Adams-Mushett, C. (1984). Fourth national cerebral palsy games: Sports by ability . . . not disability. *Palaestra*, **1**(1), 24-27, 49-51.

Sherrill, C., Adams-Mushett, C., & Jones, J.A. (1986). Classification and other issues in sports for blind, cerebral palsied, les autres and amputee athletes. In C. Sherrill (Ed.), *Sport and disabled athletes*. Champaign, IL: Human Kinetics.

Sherrill, C., Adams-Mushett, C., & Jones, J.A. (1988). Cerebral palsy and the CP athletes. *Training Guide to Cerebral Palsy Sports* (3rd ed.). Champaign, IL: Human Kinetics.

Smith, R.G., Cruikshauk, J.G., & Dunbar, S. (1982). Malalignment of the shoulder after stroke. *British Medical Journal*, **284**, 1224-1226.

Snyder-Smith, S. (1985). Traumatic head injuries. *Neurological Rehabilitation* (Vol. 3). St. Louis: Mosby.

Stern, P.H. (1970, September). Effects of facilitation exercise techniques in stroke rehabilitation. *Archives of Physical Medicine and Rehabilitation*, pp. 521-526.

Thompson, G., Rubin, I., & Bilenken, R. (Eds.) (1983). *Comprehensive management of cerebral palsy*. New York: Grune & Stratton.

United States Cerebral Palsy Athletic Association. (1990). *United States Cerebral Palsy Athletic Association classification manual*. Dallas: Author.

Van Ouwenaller, C., Laplace, P.M., & Chantraine, A. (1986). Painful shoulder in hemiplegia. *Archives of Physical Medicine and Rehabilitation*, **6**, 23-26.

Wall, J.C., & Asburn, A. (1974). Assessment of gait disabilities in hemiplegics. *Scandinavian Journal of Rehabilitation Medicine*, **11**, 95.

Whisnaut, J.P. (1984). The decline of stroke. *Stroke*, **15**, 160-168.

Wolf, P.A., Kannel, W.B., & Vester, J. (1983). Current status of risk factors for stroke. *Neurologica Clinical*, **1**, 317-343.

Chapter 6

Abramson, A.S. (1948). Bone disturbances in injuries to the spinal cord and cauda equina: Their prevention by ambulation. *Journal of Bone and Joint Surgery*, **30A**, 982.

Abramson, A.S., & Delagi, E.F. (1961). Influence of weight-bearing and muscle contraction on disuse osteoporosis. *Archives of Physical Medicine and Rehabilitation*, **42**, 147.

Agre, J.C., Rodriguez, A.A., & Sperling, K.B. (1989). Symptoms and clinical impressions of patients seen in a postpolio clinic. *Archives of Physical Medicine and Rehabilitation*, **70**, 367-370.

Asher, M. (1979). The myelomeningocele patient: A multidisciplinary approach to care. *Journal of the Kansas Medical Society*, **80**(7), 403-408, 413.

Bhambhani, Y.N., Eriksson, P., & Steadward, R.D. (1991). Reliability of peak physiological responses during wheelchair ergometry in persons with spinal cord injury. *Archives of Physical Medicine and Rehabilitation*, **72**, 559-562.

Blocker, W.P., Merrill, J.M., Krebs, M.A., Cardus, D.P., & Ostermann, H.J. (1983). An electrocardiographic survey of patients with chronic spinal cord injury. *American Correctional Therapy Journal*, **37**, 101-104.

Brocklehurst, G. (1976). *Spina bifida for the clinician, clinics in developmental medicine* (Vol. 57). Philadelphia: Lippincott.

Carr, J., & Shepherd, R. (1980). Physiotherapy. In *Disorders of the brain* (pp. 16, 25-27, 50, 51, 249, 278). London: William Heinemann Medical Books.

Chantraine, A. (1971). Clinical investigation of bone metabolism in spinal cord lesions. *Paraplegia*, **8**, 253-259.

Claus-Walker, J., Campus, R.J., Carter, R.E., Vallbona, C., & Lipscomb, H.S. (1972). Calcium excretion in quadriplegia. *Archives of Physical Medicine and Rehabilitation*, **53**, 14.

Claus-Walker, J., & Halstead, L. (1981). Metabolic and endocrine changes in spinal cord injury, I. The nervous system before and after transection of the spinal cord. *Archives of Physical Medicine and Rehabilitation*, **62**, 595-601.

Claus-Walker, J., & Halstead, L. (1982). Metabolic and endocrine changes in spinal cord injury, IV. Compounded neurologic dysfunctions. *Archives of Physical Medicine and Rehabilitation*, **63**, 632-638.

Cooper, R.A., & Baldini, F. (1991, Spring). What do VO_2max and body composition assessment mean to the wheelchair athlete? *National Wheelchair Athletic Association*, pp. 4-5.

Cooper, R.A., Horvath, S., Bedi, J., Drechsler-Parks, D., & Williams, R. (1992). Maximal exercise response of paraplegic wheelchair roadracers. *Paraplegia*, **30**, 573-581.

Corcoran, P.J., Goldman, R.F., Hoerner, E.F., Kling, C., Knuttgen, H.G., Marquis, B., McCann, B.C., & Rossier, A.G. (1980). Sports medicine and physiology of wheelchair marathon racing. *Orthopedic Clinics of North America*, **11**, 697-716.

Cowell, L.L., Squires, W.G., & Raven, P.R. (1986). Benefits of aerobic exercise for the paraplegic: A brief review. *Medicine and Science in Sports and Exercise*, **18**, 501-508.

Curtis, K.A. (1981). Part 1: Basics of exercise physiology: Wheelchair Sports Medicine. *Sports 'N Spokes*. Reprint.

Curtis, K.A., Hall, K.M., McClanahan, S., Dillion, D., & Brown, K.F. (1986). Health, vocational, and functional status in spinal cord injured athletes and nonathletes. *Archives of Physical Medicine and Rehabilitation*, **67**, 862-865.

Curtis, K.A. (1991, July/August). Sport-specific functional classification for wheelchair athletes. *Sports 'N Spokes*, pp. 45-48.

Dangelmaler, B., & Ridgway, M. (1993, Winter). Winter training: Should I go out or sit inside and watch Oprah? *National Wheelchair Athletic Association Newsletter*, pp. 20-22.

Davis, R., Ferrara, M., & Byrnes, D. (1988). The competitive wheelchair stroke. *National Strength and Conditioning Association Journal*, **10**(3), 4-10.

Davis, G.M., & Shepard, R.J. (1988). Cardiorespiratory fitness in highly active versus inactive paraplegics. *Medicine and Science in Sports and Exercise*, **20**, 463-468.

Davis, G.M. (1993). Exercise capacity of individuals with paraplegia. *Medicine and Science in Sports and Exercise*, **25**(4), 423-432.

Dean, E. (1991). Clinical decision making in the management of the late sequelae of poliomyelitis. *Physical Therapy*, **71**(10), 752-761.

Dorlands illustrated medical dictionary (27th ed.) (1988). Philadelphia: Saunders.

Eriksson, P., Lofstrom, L., & Ekblom, B. (1988). Aerobic power during maximal exercise in untrained and well-trained persons with quadriplegia and paraplegia. *Scandinavian Journal of Rehab Medicine*, **20**, 141-147.

Faghri, P.D., Glaser, R.M., & Figoni, S.F. (1992). Functional electrical stimulation leg cycle ergometer exercise: Training effects on cardiorespiratory responses of spinal cord injured subjects at rest and during submaximal exercise. *Archives of Physical Medicine and Rehabilitation*, **73**, 1085-1093.

Feiwell, E. (1978). The effects of hip reduction on function in patients with myelomeningocele. *Journal of Bone and Joint Surgery*, **60A**(2), 169-173.

Figoni, S.F. (1990). Perspectives on cardiovascular fitness and spinal cord injuries. *Journal of the American Paraplegia Society*, **13**, 63-71.

Figoni, S.F. (1993). Exercise responses and quadriplegia. *Medicine and Science in Sports and Exercise*, **25**(4), 433-441.

Finestone, H.M., Lampman, R.M., Davidoff, G.N., Westbury, L., Islam, S., & Schultz, S. (1991). Arm ergometry exercise testing in patients with dysvascular amputations. *Archives of Physical Medicine and Rehabilitation*, **72**, 15-19.

Freeman, A.R. (1982). The center and autonomic nervous systems. In E.E. Selkurt (Ed.), *Basic physiology for the health sciences*. Boston: Little, Brown.

Glaser, R.M. (1989). Arm exercise training for wheelchair users. *Medicine and Science in Sports and Exercise*, **21**, 5149-5167.

Greenway, R.M., Houser, H., Lindan, O., & Weir, D. (1970). Long term changes in gross body composition of paraplegic and quadriplegic patients. *Paraplegia*, **7**, 301-318.

Halstead, L.S. (1990). Postpolio syndrome and exercise. In J.V. Basmajian & S.L. Wolf (Eds.), *Therapeutic exercise* (5th ed.) (pp. 231-240). Baltimore: Williams & Wilkins.

Hendry, J., & Geddes, N. (1978). Living with a congenital anomaly. *Canadian Nurse*, **74**(6), 29-33.

Hooker, S.P., & Wells, C.L. (1989). Effects of low— and moderate—intensity training in spinal cord injured persons. *Medicine and Science in Sports and Exercise*, **21**(1), 18-22.

Huckstep, R.L. (1975). A guide for developing countries—including appliances and rehabilitation for the disabled. In *Poliomyelitis* (p. 1). New York: Churchill Livingstone.

Kaplan, P.E., Gandhavadi, B., Richards, L., & Goldschmidt, R. (1978). Calcium balance in paraplegic patients, influence of injury duration and ambulation. *Archives of Physical Medicine and Rehabilitation*, **59**, 447-450.

King, M.L., Freeman, D.M., Pellicone, J.T., Wanstall, E.K., & Bhansah, L.D. (1992). Exertional hypotension in thoracic spinal cord injury: Case report. *Paraplegia*, **30**, 261-266.

Lal, S., Hamilton, B., Heinemann, A., & Betts, H. (1989). Risk factors for heterotopic ossification in spinal cord injury. *Archives of Physical Medicine and Rehabilitation*, **70**, 387-390.

McLaughlin, J.F., & Shurtleff, D.B. (1979). Management of the newborn with myelody-splasia. *Clinical Pediatrics*, **18**(8), 463-476.

McIone, D.G. (1980). *An introduction to spina bifida*. Chicago: Children's Memorial Hospital Myelomeningocele Service.

Menard, M., & Hahn, G. (1991). Acute and chronic hypothermia in a man with spinal cord injury. Environmental and pharmacologic causes. *Archives of Physical Medicine and Rehabilitation*, **72**, 421-422.

Menelaus, M.B. (1976). Orthopedic management of children with myelomeningocele: A plea for realistic goals. *Developmental Medicine and Child Neurology*, **6**(37), 3-11.

National Wheelchair Athletic Association. (1990). *Functional classification chart*.

Nixon, V. (1985). *Spinal cord injury*. Rockville: Aspen Publishers.

Noble, B.J. (1986). *Physiology of exercise and sport* (pp. 26, 32, 55). St. Louis: Times Mirror/ Mosby College.

Ohry, A., Shomesh, Y., Zak, R., & Herzberg, M. (1980). Zinc and osteoporosis in patients with spinal cord injury. *Paraplegia*, **18**, 174-180.

Plum, F., & Dunning, M.F. (1958). The effect of therapeutic mobilization on hypercaluria following acute poliomyelitis. *Archives of Internal Medicine*, **101**, 528.

Salter, R.B. (1983). *Textbook of disorders and injuries of the musculoskeletal system* (2nd ed.). Baltimore: Williams & Wilkins.

Schneider, F.J. (1985). Traumatic spinal cord injury. In D.A. Umphred (Ed.), *Neurological rehabilitation* (pp. 314-374). St. Louis: Mosby.

Schneider, J.W. (1985). Congenital spinal cord injury. In D.A. Umphred (Ed.), *Neurological rehabilitation* (pp. 289-313). St. Louis: Mosby.

Selkurt, E.E. (Ed.) (1982). *Basic physiology for the health sciences* (pp. 98-113, 306-308, 319-320, 536-540). Boston: Little, Brown.

Sherrill, C. (1981). *Adapted physical education and recreation* (pp. 479-481, 492-495). Dubuque, IA: Brown.

Sorg, R.J. (1993). HDL-cholesterol: Exercise formula. Results of long term (six year) strenuous swimming exercise in a middle-aged male with paraplegia. *Journal of Sports Physical Therapy*, **17**(4), 195-198.

Steinberg, F. (1980). *The immobilized patient-functional pathology and management* (p. 77). New York: Plenum.

Stenberg, J., Astrand, P., Ekblom, B., Royce, J., & Saltin, B. (1967). Hemodynamic response to work with different muscle groups, sitting and supine. *Journal of Applied Physiology*, **22**(1), 61-70.

Traravella, S. (1991, September 16). Rehabilitation hospitals share in athletes' returns. *Modern Healthcare Weekly Business News*, pp. 22-28.

Williamson, G.G. (1987). *Children with spina bifida*. Baltimore: Brookes.

Young, J.S., Burns, P.E., Bowen, A.M., & McCutchen, R. (1982). *Spinal cord injury statistics.* Phoenix, AZ: Good Samaritan Medical Center.

Zielinski, K.E. (1991). *Physiological responses to exercise in spinal cord injured individuals* (pp. 1-15). Paper presented at the meeting of the Illinois Wheelchair Classic and Workshop, University of Illinois, Champaign-Urbana.

Chapter 7

Adler, J.C., Mazzarella, N., Puzsier, L., & Aba, A. (1987). Treadmill training program for bilateral below-knee amputee patient with cardiopulmonary disease. *Archives of Physical Medicine and Rehabilitation, 68,* 858-861.

Burgess, E.M., & Rappoport, A. (1993). *Physical fitness: A guide for individuals with lower limb loss. Rehabilitation research and development service—A clinical guide.* Baltimore: Scientific and Technical Publications Section, United States Department of Veterans Affairs.

DuBow, L.L., Witt, P.L., Kadaba, M.P., Reyes, R., & Cochran, G.V.B. (1983). Oxygen consumption of elderly persons with bilateral below knee amputations: Ambulation versus wheelchair propulsion. *Archives of Physical Medicine and Rehabilitation, 64,* 255-259.

Enoka, R.M., Miller, D.I., & Burgess, E.M. (1982). Below-knee amputee running gait. *American Journal of Physical Medicine, 61*(2), 66-84.

Finestone, H.M., Lampman, R.M., Davidoff, G.N., Westbury, L., Islam, S., & Schultz, J.S. (1991). Arm ergometry exercise testing in patients with dysvascular amputations. *Archives of Physical Medicine and Rehabilitation, 72,* 15-19.

Garvey, R.S. (1989). Individuals with amputations find rehabilitation in competitive sports. *Journal of Rehabilitation Research and Development—Clinical Supplement,* January-March, 19-20.

Ghosh, A.K. (1980). *Selection of clinically suitable test/methods for ergonomic/physiological evaluation of lower extremity handicapped persons.* Unpublished doctoral dissertation. University of Calcutta, India.

Gonzalez, E.G., Corcoran, P.J., & Reyes, R.L. (1974). Energy expenditure in below knee amputees: Correlation with stump length. *Archives of Physical Medicine and Rehabilitation, 55,* 111-119.

Grundy, D.J., & Silver, J.R. (1983). Amputation for peripheral vascular disease in the paraplegic and tetraplegic. *Paraplegia, 21,* 305-311.

Hamilton, E.A., & Nichols, P.J. (1972). Rehabilitation of the elderly lower limb amputee. *British Medical Journal, 2,* 95-99.

International Sports Organization for the Disabled. (1990). Functional classification chart. In *Handbook.*

James, U., & Nordgren, B. (1973). Physical work capacity measured by bicycle ergometry (one leg) and prosthetic treadmill walking in healthy active unilateral above knee amputees. *Scandinavian Journal of Rehabilitation Medicine, 5,* 81-87.

Karacoloff, L.A., Hammersley, C.S., & Schneider, F. (1992). *Lower extremity amputation: A guide to functional outcomes in physical therapy management.* (2nd ed.) Gaithersburg, MD: Aspen.

Kavanaugh, T., & Shephard, R.J. (1973). The application of exercise testing to the elderly amputee. *Canadian Medical Association Journal. 108,* 314-317.

Kegel, B. (1985). *Sports and recreation for those with lower limb amputation or impairment.* Washington, DC: Veterans Administration Medical Center.

Kegel, B. (1986). *Sports for the leg amputee.* Redmond, WA: Medic.

Najenson, & Levy, M. (1971). Rehabilitation of amputees due to progressive vascular disease. In V. Simr (Ed.), *Sports as a means of rehabilitation.* Natanya, Israel: Wingate Institute.

Paciorek, M.J., & Jones, J.A. (1989). *Sports and recreation for the disabled: A resource manual.* Indianapolis: Benchmark Press.

Radocy, B. (1987). Upper extremity prosthetics: Considerations and designs for sports and recreation. *Clinical Prosthetics and Orthotics, 11,* 3, 131-153.

Radocy, B. (1988, Winter). Hands for all seasons: Upper extremity sports prosthetics. *Palaestra,* pp. 24-29, 46.

Roth, E.J., Weisner, S.L., Green, D., & Wu, Y. (1990). Dysvascular amputee rehabilitation: The role of continuous noninvasive cardiovascular monitoring during physical therapy. *American Journal of Physical Medicine and Rehabilitation, 69,* 1, 16-22.

Russek, A.S. (1984). Exercises for amputees. In J.V. Basmajan (Ed.), *Therapeutic exercise* (4th ed.) (pp. 421-440). Baltimore: Williams & Wilkins.

Shephard, R.J. (1990). *Fitness in special populations*. Champaign, IL: Human Kinetics.

Sherrill, C. (1981). *Adapted physical education and recreation*. Dubuque, IA: Brown.

Van Alste, D.M. (1985). Electrocardiography using rowing ergometer suitable for leg amputees. *International Journal of Rehabilitation Medicine*, **7**, 1-5.

Waters, R.L., Perry, J., Antonelli, D., & Hislop, H. (1976). Energy cost of walking of amputees: The influence of level of amputation. *The Journal of Bone and Joint Surgery*, **58A**(1), 42-46.

Winnick, J.P., & Short, F.X. (1985). *Physical fitness testing of the disabled* (Project Unique). Champaign, IL: Human Kinetics.

Chapter 8

Adams, R. (1975). *Disease of muscle: A study in pathology* (3rd ed.). Hagerstown, MD: Harper & Row.

Agre, J.C., Rodriguez, A.A., & Sperling, K.B. (1989). Symptoms and clinical impressions of patients seen in post-polio clinic. *Archives of Physical Medicine and Rehabilitation*, **70**, 367-370.

Agre, J.C., & Rodriguez, A.A. (1990). Neuromuscular function: Companion of symptomatic and asymptomatic polio subjects to control subjects. *Archives of Physical Medicine and Rehabilitation*, **71**, 545-551.

Allsop, K.G. (1981). Loss of strength and functional decline in Duchenne's dystrophy. *Archives of Neurology*, **38**, 406-411.

Anderson, A.D., Levine, S.A., & Gellert, H. (1972). Loss of ambulatory ability in patients with old anterior poliomyelitis. *Lancet*, **2**, 1061-1063.

Anderson-Price, S., & McCarty-Wilson, L. (1986). Multiple sclerosis. *Pathophysiology: Clinical concepts of disease processes* (pp. 794-795). New York: McGraw-Hill.

Bender, L.H., & Withwor, A. (1989). Arthrogryposis multiplex congentia. *Orthopaedic Nursing*, **8**(5), 29-35.

Bennett, R.L., & Knowlton, G.C. (1958). Overwork weakness in partially denervated skeletal muscle. *Clinical Orthopaedics*, **12**, 22-29

Berlly, M.H., Strauser, W.W., & Hall, K.M. (1991). Fatigue in post-polio syndrome. *Archives of Physical Medicine and Rehabilitation*, **72**, 115-118.

Bernbaum, M., Albert, S.G., & Cohen, J.D. (1989). Exercise training in individuals with diabetic retinopathy and blindness. *Archives of Physical Medicine and Rehabilitation*, **70**, 605-611.

Bohannon, R.W. (1983). Results of resistance exercise on a patient with amyotrophic lateral sclerosis. *Physical Therapy*, **63**, 905-968.

Bonsett, C.A. (1963). Pseudohypertrophic muscular dystrophy: Distribution of degenerative features as revealed by an anatomical study. *Neurology*, **13**, 728-738.

Brown, L.M., Robson, M.J., & Sharrard, W.J. (1980). The pathophysiology of arthrogryposis multiplex congenita. *Journal of Bone and Joint Surgery*, **62**, 291-296.

Bruno, R.L. (1985). Post-polio sequelae (editorial). *Orthopaedics*, **8**, 844.

Caillett, R. (1984). Multiple sclerosis. In J.V. Basmajian (Ed.), *Therapeutic Exercise* (pp. 407-421). Baltimore: Williams & Wilkins.

Campbell, A.M., Williams, E.R., & Pearce, J. (1969). Lower motor neuron degeneration following poliomyelitis. *Neurology*, **19**, 1101-1106.

Carrol, J.E., Hagberg, J.M., Brooke, M.H., & Shumate, J.B. (1979). Bicycle ergometry and gas exchange measurements in neuromuscular disease. *Archives of Neurology*, **36**, 457-461.

Cashman, N.R., Mascutti, R., Wolfman, R.D., Ross, R., & Antel, J.P. (1987). Late denervation in patients with antecedent paralytic poliomyelitis. *New England Journal of Medicine*, **317**, 7-12.

Chyatte, S.B., Viagnos, P.J., & Watkins, M. (1966, August). Early muscular dystrophy: Differential patterns of weakness in Duchenne, limb-girdle and facioscapulohumeral types. *Archives of Physical Medicine and Rehabilitation*, pp. 499-503.

Coakes, R. (1988). Visual handicap. In J. Goodwill & M. Chamberlain (Eds.), *Rehabilitation of the physically disabled adult* (pp. 253-268). New York: Sheridan Medical Books.

Cochrane, G. (1988). Multiple sclerosis. In J.C. Goodwill & A.M. Chamberlain (Eds.), *Rehabilitation of the Physically Disabled Adult* (pp. 364-378). Dobbs Ferry, NY: Sheridan House.

Codd, M.B., Mulder, D.W., Kurland, L.T., Beard, C.M., & O'Fullon, W.M. (1985). Epidemiology and long-term sequelae: Preliminary report. In L.S. Halstead & D.O. Weicher (Eds.) *Late effects of poliomyelitis* (pp. 121-134). Miami, FL: Miami Symposia Foundation.

Cohen, L., Morgan, J., Babbs, R. (1982). Statistical analysis of loss of muscle strength in Duchenne's muscular dystrophy. *Research in Community Chemical Pathology and Pharmocology*, **37**, 123-138.

Cosgrove, J.L., Alexander, M.A., Kitts, E.L., & Swan, B.E. (1987). Late effects of poliomyelitis. *Archives of Physical Medicine and Rehabilitation*, **68**, 4-7.

Dalakus, M.C., Elder, G., & Hallett, M. (1986). A long-term follow-up study of patients with post-poliomyelitis neuromuscular symptoms. *New England Journal of Medicine*, **314**(15), 459-463.

Dean, E., & Ross, J. (1988). Modified aerobic walking program: Effect on patients with post-polio syndrome symptoms. *Archives of Physical Medicine and Rehabilitation*, **69**, 1033-1038.

Denys, E.H., & Norris, F.H. (1979). Amyotrophic lateral sclerosis: Impairment of neuromuscular transmission. *Archives of Neurology*, **36**, 202-205.

Depauw, K.P. (1981). Physical education for the visually impaired: A review of literature. *Journal of Visual Impairment and Blindness*, April, 162-163.

Drachman, D.B., Murphy, S.R., Nigam, M.P., & Hills, J.R. (1967). Myopathic changes in chronically denervated muscle. *Archives of Neurology*, **16**, 14-24.

Einarsson, G., & Broberg, C. (1990). Motor impairment in late poliomyelitis in muscle adaptation and disability in late poliomyelitis. *Physical Medicine and Rehabilitation Medicine*, **2**(4), 189-200.

Einarsson, G. (1991). Muscle conditioning in late poliomyelitis. *Archives of Physical Medicine and Rehabilitation*, **72**, 11-14.

Erwin, J.H., Keller, C., Anderson, S., & Costa, J. (1991). Hand and wrist exercises during rehabilitation of a patient with hereditary distal myopathy. *Archives of Physical Medicine and Rehabilitation*, **72**, 701-702.

Eulberg, M.K., Halstead, L.S., & Perry, J. (1988, June 15). Post-polio syndrome: How you can help. *Patient Care*, pp. 131-136.

Feldman, R.M., & Soskolne, C.L. (1987). The use of non-fatiguing strengthening exercises in late effects of poliomyelitis. In L.S. Halstead & D.O Wiechers (Eds.), *Research and Clinical Aspects of the Late Effects of Poliomyelitis* (p. 335). White Plains, NY: March of Dimes. (Original article series: Birth defects)

Fillyaw, M.J., & Ades, P.A. (1989). Endurance exercise in Friedreich's ataxia. *Archives of Physical Medicine and Rehabilitation*. **70**, 786-788.

Florence, J.M., & Hagberg, J.M. (1984). Effect of training on the exercise responses of neuromuscular disease patients. *Medicine and Science in Sport and Exercise*, **16**, 460-465.

Fowler, W.M., & Gardner, G.W. (1967, December). Quantitive strength measurements in muscular dystrophy. *Archives of Physical Medicine and Rehabilitation*, pp. 629-644.

Fowler, W.M., & Taylor, M. (1982). Rehabilitation management muscular dystrophy and related disorders: Role of exercise. *Archives of Physical Medicine and Rehabilitation*, **63**, 319-321.

Fowler, W.M. (1988). Management of muscle skeletal complications in neuromuscular diseases: Weakness and the role of exercise. *Physical Medicine and Rehabilitation: State of the Art Reviews*. Philadelphia: Hanley & Belfus.

Frankel, D. (1985). Multiple sclerosis. In D.A. Umphred (Ed.), *Neurological Rehabilitation* (pp. 398-415). St. Louis: Mosby.

George, C., Patton, R., & Purdy, G. (1975). Development of an aerobics conditioning program for the visually handicapped. *Journal of Physical Education and Recreation*, **46**, 539-540.

Goodgold, J. (1988). General principles of management and evaluation of neuromuscular disease. *Physical Medicine and Rehabilitation: State of the Art Reviews*. Philadelphia: Hanley & Belfus.

Grimby, G., Einarsson, G., Hedberg, M., & Aniansson, A. (1989). Muscle adaptive changes in post-polio subjects. *Scandanavian Journal of Rehabilitation Medicine*, **21**, 19-26.

Grimby, G., & Einarsson, G. (1991). Post-polio management. *Physical and Rehabilitation Medicine*, **2**(4), 189-200.

Hagberg, J.M., Carrol, J.E., & Brooke, M.H. (1980). Endurance exercise training in patient with central core disease. *Neurology*, **30**, 1242-1244.

Hall, J.G. (1981). An approach to congenital contractions: Arthrogryposis. *Pediatrics Annuals*, **10**, 15-26.

Hall, J.G., Reed, S.D., & Driscoll, E.P. (1983). Part I. Amyoplasia. A common sporadic condition with congenital contractures. *American Journal of Medicine and Genetics*, **15**, 571-590.

Hall, J.G. (1985). *Clinical Orthopedics and Related Research*, pp. 104-109. Philadelphia: Lippincott.

Haller, R.G., & Lewis, S.F. (1984). Pathophysiology of exercise performance in muscle disease. *Medicine and Science in Sport and Exercise*, **16**, 456-459.

Halstead, L.S. (1990). Postpolio syndrome and exercise. In J.V. Basamajian & S.L. Wolf (Eds.), *Therapeutic Exercise* (5th ed.) (pp. 231-240). Baltimore: Williams and Wilkins.

Halstead, L.S., & Rossi, C.D. (1985). New problems in old polio patients: Results of survey of 539 polio survivors. *Orthopedics*, **8**, 845-850.

Halstead, L.S., & Wiechers, D.O. (1985). *Late effects of poliomyelitis*. Miami, FL: Symposium Foundation.

Halstead, L.S., Wiechers, D.O., & Rossi, C.D. (1985). Part II: Results of a survey of 201 polio survivors. *Southern Medical Journal*, **78**, 1281-1287.

Hanna, R.S. (1986, June). Effect of exercise on blind persons. *Journal of Visual Impairment and Blindness*, pp. 248-251.

Hayward, M., & Seaton, D. (1979). Late sequelae of paralytic poliomyelitis: Clinical and electromyographic study. *Journal of Neurology and Neurosurgery Psychiatry*, **42**, 117-122.

Herbison, G.J., Jaweed, M.M., Ditunno, J.F., & Scott, C.M. (1973). Effect of overwork during reinnervation of rat muscle. *Experimental Neurology*, **41**, 1-14.

Herbison, G.J., Jaweed, M.M., & Ditunno, J.F. (1983). Exercise therapies in peripheral neuropathies. *Archives of Physical Medicine and Rehabilitation*, **64**, 201-205.

Hopkins, W.G., Gaeta, H., Thomas, A.C., & McHill, P. (1987). Physical fitness of blind and sighted children. *European Journal of Applied Physiology*, **56**, 69-73.

Horstmann, D.M. (1950). Acute poliomyelitis: Relation of physical activity of the time of onset to the course of the disease. *Journal of the American Medical Association*, **142**, 236-241.

Hsu, J.D. (1988). Management of musculoskeletal complications: Spinal deformity and the role of bracing and surgery. *Physical Medicine and Rehabilitation: State of the Art Reviews*. Philadelphia: Hanley & Belfus.

Janiszewski, D.W., Caroscio, J.T., & Wisham, L.H. (1983). Amyotrophic lateral sclerosis: A comprehensive rehabilitation approach. *Archives of Physical Medicine and Rehabilitation*, **64**, 304-307.

Jankowski, L.W., & Evans, J.D. (1981). The exercise capacity of blind children. *Journal of Visual Impairment and Blindness*, June, 248-251.

Jaweed, M.M., Herbison, G.J., & Pitnanno, J.F. (1974). Effect of swimming on compensatory hypertrophy of reinnervating soleus and plantaris muscles. *American Journal of Physical Medicine*, **53**(1), 35-40.

Johnson, E.W., & Braddom, R. (1971, July). Overwork weakness in facioscapulohumeral muscular dystrophy. *Archives of Physical Medicine and Rehabilitation*, pp. 333-336.

Jones, D.R., Speier, J., & Canine, K. (1989). Cardiorespiratory responses to aerobic training by patients with post-poliomyelitis sequelae. *Journal of the American Medical Society*, **261**(22), 3255-3258.

Jones, J., & Paciorek, M. (1986). *Sports and recreation for the physically disabled*. Indianapolis: Benchmark Press.

Katz, J., & Temple, A.P. (1987). Surgery for achondroplasia: Perioperative challenges of dwarfism. *AORN Journal*, **46**, 96-105.

Kayser-Gatchalian, M.C. (1973). Late muscular atrophy after poliomyelitis. *Eur Neurol*, **10**, 371-380.

Klingmon, J., Chui, H., Conrat, M., & Perry, J. (1988). Functional recovery: A major risk factor for the development of post-poliomyelitis. *Archives Neurol*, **45**, 645-647.

Lai, M.M., Tettenborn, M.A., & Hall, J.G. (1991). A new form of autosomal dominant arthrogry-posis. *Journal of Medical Genetics*, **28**, 701-703.

Lateur, B.J., & Giaconi, R.M. (1979). Effect of maximal strength of submaximal exercise in Duchenne muscular dystrophy. *American Journal of Physical Medicine*, **58**, 26-36.

Laureano, A.N., & Rybak, L.P. (1990). Severe otolarygologic manifestations of arthrogryposis multiplex congenita. *Annals of Otolaryngology Laryngology*, **99**, 94-97.

Lenman, J.A. (1959). A clinical and experimental study of the effects of exercise on motor weakness in neuromuscular disease. *Journal of Neurology and Neurosurgery Psychiatry*, **22**, 182-194.

Lewis, S.F. (1984). Exercise and human neuromuscular diseases: A symposium overview. *Medicine and Science in Sport and Exercise*, **16**, 449-450.

Match, R.M., Corrylos, E.V., & Corrylos, F. (1983). Bilateral avulsion fracture of the triceps tendon insertion from skiing with osteogenesis imperfecta tarda. *American Journal of Sports Medicine*, **11**, 99-102.

Maynard, F.M. (1985). Post-polio sequelae—differential diagnosis and management. *Orthopedics*, **8**, 857-861.

McCartney, N., Moroz, D., Gamer, S.H., & McComas, A.J. (1988). The effects of strength training in patients with selected neuromuscular disorders. *Medicine and Science in Sport and Exercise*, **20**, 362-368.

McKusick, V.A. (1972). *Heritable disorders of connective tissue*. St. Louis: Mosby.

Milner-Brown, H.S., & Miller, R.G. (1988). Muscle strengthening through high resistance weight training in patients with neuromuscular disorders. *Archives of Physical Medicine and Rehabilitation*, **69**, 14-19.

Milner-Brown, H.S., & Miller, R.G. (1990). Myotonic dystrophy: Qualification of muscle weakness and mytonia and the effect of amitriplyline and exercise. *Archives of Physical Medicine and Rehabilitation*, **71**, 983-987.

Moore, P., Major, R., Stallard, J., & Butler, P.B. (1990). Contracture correction device for arthrogryposis. *Physiotherapy*, **76**, 5, 303-305.

Mueller, E.A. (1970). Influence of training and inactivity on muscle strength. *Archives of Physical Medicine and Rehabilitation*, **51**, 449-462.

Mulder, D.W., Rosenbaum, R.A., & Leyton, D.D. (1972). Late progression of poliomyelitis or forme fruste amyotrophic lateral sclerosis. In *Mayo Clinic Proceedings* (pp. 47, 745).

Paciorek, M.J., & Jones, J.A. (1989). *Sports and recreation for the physically disabled* (pp. 4-5). Indianapolis: Benchmark Press.

Peach, P.E. (1990). Overwork weakness with evidence of muscular damage in a patient with residual paralysis from polio. *Archives of Physical Medicine and Rehabilitation*, **71**, 248-250.

Perloff, J.K., Delean, A.C., & O'Doherty, D. (1966). The cardiomyopathy of progressive muscular dystrophy. *Circulation*, **64**, 625-648.

Perloff, J.K. (1971). Cardiomyopathy associated with huredofamilial myopathic diseases. *Medical Concepts in Cardiovascular Disease*, **40**, 23-27.

Perry, J., & Fleming, C. (1985). Polio: Long term problems. *Orthopedics*, **8**, 877.

Pezeshkpour, G.H., & Dalakas, M.C. (1988). Long term changes in the spinal cords of patients with old poliomyelitis: Signs of continuous disease activity. *Archives of Physical Medicine and Rehabilitation*, **45**, 505-508.

Porretta, D.L. (1990). Osteogenesis imperfecta. In J. P. Winnick (Ed.), *Adapted physical education and sport* (p. 237). Champaign, IL: Human Kinetics.

Rodriguez, A.A., & Agre, J.C. (1991). Correlation of motor units with strength and spectral characteristics in polio survivors and controls. *Muscle & Nerve*, **14**, 429-434.

Rodriguez, A.A., & Agre, J.C. (1991). Physiologic parameters and perceived exertion with local muscle fatigue in post-polio subjects. *Archives of Physical Medicine and Rehabilitation*, **72**, 305-308.

Roos, R.P., Viola, M.V., Wollman, R., Hatch, M.H., & Antel, J.P. (1980). Amyotrophic lateral sclerosis with antecedent poliomyelitis. *Archives of Neurology*, **37**, 312-313.

Russell, W.R. (1947). Poliomyelitis: The pre-paralytic stage, and the effect of physical activity on the severity of paralysis. *British Medical Journal*, **2**, 1023-1028.

Russell, W.R., & Fischer-Williams, M. (1954). Recovery of muscular strength after poliomyelitis. *Lancet*, **1**, 330-336.

Ryniewicz, B., Rowinska-Marcinska, K., Emeryk, B., & Housmanowa-Petrueswicz, I. (1990). Disintegration of the motor unit in postpolio syndrome. Part I: *Electromyography Clin. Neurophysiology*, **30**, 423-427.

Saleh, M., & Burton, M. (1991). Leg lengthening: Patient selection and management in achondroplasia. *Orthopaedic Clinics of North America*, **22**(4), 589-599.

Salter, R.B. (1983). *Textbook of disorders and injuries of the musculoskeletal structure* (2nd ed.). Baltimore, MD: Williams & Wilkins.

Saltin, B., Blomquist, G., & Mitchell, J.H. (1968). Response to exercise after bed rest and training: Longitudinal study of adaptive changes in transport and body composition. *Circulation*, **38**(7), 1-78.

Sarwark, J.F., MacEwen, D.G., & Scott, C.I. (1990). Current concepts review—amyoplasia. *Journal of Bone and Joint Surgery*, **72-A**, 465-469.

Scheinberg, L.C., & Holland, N.J. (Eds.) (1987). *Multiple sclerosis: A guide for patients and their families* (2nd ed.). New York: Raven Press.

Scott, O.M., Hyde, S.A., Goddard, C., & Jones, M.B. (1981). Effect of exercise in Duchenne muscular dystrophy. *Physiotherapy*, **67**, 174-176.

Scott, O.M., Hyde, S.A., Goddard, C., & Dubowitz, V. (1982). Quantification of muscle function in children: A prospective study in Duchenne muscular dystrophy. *Muscle and Nerve*, **5**, 291-301.

Seele, W. (1983). Physical fitness of the visually impaired in Detroit public schools. *Journal of Visual Impairment and Blindness*, **77**, 117-118.

Sherrill, C. (1981). Blind and visually impaired. In *Adapted physical education and recreation: A multi-disciplinary approach* (pp. 554-569). Dubuque, IA: Brown.

Sherrill, C. (1982). Dwarfism. In *Adapted physical education and recreation* (2nd ed.) (p. 484). Dubuque, IA: Brown.

Shindo, M., Kumagai, S., & Tanaka, H. (1987). Physical work capacity and effect of endurance training in visually handicapped boys and young male adults. *European Journal of Applied Physiology*, **56**, 501-507.

Siegel, I.M. (1978). Management of muscular dystrophy: A clinical review. *Muscle and Nerve*, **1**, 453-460.

Sillence, D.O., Rimoin, D.L., & Banks, D.M. (1979). Genetic heterogeneity in osteogenesis imperfecta. *Journal of Medical Genetology*, **16**, 101-116.

Sinaki, M., & Mulder, D.W. (1978). Rehabilitation techniques for patients with amyotrophic lateral sclerosis. *Mayo Clinical Proceedings*, **53**, 173-178.

Sockolov, R., Irwin, B., Dressendorfer, G., & Bernayer, E.M. (1977). Exercise performance in 6 to 11 year old boys with Duchenne muscular dystrophy. *Archives of Physical Medicine and Rehabilitation*, **50**, 195-201.

Speier, J.L., Owen, R.R., Knapp, M., & Canine, J.K. (1987). Occurrence of post-polio sequelae in an epidemic population. In L.S. Halstead & D.O. Weichers (Eds.), Research and clinical aspects of the late effects of poliomyelitis. *Birth Defects*, **23**(4), 39-48.

Vignos, P.J., & Watkins, M.P. (1966). The effect of exercise in muscular dystrophy. *Journal of the American Medical Association*, **197**, 843-848.

Waring, W.P., & Werner, R.A. (1989). Clinical management of carpal tunnel syndrome in patients with long-term sequelae of poliomyelitis. *Journal of Hand Surgery*, **14A**, 865-869.

Waring, W.P., Maynard, R., Grady, W., Grady, R., & Boyles, C. (1989). Influence of appropriate lower extremity orthotic management on ambulation, pain, and fatigue in a post-polio population. *Archives of Physical Medicine and Rehabilitation*, **70**, 371-375.

Weichers, D.O., & Hubbell, S.L. (1981). Late changes in the motor unit after acute poliomyelitis. *Muscle & Nerve*, **4**, 524-528.

Weichers, D.O. (1985). Acute and latent effect of poliomyelitis on the motor unit as revealed by electromyography. *Orthopedics*, **8**, 870-872.

Weichers, D.O. (1988). New concepts of the reinnervated motor unit revealed by vaccine-associated poliomyelitis. *Muscle & Nerve*, **11**, 356-364.

Winnick, J., & Short, F. (1985). *Physical fitness testing of the disabled: Project Chicago.* Champaign, IL: Human Kinetics.

Wohlfart, G. (1958). Collateral regeneration in partially denervated muscles. *Neurology*, **8**, 175-180.

Wratney, M.J. (1958). Physical therapy for muscular dystrophy children. *Physical Therapy Review*, **38**, 20-32.

Ziter, F.A., Allsop, K.G., & Tyler, F.H. (1977). Assessment of muscle strength in Duchenne muscular dystrophy. *Neurology*, **27**, 981-984.

Additional Readings

Frankel, D., & Baxbaum, R. (1987). *Maximizing your health: A program of graded exercise and meditation for persons with multiple sclerosis.* New York: National Multiple Sclerosis Society.

Gehlsen, G., Beckman, K., & Assmann, N. (1986). Gait characteristics in multiple sclerosis: Progressive changes and effects of exercise on parameters. *Archives of Physical Medicine and Rehabilitation*, **67**, 536-539.

Russell, R.W. (1976). Disseminated sclerosis: Rest-exercise therapy. In R.W. Russell (Ed.), *Multiple Sclerosis: Control of Disease* (pp. 67-76). New York: Pergamon Press.

Evaluation of the Book

Please answer the following questions and send them to the address on page 260. Your responses will be used to assist us with revisions and future editions of the manual.

Disability (if applicable) _____

Affiliation with sport or fitness _____

Age _____ Educational background _____

1. Is the manual organized so that you can easily implement a beginning exercise program? Please explain:

_____

_____

_____

_____

2. If you are interested in one particular disability, is the manual organized so that you can access the information you need easily? Please explain:

_____

_____

_____

_____

3. Is there sufficient information in the introductory chapters (1. Exercise Readiness, 2. Strength Training, 3. Aerobic Training, 4. Flexibility Training) regarding training in general? Please explain:

_____

_____

_____

_____

4. Is there sufficient information in the disability-specific chapters? Please explain:

_____

_____

_____

_____

5. Is the manual written in language you can understand, or was it too technical? Please explain:

_____

_____

_____

_____

6. Are the precautions and contraindications clearly given for each disability? Please explain:

_____

_____

_____

_____

_____

7. Did you have any problems applying the disability-specific exercise program protocols? Please explain:

_____

_____

_____

_____

_____

8. Please make any additional comments:

_____

_____

_____

_____

_____

_____

_____

_____

_____

_____

_____

_____

_____

_____

_____

_____

_____

_____

_____

_____

Send evaluation to:

Don Olson, PhD
Rehabilitation Institute of Chicago
345 E. Superior Street
Chicago, IL 60611

Index

A

AAROM (active-assisted range of motion) technique, 52

Abdominal crunches (exercises), 202-204

Abdominal muscles
  anatomical exercise selection chart, 31-32
  exercise instructions, 195-207

Achondroplasia, 151

ACSM (American College of Sports Medicine), 45, 47

Active-assisted range of motion (AAROM) technique, 52

Active range of motion (AROM) technique, 52

Adolescents, training guidelines for, 4-5

Aerobic capacity ($\dot{V}O_2$max)
  with amputations, 122
  with spinal cord injury, 92, 93, 102

Aerobic endurance assessment, 11-12

Aerobic metabolism, 40

Aerobic training
  for adolescents, 5
  with amputations, 121
  basic guidelines, 41-48
  duration and frequency for, 46
  intensity for, 42-46
  maintenance of gains from, 47-48
  modes of, 41-42
  with multiple sclerosis, 42, 45, 47, 142
  with neuromuscular disease, 45
  physiological response to, 39-41, 42
  with poliomyelitis, 106
  with postpolio syndrome, 45, 149-150

program design, 46
progression in, 47-48
with quadriplegia, 42
readiness assessment for, 10-12, 98
with spinal cord injury, 45, 93, 94, 98, 101-102
with stroke, 45, 77
for wheelchair users, 42

Age, and readiness, 4-6

Agre, J.C., 148

ALS (amyotrophic lateral sclerosis), 143, 144, 146

American College of Sports Medicine (ACSM), 45, 47

American Heart Association, 43

Amputations
  aerobic training with, 121
  characteristics of, 4, 117-119
  classification chart, 124
  effect of exercise on associated conditions, 118-119
  flexibility training with, 118, 120
  lists of suggested exercises, 126-134
  log form, 125
  modification of exercise with, 120-121, 126-134
  precautions for exercise with, 123
  program design with, 123, 126-134
  readiness assessment with, 119
  response to exercise with, 121-123
  strength training with, 119, 120-121, 122, 123

Amyotrophic lateral sclerosis (ALS), 143, 144, 146. *See also* Neuromuscular disease (NMD)

About the Authors

Kevin F. Lockette and **Ann M. Keyes** are the developers of a renowned strength and conditioning program for people with physical disabilities. Created at the Rehabilitation Institute of Chicago, named by experts as the best rehabilitation facility in the United States, their program is now the largest of its kind in the country. It promotes wellness and the prevention of medical complications, allowing people with physical disabilities to live more active lives.

Trained as a physical therapist and certified strength and conditioning specialist, Kevin Lockette is also a leading coach in disabled sports. Since 1990 he has held international coaching positions in weightlifting and powerlifting, including duties as head powerlifting coach for the Disabled Sports Team representing the United States at the 1992 Paralympics. Kevin lectures at national and international conferences in the fields of medicine, adapted physical activity, and strength and conditioning. His knowledge in these areas has allowed him to bridge the gap between medicine and exercise and develop effective exercise programs for people with physical disabilities.

Kevin earned his bachelor's degree in physical therapy from the University of Missouri. He and his wife, Ginger, live in Honolulu, Hawaii, where he works at the Rehabilitation Hospital of the Pacific. Kevin likes to spend his leisure time lifting weights, jogging, and playing the blues harmonica.

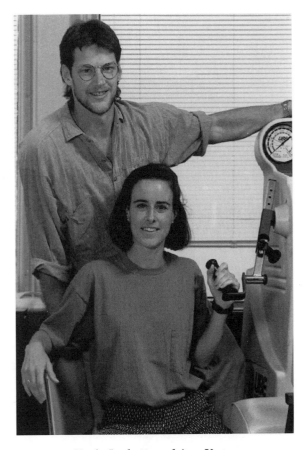

Kevin Lockette and Ann Keyes

Ann Keyes is a physical therapist and certified strength and conditioning specialist. Since 1989 she has combined these areas of expertise as a head coach and consultant for the highly acclaimed strength and conditioning program at the Rehabilitation Institute of Chicago (RIC). Her administrative and clinical positions at RIC have allowed her to research and develop fitness assessments and exercise programs for people with a variety of physical disabilities. She also has updated several exercise programs in the physical therapy departments at Northwestern Memorial Hospital and at RIC.

Ann graduated with Academic Merit Recognition from Indiana University School of Medicine in 1987. She is a member of the American Physical Therapy Association and the National Strength and Conditioning Association. Her interests include reading, running, working out, and traveling.